ACT for Anorexia Nervosa

ACT for Anorexia Nervosa

A Guide for Clinicians

Rhonda M. Merwin

Nancy L. Zucker

Kelly G. Wilson

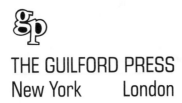

THE GUILFORD PRESS

New York   London

The authors have checked with sources believed to be reliable in their efforts to provide information
that is complete and generally in accord with the standards of practice that are accepted at the time of
publication. However, in view of the possibility of human error or changes in behavioral, mental health,
or medical sciences, neither the authors, nor the editors and publisher, nor any other party who has been
involved in the preparation or publication of this work warrants that the information contained herein
is in every respect accurate or complete, and they are not responsible for any errors or omissions or the
results obtained from the use of such information. Readers are encouraged to confirm the information
contained in this book with other sources.

Library of Congress Cataloging-in-Publication Data

Names: Merwin, Rhonda M., author. | Zucker, Nancy L., author. | Wilson, Kelly G., author.
Title: ACT for anorexia nervosa : a guide for clinicians / Rhonda M. Merwin, Nancy L. Zucker,
    Kelly G. Wilson.
Description: New York : The Guilford Press, [2019] | Includes bibliographical references and index.
Identifiers: LCCN 2018060285| ISBN 9781462540341 (pbk. : alk. paper) |
    ISBN 9781462540358 (hardcover : alk. paper)
Subjects: | MESH: Anorexia Nervosa—therapy | Acceptance and Commitment Therapy—methods
Classification: LCC RC552.A5 | NLM WM 175 | DDC 616.85/262—dc23
LC record available at *https://lccn.loc.gov/2018060285*

To my daughter, Maelyn,
who at age 6 is unencumbered by the word machine:
May you always know the light that you bring to the world

—R. M. M.

To the parents, whose commitment
never ceases to inspire one to work better

—N. L. Z.

To my many wonderful students,
who have taught me and lifted me,
even through my deepest, darkest times

—K. G. W.

In gratitude to the clients who are teaching us
how to be useful to them—*Namaste*

About the Authors

Rhonda M. Merwin, PhD, is Associate Professor in the Department of Psychiatry and Behavioral Sciences at Duke University Medical Center. She is Director of the ACT at Duke Program, which conducts training, clinical services, and research in acceptance and commitment therapy (ACT), and is a core clinical, research, and teaching faculty member at the Duke University School of Medicine. Dr. Merwin's career has focused on using contextual behavioral science to understand and treat anorexia nervosa and maladaptive eating and weight control among individuals with type 1 diabetes. She is recognized as an ACT trainer and has collaborated with the Duke Center for Eating Disorders since 2006.

Nancy L. Zucker, PhD, is Associate Professor in the Department of Psychiatry and Behavioral Sciences at Duke University Medical Center. She is Director of the Duke Center for Eating Disorders and a core clinical, research, and teaching faculty member at the Duke University School of Medicine. Widely published, Dr. Zucker is an author of the American Psychiatric Association's revised practice guidelines for the treatment of eating disorders, currently under development. Her clinical work and research focus on how to help young people develop a healthy awareness of their bodies' signals, and learn to match these signals to actions that allow them to flourish.

Kelly G. Wilson, PhD, is Professor of Psychology at the University of Mississippi and a cofounder of ACT. He is coauthor of *Acceptance and Commitment Therapy, Second Edition*, and has published numerous other books, articles, chapters, treatment manuals, and technical reports. Dr. Wilson trains and consults internationally on the design and implementation of behavioral treatments. His work includes the investigation of acceptance-, mindfulness-, and values-oriented strategies in the treatment of a variety of problems in living, as well as in the basic behavioral science underlying therapeutic change.

Acknowledgments

Thank you to Ashley A. Moskovich, PhD, and Lisa K. Honeycutt, LPC, LMFT, for their assistance in the preparation of the manuscript and original content contributions. And to Jan Mooney, MA, for her assistance in preparing Table I.1.

Contents

Introduction
WHAT IS ACT?

Words are powerful.

"You are fat."

"You need to be perfect."

"You don't deserve it; you haven't worked hard enough."

"You are over your limit; it doesn't matter if you are hungry."

"Feelings are a sign of weakness and a lack of personal control."

The same meal that was fine is not anymore. The same meal, cooked in exactly the same way, is different now. Although individuals sometimes have direct conditioning experiences that contribute to disgust or fear responses to food, for individuals with anorexia nervosa (AN), eating has become aversive primarily through a verbal process (i.e., what food and eating represent and the importance of making the right decisions about what to eat and how much). Faced with a meal, the emotional load feels unbearable.

Words dominate over experience. Instead of food, the plate is covered with numbers that the mind is busy computing. Should I eat, not eat? How much? The smell, the texture, the sensation on the tongue, preferences or other associations, such as the childhood memory of a warm breakfast on a Saturday morning, are lost from awareness. The anticipated feeling of being satisfied is a sign of fatness and of being and wanting too much. In this moment, it seems impossible to allow eating. There is only avoidance and escape, and the immediate relief provided by pushing away the plate to proclaim, "I am not hungry," which stands in for deeper communications like "I am not bad, needy, greedy, or out of control."

This is the human condition. Although not everyone will manifest AN, we all get hooked by our thoughts and start doing things that provide short-term relief from emotional pain, even when those things ultimately cause us harm. For individuals with AN, the effects can be devastating. AN is a leading cause of premature death due to a mental health condition (standardized mortality ratio of 5.9; 4.2–8.3, 95th% confidence interval) (Arcelus, Mitchell,

Wales, & Nielsen, 2011; Chesney, Goodwin, & Fazel, 2014). Suicide is particularly common (standardized mortality ratio of 31; 21–44, 95th% confidence interval) (Preti, Rocchi, Sisti, Camboni, & Miotto, 2011), highlighting the profound suffering of these individuals.

Acceptance and commitment therapy (or ACT) helps individuals with AN reverse life-threatening starvation and enhance life vitality by increasing psychological flexibility. Individuals with AN move from a rigid, punitive style of self-regulation based on rules of what is "good" or "right," to a more flexible, responsive approach to meeting their physical and emotional needs. The result is not only improved weight, but also greater self-care and participation in activities that are personally meaningful. Life becomes less of a list of tasks to accomplish or standards to meet, and more vital and fulfilling.

What Is ACT?

ACT is a third-wave cognitive-behavioral therapy (CBT) and a clinical extension of relational frame theory (RFT; Hayes, Barnes-Holmes, & Roche, 2001), a theoretical and empirical account of human verbal behavior. RFT describes how the unique human ability for *arbitrarily applicable derived relational responding* perpetuates *cognitive fusion* (overattachment to the content of mental activity) and *experiential avoidance* (attempts to change or control internal events even when doing so causes psychological harm). ACT improves human functioning and adaptability by increasing *psychological flexibility* (the ability to have thoughts and feelings as they are and move in the direction of personally chosen values).

ACT is a functional-contextualistic intervention. Thus, the focus is on how behavior functions for the individual, and events are formulated as acts in context. Rather than attempt to change the form (or *content*) of thoughts and feelings themselves, as in more traditional CBT, interventions aim to shift the *context* in which psychological events are situated or how individuals relate or respond to their thoughts and feelings. Interventions specifically aim to disrupt the social–verbal contexts of *literality*, *reason giving*, and *experiential control*, which encourage us to treat thoughts as the literal events they represent (rather than mental activity), give reasons for our behavior, and control our thoughts and feelings. When these contexts are disrupted, and internal experiences can be held lightly, behavior is freer to vary in accordance with values and the demands of the situation.

In practice, ACT engages six interrelated therapeutic processes to facilitate psychological flexibility. These include *Acceptance, Defusion, Present-Moment Awareness, Self-As-Context, Values,* and *Committed Action.*

> *Acceptance* helps individuals let go of unnecessary attempts to avoid or escape unwanted thoughts, feelings, and body sensations.
> *Defusion* deliteralizes thoughts so that they can be observed as events in the mind (rather than the literal events they represent).
> *Present-Moment Awareness* increases an individual's capacity to flexibly attend to internal and external events as they occur and "be here now."
> *Self-as-Context* enhances the individual's capacity to take the perspective of the

observer (that is "more than" any particular experience) and disentangle from unhelpful self-narratives.

Values clarification provides the individual with life direction and a guide for momentary decision making.

Committed Action helps individuals define and take action consistent with their personal values in daily life.

ACT is recognized as an evidence-based practice by APA Division 12, Society of Clinical Psychology, of the American Psychological Association and the National Registry of Evidence-Based Programs and Practices (NREPP) of the Substance Abuse and Mental Health Services Administration. There are currently over 300 randomized controlled trials testing ACT for a wide array of presenting issues and many more open trials and clinical case reports. Data on ACT with eating disorders is preliminary but promising (see Table I.1). There are two randomized controlled trials and 12 other treatment studies examining ACT with eating disorders, with the majority focused on adults ($n = 11$), AN ($n = 7$), and an outpatient setting ($n = 13$) (see Table I.1). There are several studies utilizing subclinical eating disorder populations or specifically targeting body dissatisfaction. Studies show improvements in eating disorder behavior and body mass index (BMI) among individuals with AN, which are largely maintained over brief periods of follow-up. Long-term effects are unknown.

This text describes how to apply ACT to AN and the spectrum of AN behavior. It is designed for clinical and training purposes, as well as to guide clinical research. It is informed by our experience treating individuals with AN and their families at the Duke Center for Eating Disorders within Duke University Medical Center. This program includes traditional outpatient individual, group, and family therapy, as well as an intensive outpatient program (comprising multiple group and individual appointments per week with members of the treatment team). Working with parents is a particular specialty of the program.

Although we provide all the essential information for taking an ACT approach to the treatment of AN, an ACT novice will find it useful to study a seminal text (e.g., Hayes, Strosahl, & Wilson, 1999, 2011; Wilson, 2009) and engage other intensive training experiences, such as ACT BootCamp® or annual conferences of the Association for Contextual and Behavioral Science (ACBS).

The text is appropriate for use with individuals with AN of all ages. However, we spend the most time discussing the application of ACT to adolescents and young adults, as this is the typical age of onset for AN (Halmi, Casper, Eckert, Goldberg, & Davis, 1979; Hudson, Hiripi, Pope, & Kessler, 2007), and it is rare to have an older adult present for treatment of AN. We also use "she" throughout the text as the pronoun reference to the individual with AN. This pronoun was chosen due to the increased prevalence of AN among women and girls, but is not meant to suggest that AN is isolated to females and female-identified persons. The text focuses primarily on restrictive behaviors that are central to AN phenomenology, although some individuals with AN relinquish their restraint at times and engage in more dysregulated patterns, for example, binge eating in defiance of their self-imposed rules.

In Chapters 1 and 2, we provide a framework for understanding AN that facilitates application of the ACT model and provide an overview of the treatment approach. In

TABLE I.1. Treatment Studies on ACT for Anorexia Nervosa, Bulimia Nervosa, Binge-Eating Disorder, and Eating Disorder Not Otherwise Specified

Author (year)	Study design	Sample size	Population	Treatment setting	Main outcome
Heffner, Sperry, Eifert, and Detweiler (2002)	Case study	$N = 1$	Adolescent (AN)	Outpatient	Improved BMI, decreased eating disorder behaviors.
Berman, Boutelle, and Crow (2009)	Case series	$N = 3$	Adults (previously treated but unremitted AN)	Outpatient	One improved BMI at EOT and showed continued improvement at 1-year follow-up (the other two maintained baseline BMI); sporadic declines in eating disorder behaviors.
Wildes and Marcus (2011)	Case series	$N = 5$	Adults (AN)	Outpatient	Three with modestly improved BMI; one with decreased eating disorder behaviors.
Merwin, Zucker, and Timko (2013)	Case series	$N = 6$	Adolescents (AN)	Outpatient	Five with improved BMI; four with decreased eating disorder behaviors.
Juarascio et al. (2013)	Other design with comparison condition (ACT + TAU vs. TAU)	$N = 140$ ACT + TAU: $n = 66$ TAU: $n = 74$	Adults (AN, BN, ED-NOS in AN/BN spectrum)	Residential (group format)	ACT + TAU trended toward outperforming TAU on decreasing eating disorder behaviors at EOT and lowering rehospitalization rates at 6-month follow-up.
Wildes, Marcus, Cheng, McCabe, and Gaskill (2014)	Open trial	$N = 24$	Adults (AN)	Outpatient	Improved BMI and decreased ED behaviors at EOT. Improvements maintained at 6-month follow-up.
Hill, Masuda, Melcher, Morgan, and Twohig (2015)	Case series	$N = 2$	Adults (BED)	Outpatient	Decreased eating disorder behaviors, including binge eating, at EOT. Declines in ED behaviors largely maintained at 3-month follow-up.

Study	Design	N	Population	Setting	Findings
Hill, Masuda, Moore, and Twohig (2015)	Case series	$N = 2$	Adults (BED, ED-NOS)	Outpatient	Decreased eating disorder behaviors, including emotional/binge eating, at EOT. Declines in eating disorder behaviors largely maintained at 3-month follow-up.
Timko, Zucker, Herbert, Rodriguez, and Merwin (2015)	Open trial	$N = 47$	Adolescents (AN)	Outpatient	Improved BMI and decreased eating disorder behaviors; 49% met criteria for full remission and 30% met criteria for partial remission at EOT.
Masuda, Ng, Moore, Felix, and Drake (2016)	Case study	$N = 1$	Adult (OSFED: purging disorder)	Outpatient	Decreased eating disorder behaviors, including self-induced vomiting, at EOT. Continued decline in eating disorder behaviors and abstinence from self-induced vomiting through 12-month follow-up.
Parling, Cernvall, Ramklint, Holmgren, and Ghaderi (2016)	RCT (ACT vs. TAU)	$N = 43$ ACT: $n = 24$ TAU: $n = 19$	Adults (AN)	Outpatient (post-day care)	ACT and TAU demonstrated similar improvements in BMI and eating disorder behaviors at EOT and through 5-year follow-up.
Juarascio et al. (2017)	Open trial	$N = 19$	Adults (BED)	Outpatient (group format)	Decreased ED behaviors, including binge eating, at EOT. Continued decline in binge eating at 3-month follow-up, with 60% reporting abstinence.
Strandskov et al. (2017)	RCT (ACT vs. WLC)	$N = 92$ ACT: $n = 46$ WLC: $n = 46$	Adults (BN, ED-NOS)	Outpatient (Internet-based)	ACT outperformed WLC on decreasing eating disorder behaviors; 37% made clinically significant improvements in eating disorder behaviors in ACT versus 7% in WLC.
Pinto-Gouveia et al. (2017)	Other design with comparison condition (ACT vs. WLC)	$N = 36$ ACT: $n = 19$ WLC: $n = 17$	Adults (BED)	Outpatient	ACT outperformed WLC on decreasing eating disorder behaviors, including binge eating, at EOT. Improvements in ACT group maintained through 6-month follow-up.

Note. AN, anorexia nervosa; BN, bulimia nervosa; BED, binge-eating disorder; ED-NOS, eating disorder not otherwise specified; OSFED, other specified feeding or eating disorder; BMI, body mass index; RCT, randomized controlled trial; EOT, end of treatment; TAU, treatment as usual; WLC, wait-list control.

Chapter 3, we provide guidance on formulating cases from an ACT perspective, including an in-depth description of the functional assessment and evaluation of client capacities in the six core process domains mentioned earlier. Chapter 3 is essential for treatment planning. It also functions as early intervention as clients review their life history, practice taking their own perspective at different times and places, and begin to identify the function of AN and its consequences and costs (an issue to which we return in Chapter 6).

Chapters 4 and 5 cover issues specific to weight restoration and the engagement of parents, family, and significant others in AN treatment. Some interventions in Chapter 5 are also useful in working with individual clients, and the reader is encouraged not to skip this content. Chapter 6 describes creating a context for change (or *creative hopelessness*). This work is critical for acceptance interventions and begins the process of clarifying personal values. Chapter 7 describes strategies for building acceptance of unwanted internal experience. This work begins with increasing awareness of the presence of unwanted feelings. In Chapter 8, we outline strategies to help clients author and engage values, which is often facilitated by increased openness to experience. Chapter 9 describes strategies to decrease attachment to the content of mental activity (*defusion* processes) and increase present-moment awareness. Chapter 10 describes strategies to further address self issues in AN, including overidentification with outward appearance and deficits in perspective taking. We close with Chapter 11, which discusses treatment progress and termination and provides some final thoughts for the therapist.

Chapters are organized by clinical goals, when appropriate. See Figure I.1 for a complete list. Therapist scripts are provided to illustrate the clinical approach. Dialogues are also included to put the scripts in the context of a therapeutic encounter. Some dialogues and scripts reference common ACT metaphors. These metaphors are not explained in the text. The reader is assumed to have some familiarity with these interventions. Throughout the text, tables summarize content or provide additional details, descriptions, and/or examples of concepts or interventions. Key resources for the therapist also include a case formulation form (Form 3.1) and a form to assess client capacities in the ACT core process (or functional) domains (Form 3.2). Both forms can be photocopied or downloaded and printed from the publisher's website (see the box at the end of the table of contents).

Several handouts are also available for clients. Handouts are given to clients between sessions to increase their awareness of their behavior patterns and help them relate differently to their thoughts and feelings. Handouts also help clients practice and track value-guided action. Client handouts can be found at the ends of Chapters 7, 8, 9, and 10. They can be photocopied or downloaded and printed from the publisher's website (see the box at the end of the table of contents).

Chapter 6

- Clinical Goal 1: Appreciate the Immense Emotional Benefits of AN
- Clinical Goal 2: Validate the Fear of Losing the Emotional Benefits of AN
- Clinical Goal 3: Appreciate How Rigid, Punitive Self-Regulation Has Been Helpful
- Clinical Goal 4: Invite Curiosity about Whether Rigid Self-Regulation Is Optimal in All Situations
- Clinical Goal 5: Acknowledge Clients' Fear in Experimenting with a Less Rigid Approach
- Clinical Goal 6: Encourage a Separation between AN and the Person
- Clinical Goal 7. Increase Contact with the Undesirable Consequences of AN
- Clinical Goal 8: Contact Consequences for Personal Values
- Clinical Goal 9: Expand to Other Behaviors That Serve a Similar Purpose as AN and Offer an Alternative

Chapter 7

- Clinical Goal 1: Help the Client Notice Unwanted Feelings
- Clinical Goal 2: Provide a Frame for Acceptance Work
- Clinical Goal 3: Teach the Client to Discriminate Initial Reactions from Secondary Responses
- Clinical Goal 4: Continue to Shape Acceptance of Unwanted Internal Experience
- Clinical Goal 5: Leverage Acceptance to Meet Needs
- Clinical Goal 6: Help Clients Discriminate the Motivations of Their Actions
- Clinical Goal 7: Expand the Client's Capacity for Acceptance with Behavioral Challenges

Chapter 8

- Clinical Goal 1: Introduce the Concept of Values and Set the Context for Values Authorship
- Clinical Goal 2: Help the Client Author Personal Values
- Clinical Goal 3: Leverage Values to Restore Energy Balance/Meet Needs
- Clinical Goal 4: Offer Valuing Oneself (Kindness, Compassion, and Attunement to One's Needs)
- Clinical Goal 5: Clarify Values Related to Others
- Clinical Goal 6: Help the Client Use Values to Guide Momentary Decisions
- Clinical Goal 7: Help the Client Use Values to Enhance Life

Chapter 9

- Clinical Goal 1: Increase Client Awareness of Ongoing Mental Activity and Discriminate this Activity from Direct Experience
- Clinical Goal 2. Identify AN as Content the Mind Produces in Times of Stress/Distress
- Clinical Goal 3: Introduce Workability as the Metric
- Clinical Goal 4: Identify Choice and Reinforce the Person as a Choice-Maker
- Clinical Goal 5: Practice Defusion with Thoughts Exerting Undue Influence over Behavior
- Clinical Goal 6: Diversify the Psychological Functions of Food, Eating, and the Body or Meeting Needs
- Clinical Goal 7: Practice Being in the Present Moment
- Clinical Goal 8: Practice Broad and Flexible Attention

Chapter 10

- Clinical Goal 1: Enhance Self-Awareness (or Strengthen the Knowing Self)
- Clinical Goal 2: Decrease Attachment to a Narrow Conceptualized Self and Build Self-Content
- Clinical Goal 3: Increase Capacity to Experience the Self as Transcending Any Particular Experience
- Clinical Goal 4: Practice Flexible Perspective Taking
- Clinical Goal 5: Help the Client Practice Self-Compassion

FIGURE I.1. List of clinical goals.

CHAPTER 1

The Phenomenology and Conceptualization of Anorexia Nervosa from an ACT Perspective

Motivational states (e.g., hunger, pain) direct and organize behavior in a way that ensures survival. Human beings are the only animals that override these signals and starve themselves to death. The reasons for this are rich and complex but are driven in part by the meaning human beings assign to self-imposed restraint.

The notion that overcoming human motivational states is somehow virtuous is deeply embedded in the human psyche. In early accounts of self-starvation, women who denied themselves food were viewed as pure, divine, and as possessing a special gift from God. As society began to view phenomena more secularly, these women were no longer deified in a literal sense, but continued to be held in extremely high regard: They were "miraculous maids" receiving money and fame. Self-starvation was medicalized in 1689 and AN was identified as a syndrome in the late 1800s. However, the notion that overriding biological drives or needs (particularly in the context of abundance) is virtuous is an element of modern human life.

Appreciating this fact is essential in understanding the phenomenology of AN. Extreme dietary restraint, while destructive in many ways, also evokes strong feelings of effectiveness, mastery, and pride. This stands in stark contrast to most other mental health conditions in which characteristic behaviors may provide relief but do not make the individual feel particularly good about herself. Consider the example of social phobia. Individuals who experience extreme anxiety in social situations experience relief when they avoid interactions, but they do not feel particularly good about it. More likely, they feel ineffective and shameful about their inability to interact with others. The ability to override hunger is also highly visible, and thus it serves social functions, solidifying the individual's status, or otherwise affecting the behavior of other people. Individuals with AN often describe receiving compliments, attention, caretaking, and other social benefits. Thus, they feel like a good or better person and their behavior is reinforced by other people. Together, these more *immediate and emotionally charged* contingencies are often far more compelling than the delayed negative consequences of low weight (e.g., decreased bone density).

Although AN might be driven initially by psychological factors, it may persist because of the incredible impact of starvation on the brain and the body. In the famous case of Saint Catherine (one of the earliest well-documented cases of self-starvation), the church became concerned about her safety and urged an end to her fast, stating that it was inconsistent with biblical tenets. However, she continued to withhold food and eventually died. Like a ball rolling downhill, starvation begets starvation as undernourishment impairs the individual's ability to change course. Individuals who are nutritionally depleted evidence structural brain abnormalities (e.g., enlarged ventricles) and have difficulty reasoning, shifting attention flexibly, and adapting behavior to changing contingencies, with increased rigidity and obsessionality often beyond premorbid levels. Biological adaptations to starvation further perpetuate the problem. Attention narrows to food and the individual experiences less interest and pleasure in social interactions or other activities. Thus, the world becomes increasingly centered on the next meal (as a biological imperative) and there is limited contact with competing reinforcers. Menses cease, body temperature drops, and metabolism and heart rate slow. Hunger cues and the somatic constituents of emotions, initially intensified by restricted food intake, mute. While individuals with AN may welcome the newfound quietness of their bodies, these signals provide essential information to make decisions. Thus, it becomes *more difficult* for the individual to know and respond to her physical and emotional needs. The mind also makes sense of the individual's experience: The quietness of the body is interpreted as having "more control." The drive toward food and the ease of weight gain is viewed as evidence that they need to be restrained. Thus, the initial factors that contributed to the onset of AN behaviors are joined by biological and psychological changes that further entrench the individual in AN (see Figure 1.1).

Prevalence and Age of Onset of AN

AN is relatively rare. The National Comorbidity Study reported a lifetime AN prevalence rate of 0.6% (Hudson et al., 2007) based on the diagnostic criteria of the fourth edition of the *Diagnostic and Statistical Manual of Mental Disorders* (DSM-IV). The fifth edition of the DSM (DSM-5) casts a wider net for AN, no longer requiring the cessation of menses or the

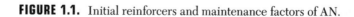

FIGURE 1.1. Initial reinforcers and maintenance factors of AN.

direct endorsement of fear of weight gain (American Psychiatric Association, 2013). In one study, this resulted in a 60% increase in incidence of AN, although cases identified using the new criteria were characterized by a higher BMI, shorter duration of AN, and higher rate of improvement (Mustelin et al., 2016). They also had a slightly later average age of onset (18.8 years compared to 16.5 years) (Mustelin et al., 2016).

Risk for AN is higher among women and girls (0.9%), about three times that of their male counterparts (Hudson et al., 2007), although other studies indicate that estimates are higher in some male subgroups, such as gay men (e.g., Feldman & Meyer, 2007). AN typically emerges in adolescence and young adulthood, and a first episode of AN rarely occurs after age 25 (Hudson et al., 2007).

Prognosis, Mortality, and Morbidity of AN

Intervention within short duration of AN onset is associated with a better prognosis (Steinhausen, 2002). Factors such as lowest BMI, obsessionality, and expressed emotion in families predict worse outcomes (Berkman, Lohr, & Bulik, 2007). Individuals with a more chronic course are more likely to be seeking treatment for a problem other than eating (e.g., depression) (e.g., Hall, 1982; Noordenbos, Oldenhave, Muschter, & Terpstra, 2002).

Researchers estimate that 50% of individuals with AN fully recover, 30% partially recover, and the rest suffer with chronic difficulties or premature death (Steinhausen, 2002). In one study of 84 individuals who were hospitalized for AN, 21 years later (average age = 42.0, SD = 6.5), 51% were fully recovered, 21% were partially recovered, 10% still met full diagnostic criteria for AN, and 16% had died due to causes related to AN or suicide (Löwe et al., 2001). AN has the highest mortality rate of any psychiatric condition (excluding opioid, amphetamine, and cocaine use) (Chesney, Goodwin, & Fazel, 2014). Mortality in AN is twice as high as that in other mental health conditions in women and 12 times the number of deaths expected for women ages 15–24 (Sullivan, 1995). In a meta-analysis of 36 studies conducted by Arcelus, Mitchell, Wales, and Nielsen (2011), suicide was the reported cause of death for 20% of individuals with AN.

AN is also associated with significant morbidity related to (1) psychiatric comorbidities (e.g., depression, anxiety) (Halmi et al., 1991; O'Brien & Vincent, 2003), (2) avoidance of situations that involve eating (or would challenge eating or exercise routines, or reveal low weight), and (3) the physical sequelae of starvation (Katzman, 2005; Mitchell & Crow, 2006; Pomeroy & Mitchell, 2002; Sharp & Freeman, 1993). The physical sequelae of starvation are vast and include changes or damage to the nervous system (e.g., enlarged brain ventricles); circulatory and respiratory systems (e.g., heart damage, low blood pressure, slowed breathing and pulse); integumentary system (e.g., brittle hair and nails, dry and yellowish skin, *lanugo* [growth of fine hair on the body] to conserve body heat); gastrointestinal system (e.g., constipation, delayed gastric emptying); skeletal system (e.g., osteopenia or osteoporosis); muscular system (e.g., muscle wasting and weakness); endocrine and reproductive systems (e.g., hypogonadism, infertility); and urinary system (e.g., chronic kidney disease) (Katzman, 2005; Mitchell & Crow, 2006; Pomeroy & Mitchell, 2002; Sharp & Freeman, 1993).

Subtypes and Comorbidity

There are two subtypes of AN: restricting and binge-eating/purging subtypes. For individuals with the restricting subtype, primary behaviors are restrictive eating and excessive exercise. Individuals with the restricting subtype tend to be anxious, inhibited, and obsessional (Lock, Garrett, Beenhakker, & Reiss, 2011; Pollice, Kaye, Greeno, & Weltzin, 1997; Rommel et al., 2015; Strober, 1980). The binge-eating/purging subtype is characterized by the presence of breaks in restrained eating and/or purging behaviors, including self-induced vomiting and the misuse of laxatives, diuretics, and weight-impacting medications (e.g., thyroid hormone or insulin among individuals with type 1 diabetes). Individuals with the binge-eating/purging subtype may have similar temperament features as individuals with the restricting subtype, but with more labile affect and greater impulsivity (Hoffman et al., 2012; Strober, 1980). Recent studies suggest that diagnostic crossover from AN–restricting subtype to AN–binge/purge subtype is high (Eddy et al., 2002, 2008) and that some individuals with AN cross over to bulimia nervosa, although the reverse is rare (Bulik, Sullivan, Fear, & Pickering, 1997; Eddy et al., 2008).

Anxiety is common among individuals with AN and often far predates onset of the eating disorder (Deep, Nagy, Weltzin, Rao, & Kaye, 1995; Godart, Flament, Lecrubier, & Jeammet, 2000; Kaye, Bulik, Thornton, Barbarich, & Masters, 2004; Toner, Garfinkel, & Garner, 1989). This includes general trait anxiety, as well as generalized anxiety disorder, obsessive–compulsive disorder, and social phobia. Depression is also common and may predate eating concerns or emerge after AN onset (as the individual becomes increasingly starved, experiences low energy, and disengages from activities that would be rewarding or vital) (Deep et al., 1995; Halmi et al., 1991; Ivarsson, Råstam, Wentz, Gillberg, & Gillberg, 2000; Toner et al., 1989). Individuals with AN (particularly binge/purge subtype) might also evidence personality disorder features or have issues with substance use or self-harm or have a history of trauma (Carter, Bewell, Blackmore, & Woodside, 2006; Pawlowska & Masiak, 2007).

Treatment Options

Second-Wave CBT and Family-Based Treatment

Treatment development has been slower for AN than for other mental health issues, particularly for adults over the age of 18 (Agras et al., 2004; Le Grange & Lock, 2005). A recent review of treatment options for adults with AN concluded that there is no appreciable empirical evidence for any particular treatment option (Brockmeyer, Friederich, & Schmidt, 2018). High dropout rates are also a significant problem for adults with AN, commonly ranging between 33 and 50% for outpatient treatment (Della Grave, El Ghoch, Sartirana, & Calugi, 2016; Galsworthy-Francis & Allan, 2014).

Second-wave cognitive-behavioral therapy (CBT) is less effective for adults with AN than for individuals with bulimia nervosa or binge-eating disorder (Brown & Keel, 2012), although outcomes for AN are better with "enhanced CBT" (CBT-E; Fairburn, Cooper, & Shafran, 2008; Fairburn et al., 2013). Studies of CBT-E that include low-weight individuals are 40 sessions; in these studies, about 60% of individuals complete treatment, and 60% of treatment completers show improvement (Murphy, Straebler, Cooper, & Fairburn, 2010). A few studies have examined exposure and response prevention to decrease food-related anxiety and increase caloric intake during meals among adults with AN (Boutelle, 1998; Steinglass et al., 2012, 2014). ExRp seems to be effective for this narrowly defined goal, but it has only been tested with a couple dozen participants across three studies. Cognitive remediation therapy has also been explored, based on studies that suggest individuals with AN have neurocognitive deficits including weak central coherence (i.e., extreme attention to detail to the neglect of context) and impaired cognitive flexibility (Lindvall Dahlgren & Rø, 2014; Tchanturia, Lounes, & Holttum, 2014). Cognitive remediation seems to improve central coherence and cognitive flexibility among individuals with AN, but it does not appear to have a major impact on eating-related outcomes and is considered a preintervention or adjunct to ongoing intervention (Lindvall Dahlgren & Rø, 2014; Pitt, Lewis, Morgan, & Woodward, 2010; Tchanturia, Giombini, Leppanen, & Kinnaird, 2017; Tchanturia, Lloyd, & Lang, 2013; Tchanturia et al., 2014). More recently, a cognitive-interpersonal treatment has been tested, with effects comparable to CBT-E (Byrne et al., 2017).

There has been relatively more progress in the treatment of adolescents with AN with the emergence of family-based treatment (FBT). This was a slow development and a brief history may be useful in appreciating its significance. Until fairly recently, parents and caregivers were purposefully excluded in the treatment of adolescent AN. Exclusion was based on early formulations that AN was due to parental overregulation of the child's behavior or parent–child enmeshment that resulted in a failure of the child to develop a sense of herself as an individual, including her opinions, beliefs, or emotional experience (Bruch, 1962, 1982). Control over eating was hypothesized to represent a unique display of autonomy on the part of the child, and was therefore a concrete attempt to separate and individuate from parental influence. It was feared that parent involvement in treatment would stymie this process. This conceptualization lacked empirical evidence. Furthermore, while parental overcontrol, parent–child enmeshment, or other unhelpful family dynamics were sometimes observed clinically, this formulation failed to appreciate the potential transactional process between the child's temperament and parent behavior (e.g., a highly anxious child might elicit greater parental involvement) and that some of the observed patterns might be the result of having a child who is struggling rather than the impetus for AN.

The shift to include parents in treatment was initially driven by necessity. At least in the United States, changes in mental health care reimbursement forced inclusion of families in the treatment of adolescent AN. In 1984, the length of stay in long-term inpatient treatment facilities for eating disorders was 149.5 days (Wiseman, Sunday, Klapper, Harris, & Halmi, 2001). This was long enough to restore a child to a healthy weight before returning home. By 1998, the average stay was 23.7 days (Wiseman et al., 2001). This dramatic decrease in inpatient stay meant children were being returned to their parents while still at a dangerously low body weight (Wiseman et al., 2001).

In the late 1980s, a series of clinical trials tested FBT developed at the Maudsley Hospital in London (Lock, Le Grange, Agras, & Dare, 2001). This model integrated parents into treatment by centering intervention on present-day symptom management and deemphasizing AN etiology. FBT focused almost exclusively on supporting parents assuming temporary control over mealtimes until their child was able to resume eating on her own. Little to no attention was given to contributing factors, and it was assumed that once restriction remitted, adolescents would return to their normal developmental trajectory. FBT outperformed individual adolescent therapy and was particularly good at reversing starvation (Le Grange, 2005; Lock, 2011; Lock et al., 2010). Including parents and family became a standard of care for adolescent AN. While the majority of adolescents treated with FBT (as manualized by Lock & Le Grange, 2015; Lock et al., 2001) benefit, studies show that greater than 45% achieve suboptimal outcomes (Lock, 2015; Lock et al., 2010). Factors that limit FBT effectiveness include adolescent rigidity or obsessionality and familial expressed emotion (i.e., emotional overinvolvement and critical communication, although data are mixed, and at least one study suggests that parental warmth may be a better indicator) (Le Grange, Eisler, Dare, & Hodes, 1992; Le Grange, Hoste, Lock, & Bryson, 2011; Le Grange et al., 2012).

Several studies have examined strategies to enhance the effectiveness of FBT for adolescents who show improvement and reach those who do not. For example, researchers have varied FBT intervention parameters, changing the length of treatment or treatment format (separated vs. combined family sessions), and increased parental education and support (Eisler et al., 2000; Lock, Agras, Bryson, & Kraemer, 2005; Rhodes, Baillee, Brown, & Madden, 2008; Rhodes, Brown, & Madden, 2009). Others, hypothesizing that FBT may work through parent-facilitated food exposure, have suggested broadened adolescent exposure to fear, worry, and disgust associated with interoceptive cues (e.g., fullness), weight and shape, and social evaluation (Hildebrandt, Bacow, Markella, & Loeb, 2012). Some individual treatments are also being tested as an alternative to family-based intervention for adolescents with AN, including CBT-E (Della Grave, Calugi, Doll, & Fairburn, 2013).

Third-Wave CBT and ACT for AN

Over the last decade, contemporary (or third-wave) CBTs have emerged, with good supportive evidence for a variety of presenting issues (Powers, Zum Vörde Sive Vörding, & Emmelkamp, 2009; Thoma, Pilecki, & McKay, 2015). This includes not only ACT but also dialectical behavior therapy (DBT) and mindfulness-based cognitive therapy (MBCT), among others. These therapies, while diverse, share an emphasis on acceptance and mindfulness, functional formulations, and second-order change (i.e., changing how individuals relate or respond to their thoughts and feelings). They also tend to engage strategies typical of humanistic or existential approaches, as well as more frequent exposure (Brown, Gaudiano, & Miller, 2011). Of the third-wave therapies, ACT is the most researched for AN. Seven studies have examined ACT for AN, including four case studies (Berman et al., 2009; Heffner et al., 2002; Merwin et al., 2013; Wildes & Marcus, 2011), two open trials (Timko et al., 2015; Wildes et al., 2014), and one randomized controlled trial (Parling et al., 2016); see Table I.1 in the Introduction. Studies of ACT for AN have examined both adolescents (n = 54) and adults (n = 75), and all have occurred in an outpatient setting (for a total of 129 participants). DBT has also recently been adapted to address constricted affect and piloted with individuals with AN (Chen et al., 2015; Lynch et al., 2013; Robertson, Alford, Wallis, & Miskovic-Wheatley, 2015; Salbach, Klinkowski, Pfeiffer, Lehmkuhl, & Korte, 2007).

While the empirical evidence of ACT for AN is still in its infancy, outcomes are positive. Studies show improvements in BMI and reduction in AN behaviors among individuals completing treatment (Berman et al., 2009; Heffner et al., 2002; Merwin, Zucker, et al., 2013; Parling et al., 2016; Timko et al., 2015; Wildes & Marcus, 2011; Wildes et al., 2014).

Conceptually, the ACT model is well suited to address the emotional avoidance and overregulation that characterizes AN. ACT focuses on acceptance or willingness to have unwanted thoughts, feelings, or body sensations. This goes to the heart of the struggle of individuals with AN who have difficulty allowing feelings or drives that feel out of their control and tolerating variation in experience and their body and internal states. By increasing acceptance of unwanted internal experiences, it might be possible for individuals with AN to meet their physical and emotional needs and pursue elements of life that are vital and meaningful, even if not predictable or well controlled.

ACT's functional-contextualistic approach to cognition might also be advantageous for treating individuals with AN. Rather than aim to change the form (or the *content*) of thoughts/feelings, ACT aims to decrease the extent to which they exert undue influence over behavior. Thus, unlike more traditional CBT, there is no need for eating disorder thoughts to change in order for behavior to change. Given that cognitions in AN tend to be highly intractable (and individuals with AN tend to exhibit high cognitive rigidity, premorbidly and after onset of starvation), this might be a more efficient way to achieve behavior change. It might also be better matched to the client's experience. Rather than having the expectation that AN thoughts will resolve, clients might expect that these thoughts will be present indefinitely, and particularly at times of stress. Furthermore, because clients learn to view cognitions in AN functionally (as a signal of emotional distress), and have learned to behave differently in their presence, they might have a lower risk of relapse (which is extremely high in AN) (Carter, Blackmore, Sutandar-Pinnock, & Woodside, 2004).

ACT's functional approach might also broadly improve client adaptability by targeting behaviors that are functionally equivalent to AN (or serve a similar purpose). These behaviors, while not life threatening, limit life vitality. This includes, for example, excessive devotion to work or people pleasing (to the neglect of one's own needs).

The ACT model also centers on personal values as a guide for behavioral choices. This could be extremely helpful for individuals with AN who tend to be low in self-directedness and make decisions based on external systems of control (e.g., rules). By clarifying personal values, individuals with AN might come to know themselves more deeply and choose actions that enhance their lives (rather than doing what they think is good, right, or expected of them). Values might also serve an adaptive organizing function for individuals with AN who may be overwhelmed by a lack of structure. Values may replace rigid rules, providing flexible guidelines from which to choose actions.

Personal values may also be a powerful motivator of behavior change and more effective than identifying the "cons" of restrictive eating and low weight, which tend to be more logic based (e.g., "Being cold all the time") or focused on future goals ("It might affect my ability to have children").

Finally, ACT specifically addresses issues of self-awareness and flexible perspective taking. Thus, it may be well suited to help individuals with AN establish a sense of self beyond outward appearance, achievements, and goals and develop a greater capacity for a compassionate (rather than judgmental) approach to themselves and their experiences.

An Alternative Framework: AN as Maladaptive Self-Regulation

AN is typically formulated as pathological weight regulation, driven by a distorted view of the body. Below, we offer an alternative framework of AN as *verbally mediated punitive self-regulation*, which may facilitate application of the ACT model.

From the broader vantage point of self-regulation, it may be less likely that the therapist will be hooked by the particularly evocative topography of self-starvation and maintain a functional view. This framework might also clarify the continuum and severity of AN behavior and the goal of intervention, which is to move individuals from rigid, rule-based self-regulation to more flexible responding to their physical and emotional needs.

Importantly, this formulation is grounded in pragmatic truth rather than the assumptions of scientific realism; that is, it is only "true" inasmuch as it guides the therapist and the clinical encounter in an effective manner to produce meaningful behavior change.

When we are very young, other people have a major role in meeting our basic physical and emotional needs. To do this, our parents (or caregivers) observe our behavior and elements of the situation and infer our private experience. For example, they may observe us crying and rubbing our eyes, note that we have been awake for hours, and infer that we tired. They might even say to us, "Are you tired? You look tired." If the situation is suitable for it, they might create conditions for us to sleep. Similarly, they may observe signals that we are hungry and provide food, or that we are scared or sad, and comfort us. As we get older, we take on the responsibility of caring for ourselves. It becomes our job to notice how we are feeling and take actions to meet our needs. Ideally, we establish a respectful, reciprocal relationship between signals originating from our body and our actions. For example, when our stomachs rumble, we recognize this feeling as the need for food and respond accordingly. As we do so, we come to know ourselves and our signals and establish a sense of safety and self-trust. We may even come to have warm feelings for ourselves as the caretaker and the one being taken care of.

Rather than warmth and reciprocity, individuals with AN have adopted a rigid, punitive approach to managing themselves and their needs. They behave like an *authoritarian* parent, imposing rigid rules and demanding obedience, without regard for their own feelings or extenuating circumstances. Rules prioritize work and performance to the neglect of the individual. While emergencies may call for such driven behavior, as a lifestyle, it takes a toll. Individuals with AN exist in a profound state of physical and emotional deprivation. They are not fed when they are hungry or comforted when they are sad. For some individuals with AN, the situation is worse, and they not only ignore their needs, but also berate themselves for having them, calling themselves *weak*, *lazy*, or *pathetic* for being tired, hungry, or upset. Although rigid rules might be most poignant in the areas of eating and exercise, they typically occur across life domains (e.g., relationships) and disregard the individual based on rules of what is "good" or "right" or what will make them a good or better person (see Figure 1.2 on p. 18).

> From a client with AN binge/purge subtype:
>
> "Do not sleep tonight and do not eat that grape. 566 sit-ups, not 565. If it burns, it's not good enough, it needs to kill. Go until you can feel no more and then you can go even harder. Push it, come on, run another mile. No wait, run 3 more. Do some stairs. Don't eat that. Damn it, she's in the bathroom. Hurry up. OK, OK, go throw up. There's some left, you're not throwing up pure bile yet. Throw up more. More. More. What, your throat hurts? No it doesn't. Shove your fingers deeper. Ignore the tingling, it will go away. You're not puffy from puking, no your face is just fat. Why did you have to eat that banana? Get it out, NOW. Why are you sleeping, you lazy bastard. Get up and jump on the trampoline. Look at you, you're so fat. They don't know what they're talking about, you're not sick, they're just trying to stop you from being good. This isn't hurting me. I can't die from this. Look, I can go run 5 miles and you want to tell me I'm sick? Your clothes aren't getting baggy; no you're so fat that you're stretching them out."

Another important element of this approach to (self-)parenting is that no performance is ever really *good enough*. As individuals with AN meet their self-imposed demands, rules for behavior become more extreme, with greater mandates on the individual despite increasing personal costs (e.g., less food or rest is allowed and more work is demanded). In the domain of academics, if an A is achieved, an A+ is expected next time. In the domain of eating, less than 500 calories becomes less than 400, and then 300.

Inflexibility in outcome also occurs alongside inflexibility in approach. Rather than experiment with different strategies to meet their increasing demands of themselves with less sacrifice, individuals with AN simply do more to achieve more. Thus, if studying all night for an exam resulted in an A, the next time they will stay up two or three nights. From this perspective, low weight *is but one outcome* of this verbally mediated, punitive system of self-regulation.

Punitive overcontrol and self-sacrifice are seductive because they work well for conventional measures of success. Individuals with AN excel in almost everything they do: They are valedictorian; they have the fastest running times or the first chair in the orchestra, and they achieve the thin-ideal. They may even seem to excel socially, at least when social activities have a clear structure that outlines how to succeed (e.g., club president). However, it is not a kind way to live or to treat oneself, and it comes with a significant cost to their health and well-being. Over time, relentlessly pursuing difficult-to-attain goals using a "push harder" approach depletes the individual, and it results in a lack of personal meaning or vitality. Life becomes a list of tasks to accomplish. Individuals with AN have limited free time to develop personal interests, and they avoid activities that they would enjoy because they feel frivolous or self-indulgent.

The Continuum of Self-Regulation

Thus far, we have only outlined one end of the spectrum of self-regulation that we think differentiates AN from other problems of living. It also points to the overlap between AN and high-functioning autism, obsessive–compulsive personality disorder (OCPD), obsessive–compulsive disorder (OCD), or other conditions characterized by rule-governed rigidity.

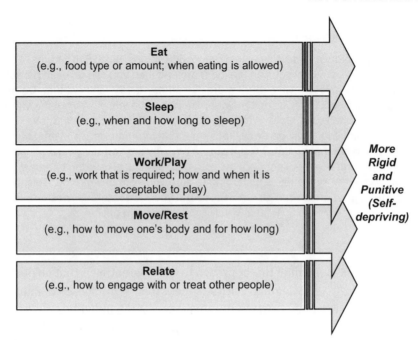

FIGURE 1.2. AN as a functional class of behavior of imposing rules to maintain emotional and behavioral control and be a good or better person. Moving from left to right, behavior becomes increasingly dictated by harshly imposed rules that disregard the individual and her needs. This continuum reflects the progression of AN over time and its severity. The clinician targets rigid self-regulation and, in doing so, impacts the larger functional class in which restrictive eating is one element.

However, expanding our perspective, we extend this continuum in both directions (see Figure 1.2). On one end of the continuum is the rigid, rule-based regulation that we have outlined thus far. On the other end is self-regulation determined only by one's feelings in the moment, disregarding rules or the consequences of more immediate impulses ("mood-dependent" behavior).

Extending the self-regulation continuum in both directions has two distinct benefits. First, it allows us to situate clients at different stages of recovery or with different clinical presentations. This might include, for example, an individual with AN who is typically restrained but abandons all self-control, eating indiscriminately and vomiting, or the individual with AN who vacillates between driven rigid perfectionism and boundless procrastination. These individuals may be described as moving rapidly from opposite ends of the continuum. Second, extending the continuum in both directions, we can also see more clearly that optimal regulation is positioned in the middle, with somatic–affective signals integrated flexibly with other sources of information to determine behavior (see Figure 1.3).

Factors That Contribute to Rigid Self-Regulation

A significant body of literature has identified individual differences (e.g., temperament) that are reliably associated with AN. These individual differences may function as establishing

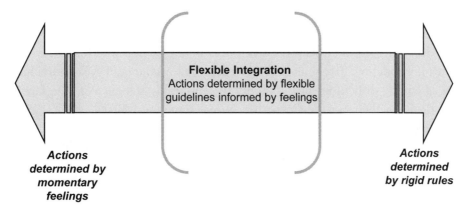

Flexible Integration
Actions determined by flexible
guidelines informed by feelings

*Actions
determined by
momentary
feelings*

*Actions
determined
by rigid rules*

FIGURE 1.3. Continuum of self-regulation. On one end is rigid regulation by rules to the neglect of feeling or extenuating circumstances. At the other end, behavior based only in momentary feelings, without regard for verbally articulated values or long-term goals.

operations for rule following and/or make it difficult to deviate from rules when conditions change.

Temperament

Decades of research indicate that individuals with AN are harm avoidant and perfectionistic (Bardone-Cone et al., 2007; Cassin & von Ranson, 2005; Farstad, McGeown, & von Ranson, 2016). Thus, they tend to be inhibited, obsessional individuals that are afraid of making mistakes. They also tend to be interpersonally sensitive (Schmidt & Treasure, 2006). As such, they are often hyperaware of how others perceive them and specifically sensitive to signals that they have not met the expectations of other people. For individuals with this temperament, societal messages about the importance of self-discipline/self-control and rule following may be powerful determinants of behavior. These messages may be further reinforced by an individual's immediate social environment (i.e., families and communities), which may differ in their expectations for behavior.

The temperament of individuals with AN might also increase rejection of somatic-effective cues and reliance on rules to make self-care decisions. Felt states are amorphous and fluctuate, sometimes in unpredictable ways. For example, on any given day, our energy needs vary due to factors that we do not determine and cannot fully know (e.g., subthreshold disease processes, temperature regulation, the stage of one's menstrual cycle). Thus, a meal that was completely sufficient on Monday may on Tuesday be followed by hunger pangs only an hour later. For individuals with a more cautious temperament, afraid of being wrong, this is extremely unsettling. There is no objective measure on which to base how we feel ("Am I really hungry?") or the appropriate response to these feelings ("Should I eat?"). Making decisions based on feelings is overwhelming and risky. Uncertain or unsure, individuals with AN may impose rules and cautiously err on the side of eating (much) less and doing (much) more, rather than risk momentary decisions that may be "wrong."

Interoceptive Awareness

Individual differences in interoceptive awareness might further interfere with the use of feelings to inform action. In the earliest psychological accounts of AN, individuals were described as having difficulties in the ability to sense body signals (e.g., the face turning hot) and to decipher their meaning (e.g., discriminate emotions) (Bruch, 1962, 1982). While researchers have consistently observed difficulties in deciphering feelings (e.g., poor interoceptive awareness, alexithymia) in individuals with AN, the data on the ability to sense body signals (i.e., somatic sensitivity) are mixed. Some studies suggest hyposensitivity, while others suggest that individuals with AN may be hypersensitive prior to eating disorder onset. For example, Pollatos and colleagues (2008) found that individuals with AN are less able to detect their own heartbeat than are healthy controls, and that this deficit is associated with BMI, suggesting that it may be an outcome of low weight. Other researchers have found that individuals with AN who are weight-restored have superior heartbeat detection and report greater sensory and emotional sensitivity (e.g., having an exaggerated startle response to both positively and negatively valenced stimuli despite limited display of facial affect) (Davies, Schmidt, & Tchanturia, 2013; Erdur, Weber, Zimmermann-Viehoff, Rose, & Deter, 2017; Merwin, Moskovich, et al., 2013).

A significant body of literature also indicates that individuals with AN have fear and disdain for emotions and believe that there are negative consequences for expressing feelings (e.g., viewing emotion as a personal failing) (e.g., Davies, Schmidt, Stahl, & Tchanturia, 2011; Fox, 2009; Harrison, Sullivan, Tchanturia, & Treasure, 2009; Lavender et al., 2015; Schmidt & Treasure, 2006; Wildes, Ringham, & Marcus, 2010). Both hypersensitivity to somatic-affective cues and nonacceptance of emotions may motivate imposing rules and structure to constrain affect. It might also increase the reinforcement value of starvation, which directly mutes signals arising from the body. Hyposensitivity (or similar issues, e.g., alexithymia) might require individuals to find alternative sources of information to guide actions (i.e., rules).

Neurocognition

Some data suggest that individuals with AN have neurocognitive differences that might make it difficult for individuals with AN to deviate from rules based on feedback and/or see the "bigger picture." For example, researchers have reported that individuals with AN have difficulty shifting cognitive or behavioral sets and moving flexibly from one task or strategy to another when the immediate contingencies no longer support the action (Danner et al., 2012; Roberts, Tchanturia, Stahl, Southgate, & Treasure, 2007; Roberts, Tchanturia, & Treasure, 2010; Tchanturia et al., 2012). This difference is observed not only in individuals who are underweight, but also in individuals with AN who are at a healthy weight (Roberts et al., 2007, 2010; Tchanturia et al., 2012) and their nonaffected sisters (Roberts et al., 2010). Individuals with AN have also been found to have weak central coherence, demonstrating a local processing bias (Danner et al., 2012; Lopez et al., 2008). This difference does not appear to be as pronounced in younger individuals with AN (Lang, Stahl, Espie, Treasure, & Tchanturia, 2014), which suggests that it might be a consequence of AN and indicative of a longer duration of underweight. A local processing bias might maintain AN by encouraging a narrow focus on details (e.g., calorie counts or small changes in body experience) without appreciation for the broader context. Recent years have seen an uptick of interest in other neurobiological differences among individuals with AN that might be relevant to the value placed on stimuli (e.g., reward processing) or the integration of information about the state of the body (Kaye, Wierenga, Bailer, Simmons, & Bischoff-Grethe, 2013; Nunn, Frampton, Gordon, & Lask, 2008).

Development

AN typically emerges at key developmental periods, such as when entering puberty or young adulthood. During these times, there are not only physical changes (e.g., hormonal shifts) but also psychological changes. Individuals are developing self-awareness, and there is a change in responsibility or expectations. In this context, rules may offer an organizing frame amid the chaos and restore predictability and control (including control over the experience of the body and its impulses; Crisp, 2006).

Impact of Rigid Self-Regulation on Valued Living: Limiting Self-Knowledge and Social Connection

When decisions are based on rigid rules, they are, by definition, insensitive to day-to-day (or moment-to-moment) variation. As a result, there is a mismatch between one's actions and the needs or demands of a situation. If rules are punitive (self-depriving) or extreme, they can produce severe nutritional deficits that are life threatening or other problems in functioning or adaptability. However, using rigid rules to determine action also has broad implications for valued living.

Learning who we are, our preferences and opinions (i.e., self-knowledge), requires paying attention to our internal experience and experimenting to discover what we like or dislike. Following rigid rules based on what is "good" or "right" or what meets conventional standards of success interferes with knowing oneself and pursing activities that are personally meaningful. Among individuals with AN, even big life decisions (e.g., career choice) may be based on the perceived expectations of other people or of society, rather than on personal preference. As a result, individuals with AN may experience a lack of vitality (or chronic dissatisfaction) at the same time that they believe they "should" be happy or fulfilled.

Social connection might also be negatively impacted by an overreliance on rules. Social situations are dynamic and nuanced. The "right" way to behave is also often unclear, and it may be impossible to employ rigid rules. Social interactions are also not advanced by self-discipline. In fact, they are advanced by the opposite: contact with feeling and the willingness to express these feelings and be vulnerable, present, and spontaneous. Individuals with AN often avoid unstructured social interactions or require that social exchanges occur in a highly predictable manner (e.g., rejecting unexpected invitations, avoiding chit-chat). Using rules rather than empathetic attunement, they may also find it impossible to understand the feelings and actions of other people or relate to another person in a meaningful way. Thus, individuals with AN may appear cold and aloof and lack intimate connections with other people.

How ACT Addresses Rigid Self-Regulation

ACT helps individuals with AN reverse life-threatening restriction and build a valued, vital life via increasing *psychological flexibility* or the ability to contact the present moment fully and without defense and cease or persist in behaviors that would be effective given the individual's values and what the environment affords. Clients learn to respond flexibly and effectively to situations (using their experience rather than rigid rules as their guide). Treatment begins by determining the contingencies maintaining AN, and specifically how imposing rigid rules (or punitive overcontrol) allows the individual to avoid or escape momentary discomfort (e.g., uncertainty). The context is set for the individual to contact the ultimate unworkability of current behavior patterns and the costs for valued living. The ACT processes of Acceptance, Defusion, Present-Moment Awareness, Self-As-Context, Values, and Committed Action are then engaged to create an open, curious stance to one's feelings and increase willingness to experiment with new behaviors to meet one's physical and emotional needs. Committed actions linked to values enhance life meaning and create patterns of activity incompatible with AN.

Looking Ahead

In Chapter 2, we provide a more in-depth overview of ACT-based treatment for individuals with AN. We also discuss orienting clients to an ACT approach and forming a therapeutic alliance. Alliance building might be more challenging with individuals with AN (relative to other populations), due to their beliefs about the implications of expressing feelings and the desire to maintain restriction and low weight.

CHAPTER 2

Overview, Orienting Clients to Treatment, and Forming a Therapeutic Alliance

AN may be understood as verbally mediated, punitive self-regulation, in which actions are rigidly dictated by rules, without consideration for the individual's wants, needs, or extenuating circumstances. ACT disrupts the rigidity that characterizes AN by increasing psychological flexibility (or the ability to allow thoughts and feelings to be what they are and choose actions based on personal values and what the situation affords). Individuals move from rigid rule following to a more flexible and responsive approach to caring for themselves and engaging with the world.

Early Treatment

Treatment begins with identifying the more immediate contingencies that maintain AN, despite diminishing health and psychological harm. The context is then set such that the client can contact the full breadth of her experience, including the way in which current behavior patterns are *not* working and their costs for personal values. This stage of treatment is referred to as *creative hopelessness* because it paves the way for a creative solution to the client's pain (i.e., acceptance of unwanted internal experience as an alternative to avoidance and control).

Identifying creative hopelessness as a "stage" of treatment is really a misnomer. Rather, the therapist might return to this work again and again throughout treatment to increase willingness to experiment with new behavior. Overall, the aim is to amplify contingencies that are not currently exerting stimulus control over the client's behavior, but that if contacted would support more adaptive repertoires.

Creative hopelessness might be difficult and prolonged in the treatment of AN for a number of reasons. First and foremost, AN is highly ego-syntonic. Thus, the individual views AN as desirable and consistent with her self-concept (or with whom she wishes to be). It may take time for negative consequences of AN to reveal themselves, and the full extent may not be known until the individual clarifies personal values. Second, initial improvement in nutrition is often necessary to do this work. Improved nutrition allows the client's attention to broaden beyond food to consider the impact of AN on other life domains. Increased food intake might also be necessary for clients to have the cognitive and emotional faculties to participate in treatment.

Early in treatment, the therapist may have to leverage outside contingencies to improve the client's nutritional status. This includes, for example, engaging the family in mealtime management or working with medical providers to require weight restoration for continued participation in extracurricular activities or work (see Chapter 5). The therapist may then work with the client to loosen attachment to AN using externalizing strategies (or other interventions that differentiate the *person* from her anorectic thoughts, feelings, and behaviors). With better nutrition, and a greater distinction between herself and AN, the client may be poised for a more in-depth or honest examination of the workability of current behavior patterns. The process iterates as individuals gain greater clarity about their personal values and, subsequently, a deeper appreciation for the costs of AN and a desire for change (see Chapter 6).

Full Engagement of the Six Core Processes (or Functional Domains)

Treatment continues with full engagement of the six core ACT processes (Acceptance, Defusion, Present-Moment Awareness, Self-As-Context, Values, and Committed Action) to reverse the client's severe weight loss and improve functioning and adaptability.

Acceptance interventions increase the individual's capacity to allow internal experiences (thoughts, feelings, body sensations) to be what they are, without unnecessary attempts to change their form, frequency, or intensity. Acceptance interventions improve the clients' ability to be flexible (relinquish oppressive structure that denies their needs) and take risks (approaching situations that may generate feelings). Acceptance also enhances self-knowledge. By being open and receptive to experience, individuals with AN may learn about their wants, needs, and personal preferences, as well as what brings deep meaning or enhances life vitality (which they are then freer to pursue).

Defusion interventions decrease unhelpful attachment to the content of mental activity. As a result, thoughts such as "You need to be perfect" can be observed as thoughts rather than literal dictates for action, and even the most evocative thoughts ("You are an undeserving human being") may be observed dispassionately, reducing their influence over behavior. Less entangled with their mental activity, individuals with AN may also live less in their heads (e.g., analyzing, counting, planning) and more in the world that is directly available to them. This enhances learning from the environment and allows more adaptive repertoires to be developed and maintained.

Interventions that focus on Present-Moment Awareness processes help individuals with AN develop a greater capacity to flexibly attend to internal and external events as they occur and be in the here-and-now (rather than in the feared future or regretted past). With greater present-moment awareness, an individual with AN may be better able to navigate dynamic social situations and maintain fluid, ongoing awareness of the changing state of her body and its needs.

Self-as-Context interventions help individuals experience themselves as "more than" their content (e.g., thoughts/feelings) and engage in flexible perspective taking. When clients experience the self as transcending their thoughts, feelings, or roles, they may be less invested in the presence or absence of any particular experience and less attached to unhelpful self-narratives (about themselves, their body, or the need to maintain emotional and behavioral control). With practice perspective taking, individuals may have a greater ability to differentiate their thoughts and feelings from the experiences of other people and to experience greater self-compassion. Over time, as individuals learn to speak more from "I" (e.g., "I want," "I need," "I like"), they may build a greater sense of agency in their personal choices.

Values interventions help individuals with AN clarify what is personally and deeply meaningful and use this as a guide to choose actions. Individuals practice authoring their lives, and what they want to "be about," beyond what they think they should, ought, or must be to succeed or meet expectations. Values also facilitate willingness to experience discomfort, including the discomfort that they experience when they care for their own needs (e.g., guilt, thoughts of selfishness).

Committed Action interventions help individuals move in the direction of their chosen values in daily life. Initially, committed actions focus on stabilizing and restoring weight, which is necessary to engage fully in life and other values. Over time, the focus shifts to building life vitality and meaning that can effectively compete with the emotional benefits of AN. Clients practice letting go of oppressive structure and overcommittment and reallocate time to activities that they enjoy or that matter deeply to them.

ACT is an integrated model of behavior change. Thus, these six processes are present to some degree in all sessions, although relative emphasis might change. Processes are always in the service of behavior change, with the goal of valued vital living in the presence of any and all thoughts and feelings.

Methods of Intervention

Although nearly any *form* of intervention is acceptable (provided that it is consistent with the core tenets of the ACT model), ACT interventions emphasize experiential learning over didactic methods. This is to decrease unhelpful verbal entanglement, which is understood as contributing to clients' problems. There is also an emphasis on metaphor, which takes advantage of the human ability to relate events to one another and have some of the psychological functions of those events transformed in accordance with the relation. In this case, verbal abilities are being wielded to promote more effective responding. For example, likening a painful feeling to *a houseguest* may allow the client to welcome this experience as they would a guest in her home. Similarly, likening thinking to *a parade* may cue dispassionate observation. Because they tend to think more concretely, experiential exercises and metaphors might require greater use of props with individuals with AN than with other populations.

Homework is typically assigned between sessions to enhance learning. As treatment progresses, intervention shifts from the primary task of skills acquisition (acquiring the skills of being present, allowing internal experiences, and choosing actions based on values) to skills generalization. Skills generalization occurs as clients practice skills across a variety of settings or situations. In AN, early learning may be predominantly in the domain of eating and weight, but over time, this expands to other domains such as work or interpersonal interactions. For example, individuals may practice allowing uncertainty to consume a food of unknown calories, and later practice allowing uncertainty to pursue a new job position or engage in less structured social activities. Most sessions include concrete goals for behavior change (or committed actions).

Additional behavioral strategies may be used to increase skills generalization or address skill deficits. For example, a novel stimulus might be introduced into the natural environment to cue adaptive behavior (e.g., a values-relevant image on the mirror or refrigerator) or sessions might include appetite awareness or assertiveness skills training. When conducting ancillary skills training, the therapist should be cognizant of other factors that might motivate this intervention to the client's detriment (e.g., client or therapist avoidance of other, more difficult or less structured therapeutic activities).

Exposure is also an important element of ACT and likely occurs to some degree in most interventions. However, exposure might also be conducted in a very deliberate manner in ACT (i.e., planned exposure to evocative situations on a fear hierarchy). When conducting exposure in ACT, the aim is not fear reduction (or habituation per se), but rather a broad and flexible repertoire of behavior in the presence of fear (or other uncomfortable thoughts and feelings). Rather than gathering subjective units of distress (SUD) ratings, the therapist may track clients' openness or willingness (to allow internal experience). Exposure is framed with the client's values and might include food or mirror exposure or exposure to social situations.

Adapting Therapy for Younger Clients

Some of the challenges in conducting psychotherapy with young people may be less of an issue with adolescents with AN. Adolescents with AN tend to be mature beyond their years and have high cognitive abilities. They also do not typically have significant issues talking to adults (and may even prefer it to interacting with peers).

Other challenges in working with young people may be more pronounced among individuals with AN. Individuals with AN tend to be more concrete in their thinking, and this might be particularly true of younger clients. As mentioned previously, using props or visual aids can be helpful to make metaphors more accessible or to illustrate abstract or difficult concepts (e.g., defusion). This might include, for example, using real boxes to fill with the client's "stuff" (unwanted thoughts and feelings), an actual chessboard for the chessboard metaphor, worksheets with thought bubbles, or comic book–like illustrations (that include "the mind" as a character in the story). Interventions might also include games, which may be more engaging for younger adolescents and provide additional opportunities for experiential learning (e.g., the Game of Life [Bailey, Ciarrochi, & Hayes, 2012]). However, the therapist may keep in mind that playful interventions (e.g., "acting-out" metaphors such as "Passengers on the Bus"), which are typically well suited for young people, may be extremely challenging for adolescents with AN (who fear judgment and making mistakes). These activities should not be avoided but rather should be titrated accordingly and executed with permission.

The content of interventions might also be adapted to be more relevant to the lives and experiences of younger clients. For example, the automaticity of thoughts might be illustrated by describing thoughts as "pop-up advertisements," or defusion work might include creating a text-message exchange between the individual and "anxiety."

Prioritizing Starvation and Engaging Support People

Reversing life-threatening starvation is the priority in early treatment. This is because undernourishment not only poses a safety concern, but also interferes with an individual's ability to engage fully in treatment. In prioritizing starvation, the therapist devotes some time in session to setting goals related to systematically increasing food intake. Challenges in eating more are used as opportunities to practice acceptance, defusion, or committed action. In many cases, reversing starvation requires engaging other people in the individual's natural environment. These individuals can create a context for change by providing instrumental or emotional support or managing contingencies regarding eating and exercise. While somewhat counterintuitive, having other people insist that they eat or having clear boundaries for AN (e.g., minimum amout of food that is required) is often a relief (allowing them to break restraint with dignity and decreasing guilt or shame for choosing to eat more on their own). Later, the therapist can help clients independently *choose* to feed themselves or otherwise care for their own needs.

For younger clients, parents often provide additional support to restore nutrition. For older adolescents or adults, it might be other family members, significant others, or even the client's adult children. While ACT for AN is not absolutely an FBT, it incorporates the family when it is useful to do so, which is more commonly indicated with AN than with other clinical issues, and is the standard of care for adolescents (American Psychiatric Association, 2006; Golden et al., 2003; Lock, 2015). Guidance on including family or other support people in AN treatment is provided in Chapter 5. Additional information on weight restoration is provided in Chapter 4.

Working with a Multidisciplinary Treatment Team

AN treatment requires a multidisciplinary treatment team (American Psychiatric Association, 2006; Golden et al., 2003). In addition to a therapist, this includes a physician, a nutritionist, and, in some cases, a psychiatrist. Ideally, members of the treatment team have experience specifically with AN, which can be unique in some ways. The physician provides medical monitoring of the low weight and the complications associated with eating disorder behavior (e.g., vomiting). The physician also typically provides ideal body weight estimation, monitors weight, and makes recommendations regarding the speed of weight gain, participation in activities (e.g., sports), or the appropriateness of school/work. The nutritionist might also monitor weight and can estimate the client's caloric needs and provide specific recommendations for meals and snacks (i.e., target number of servings of particular macronutrients) and for titrating clients to their full meal plan. A psychiatrist might be useful when clients present with complex comorbidities or already have established psychotropic medications. Psychotropic medications might also be useful for a circumscribed period when the individual is evidencing severe obsessional cognitions. Some medications are not effective at exceedingly low weight and others will be resisted due to the side effect of weight gain or fear of body contamination.

Regular communication among members of the treatment team is essential for coordination of care. This includes sharing key elements of case formulation and agreeing on a treatment plan, with contingencies for lack of weight improvement. Discrepancies among treatment team members generate unhelpful confusion for clients with AN, who may already feel uncertain or fearful of change.

Treatment team members have a wide array of theoretical approaches and training backgrounds. Thus, it may be helpful for the therapist to also orient members of the team to the ACT approach. The notion that negative thoughts and feelings are "problems to be solved" runs deep in our culture and specifically in the medical model, in which the goal is often to suppress or eliminate thoughts and feelings formulated as "symptoms" of underlying pathogenesis. Communication from other members of the treatment team that the client should think or feel differently could interfere with the mindful, accepting stance to internal experiences that the therapist is working to cultivate.

Monitoring Weight

Focusing narrowly on weight is not likely to be helpful. However, ongoing information about the individual's weight is necessary to guide treatment decisions, including the need for a higher level of care. This is accomplished by regular weight checks conducted by the therapist or another member of the treatment team, such as the physician or nutritionist. In some cases, the therapist conducting weight checks (at each session) increases client accountability and provides information useful in guiding session activities. In other cases, weight checks at the time of session are disruptive and impede the therapeutic process. The general approach to weight monitoring is to respond to trends (e.g., over the course of 2–3 weeks) rather than to individual data points. Weights may be shown or blinded to the client, as clinically indicated. We expand on the topic of weight monitoring in Chapter 4.

Appropriateness of Outpatient Treatment/ Level-of-Care Considerations

There are obvious instances in which individuals who present for treatment are inappropriate for outpatient care due to the extent of undernourishment and medical compromise.

However, often, this determination is more difficult. In these cases, it may be useful to engage clients in a "trial" of outpatient care to determine whether the support offered by this modality is sufficient. A typical trial period may range from 2 to 4 weeks, based on the treatment team's current comfort regarding the client's safety. The effectiveness of outpatient intervention is indicated by some measurable improvement in nutritional status (increased calories, halting of weight loss or weight gain) over the course of the trial period. The necessary parameters for continued outpatient care (e.g., weight threshold) should be agreed upon by all members of the treatment team to maintain consistency in the message to the client. Over the course of treatment, clients may evidence weight loss that indicates outpatient care is no longer tenable. Setting a boundary for appropriateness for continued outpatient care (e.g., no additional weight loss), although painful, often creates a sense of safety or security for the client by setting a limit on AN when she is not able to do so for herself.

A higher level of care is relatively common in the treatment of AN and might include a brief medical stabilization, a longer admission to an inpatient psychiatric unit, or residential treatment (American Psychiatric Association, 2006; Anderson et al., 2017). A brief medical stabilization might occur if a client presents to a physician visit with a heart rate below 30 beats per minute or sufficiently disturbed laboratory results (e.g., electrolyte imbalances) (American Psychiatric Association, 2006). An admission to a psychiatric unit might be necessary if an individual is so physically compromised that any additional weight loss or a lack of immediate weight gain is too risky. In this case, inpatient treatment allows for more rapid weight gain, while closely monitoring metabolic parameters for refeeding syndrome. Clients may then reengage outpatient treatment after discharge. Residential treatment might be recommended if outpatient treatment has not resulted in improvements in eating behavior after several weeks to months of active engagement, and the individual is entrenched in AN. It might also be recommended when external supports are exhausted, leading to a decreased ability to behave in ways that challenge AN at home. Residential treatment facilities can take over the task of preparing and providing meals and monitoring eating for a period of time. Thus, they assume the role of the external supports and can allow clients to practice skills, without being responsible for managing their eating or food choices.

For Whom Is This Treatment, and Who Are the Treatment Providers?

AN has a bimodal typical age of onset, occurring most frequently in adolescence and young adulthood (Halmi et al., 1979). A new onset of a case of AN rarely occurs after age 25 (Hudson et al., 2007). When older clients do present, it is often for reasons other than AN (e.g., depression) (Hall, 1982; Noordenbos et al., 2002). While the content of this text is geared toward adolescents and young to middle-aged adults, there is no age limit for this manual, and interventions are relevant for individuals of all ages presenting with AN-spectrum issues. Women and girls continue to be at greater risk for AN (Hudson et al., 2007). Throughout the manual, we default to the pronoun "she" for this reason. However, interventions in this text may be used with individuals who identify as female, male, transgender, or genderqueer. The therapist should keep in mind that whereas interventions are the same at the process level for individuals of various demographics, as expected, the content of some interventions may need to be adapted to match the unique experience of the individual.

Treatment should be provided by a qualified professional licensed in counseling or psychotherapy or a licensed mental health professional. Ideally, professionals have a background in eating disorder treatment and behavioral interventions or behavior analysis.

Presenting the Treatment Approach to Clients

Unlike some presenting problems, there are few alternative empirically based treatment options to discuss with clients presenting with AN. There is no appreciable evidence for a particular approach with adults (Brockmeyer et al., 2018; Watson & Bulik, 2013), and with adolescents, we know the most about the importance of including the family (American Psychiatric Association, 2006; Le Grange, Lock, Loeb, & Nicholls, 2010; Lock, 2015) rather than the key ingredients of treatment. Therapists should inform clients that the standard of care for AN is to include parents or caregivers in the treatment of adolescents (American Psychiatric Association, 2006; Golden et al., 2003) and for all clients to be medically monitored (American Psychiatric Association, 2006). Clients should be aware that treatment of AN is an active area of development and that there is evidence for the efficacy of CBT (including newer CBTs, such as ACT), albeit preliminary (e.g., Fairburn et al., 2013; Timko et al., 2015).

Similar to how the therapist might set a trial of outpatient treatment, clients may be invited to engage in a trial period of ACT (e.g., participating in four sessions before determining whether the therapeutic approach is useful). The core premise of ACT and how it differs from second-wave CBT should be described. It might also be useful to discuss remission rates and that weight restoration reverses some of the consequences of AN. We provide a sample script below. This information should not be delivered all at once (as it is presented), but rather in a manner that allows for the client's participation in the discussion. We also provide a brief dialogue differentiating ACT from treatment strategies that focus on cognitive change. Other, more experiential introductions to ACT might also be used, although they may be less well tolerated by individuals with AN initially.

IN PRACTICE

Therapist Script

"I know it is a lot, and I imagine you have a lot of questions. I can sense some ambivalence, too, and that is completely understandable. I do want to tell you a little bit about the state of the field and our approach, if that's OK . . . and answer any questions that you might have at this point.

"Early evidence suggests that cognitive-behavioral therapy (or CBT) is useful for people with eating and weight concerns.

"As you know, the model of therapy that I use is ACT. There are a lot of therapy models under the broader CBT umbrella (and outside of it) and I am happy to tell you more about these other therapies if you think you might be interested in a different approach. ACT is a CBT, but it is a newer CBT that uses acceptance and mindfulness. It is based on the assumption that many of our thoughts and feelings do not go away—and what's important is how we respond to them.

"We tend to do a couple of things as humans that, while completely sensible in the moment, end up being less helpful in the long run. First, we try to avoid or escape uncomfortable or unwanted feelings—and this leads us to do all kinds of things that we might not otherwise choose. And the more we fight feelings, the worse it gets. When we try to make them go away, life turns upside down. Part of the solution, then, is to allow feelings (or other internal experiences that are uncomfortable), so we can behave in ways that enhance our lives.

"The other thing is that sometimes we get caught up in (or entangled with) our thoughts in a way that isn't helpful—listening to our thoughts, we lose touch with the present moment and our current experience. We start doing things that are ineffective or even cause harm. In ACT, the aim is to step out of the entanglement of our thoughts—to observe our thoughts for what they are without letting them dictate our actions. This is different than other therapies that might try to change the thoughts themselves in some way.

"Another important element of ACT is a focus on personal values—your values—as a guide for treatment and for life. Thus, we will be talking about what is important to you, deep in your heart, and our work will be about helping things line up with that . . . so that life is valued, vital, and meaningful. Values can also dignify the pain that comes from living. We are much more willing to feel uncomfortable if it is for something that matters to us.

"There are a couple of other things I need to tell you about treatment that are not related to the therapeutic approach.

"Eating issues are complicated and require a multidisciplinary team. The team must include a physician who is familiar with eating disorders, who can follow you throughout treatment. Medical monitoring is essential when individuals are undernourished or engaging in behaviors such as fasting, exercising at a low weight, or self-induced vomiting. These behaviors impact all body systems and can be dangerous. The physician can monitor your health (conduct regular weight monitoring and laboratory tests) and make recommendations regarding weight restoration and how to keep you safe.

"Also, there is a lot of evidence that young people (particularly adolescents, but likely young adults as well) do better when their parents (or family) are part of the therapeutic process. There are different ways that this may look, and this is something for us to figure out together.

"Sometimes a nutritionist and a psychiatrist are also part of the multidisciplinary team. We can decide whether it also makes sense for you to meet with these individuals.

"People sometimes have questions about whether they are 'sick.' . . . This is what I can tell you based on your initial assessment. [Therapist discusses level of severity as it is known and the risks associated with particular behaviors in which the individual is engaging.]

"Many of the effects of AN can reverse with renourishment. However, the longer that people are underweight, the more likely there will be long-term complications—for example, osteoporosis associated with persistent estrogen depletion. You may know that AN actually has the highest mortality rate of any psychiatric issue, and this is of concern.

"The other thing is that bodies are resilient, too. They adapt for a period of time, but this doesn't persist indefinitely; things start breaking down, if they haven't already. Often, people think low weight is OK because the body is not showing certain signs yet. Some signs only show themselves as people start to renourish their bodies.

"I am wondering, how all of this is sounding to you . . . and whether you would be willing to try it out for a period of time? We can then revisit whether there is something in here that feels vital or meaningful . . . useful to you.

"I'm happy to answer any questions that you have, or discuss any part of this in more detail."

Dialogue

CLIENT: I'm not sure that I understand. . . . How are we going to work on this if we are not changing my thoughts?

THERAPIST: Imagine you are moving toward things that you care about in your life (relationships, for example) and inevitably difficult thoughts and feelings show up (like "I am so ugly"; "People don't like me"). The next thing you know, you are doing things to make these thoughts and feelings go away . . . rather than doing things that matter to you. Instead of spending time with friends or getting to know people, you are at the gym, trying to feel better about yourself or the situation. Meanwhile, your relationships aren't improving. We all get stuck in these kinds of traps.

CLIENT: (*Nods.*)

THERAPIST: There are a couple of ways to work on this. One way would be to try to change your thoughts and feelings about whether you are attractive or likable, maybe by examining the validity of your thoughts: whether they are realistic, logical, overly negative. . . . Another way would be to take the power out of these thoughts and feelings . . . so they don't decide, you do. Instead of choices being rigidly determined by these experiences, they can be guided by deeply held personal values: What you want to be about, deep in your heart . . . what you want your life to be like.

The Therapeutic Alliance

The ACT Stance

While all organisms experience pain, the unique ways in which humans suffer may be understood as arising from our capacity for language—that is, our ability to have words stand in for events and compare and evaluate everything (including ourselves and the signals arising from our body) (Hayes et al., 2001). Because suffering arises from language rather than some pathogenic disease process, the ACT perspective is one of *shared vulnerability*. ACT assumes that there is no substantive difference between the client and the therapist; the only difference is vantage point: the vantage point from which we experience our own thoughts and feelings versus those of our clients. The common humanity (or shared vulnerability) of the client and therapist is deeply appreciated and directly acknowledged throughout treatment, and is an important element of the therapeutic alliance.

Challenges to the Therapeutic Alliance in AN

AN poses some unique challenges in alliance building irrespective of the therapeutic approach. First, AN is highly ego-syntonic, and individuals with AN may experience a strong sense of mastery or pride in their restraint (e.g., Serpell, Treasure, Teasdale, & Sullivan, 1999). Thus, they not only fear relinquishing food restriction or weight loss, but they are also specifically motivated to protect it. They might also be motivated to protect their critical self-talk, which they may experience as helping them stay focused, driven, and in control. This creates tension, as clients may view treatment as a threat and fear becoming lazy, greedy, or selfish if they treat themselves with more compassion. Second, individuals with AN also often have difficulty with intimacy and disclosure of feelings. They may view expression of feelings as a personal failure and fear that they will be judged as weak or uncontrolled (e.g., Davies et al., 2011; Fox, 2009; Harrison et al., 2009; Lavender et al., 2015; Schmidt & Treasure, 2006; Wildes et al., 2010). They might also be confused about how they feel and resist disclosure for fear of making a mistake (Farstad et al., 2016; Haynos & Fruzzetti, 2011; Schmidt & Treasure, 2006). Often, they have a history of having their experience invalidated by others, potentially due to masking feelings or decreased facial affect (Davies et al., 2011; Haynos & Fruzzetti, 2011), which limits the information the outside world receives about their internal experience. Therapeutic alliance is facilitated by the therapist's willingness to be genuine and vulnerable. This includes the therapist's expression of personal values related to the therapeutic encounter and being open with regard to his or her own experience in the moment (i.e., ongoing thoughts and feelings), sometimes verbalized to the client, sometimes not. Additional tips include:

- Appreciate the rich and complicated motivations for AN (or what AN "does" for the client) and how hard it might be to let go of restrictive eating and weight loss.

- Be forthcoming about the need for weight restoration, and connect weight restoration directly to values. This includes not only the therapist's value to be useful to the client (to preserve the longevity and quality of her life), but also the client's values: what is meaningful to her in the deepest sense, or what she would want for her life if she could live inside her own skin. For clients who are compelled to treatment by others, the value of reestablishing independence or autonomy may be all that is available. In this case, treatment may be initially framed as working to free the client from some of the additional unwanted oversight.

- Meet the client "where she is," while also standing for her. This includes the therapist acknowledging that the client might not want or be ready for change, and (with the client's permission) setting clear, warm, but firm boundaries around AN. Boundaries for AN paradoxically strengthen the therapeutic alliance by increasing the client's sense of safety and security (i.e., she is not abandoned to the eating disorder).

The dialogues below illustrate alliance building in initial sessions. Dialogue B also illustrates how the therapist avoids getting entangled with the content of AN thoughts.

IN PRACTICE

Dialogue A

CLIENT: I don't even know why I am here.

THERAPIST: You feel confused about this whole thing. You know your family is really concerned about your eating and weight, and so is your doctor.

CLIENT: I think that they are making something out of nothing. I'm fine. I just want to be left alone.

THERAPIST: I get that this is the last thing you feel like you need. I want you to know that as far as you and I are concerned, this is about you and your life. That doesn't mean that I can stand by and lose you to the eating disorder (that actually wouldn't be standing with you at all, and it is important to me that I do that), but it does mean that I want to find what is important in here for you. I wonder . . . what might make it worthwhile to face fears about eating . . . ?

Dialogue B

CLIENT: I just feel like everyone is trying to make me fat! Why does everyone want me to be fat?!

THERAPIST: (*compassionately*) It sounds like you feel frustrated or angry. [The therapist responds to the emotional content rather than convincing the client that this isn't so and getting entangled in the content of her thoughts.]

CLIENT: I just don't understand why I have to gain weight when that woman in the waiting room gets to walk around. I don't think I need to gain weight.

THERAPIST: I hear you. I also wonder if this is familiar to you? Something your mind says when you are feeling afraid . . . afraid of change?

CLIENT: Well, she is really thin! Thinner than me! I'm sorry. I'm not mad at you.

THERAPIST: It is totally fine to have all of this here. In fact, it is nice to see you (*smiles gently*). Like more the full range of you. Mad, that is part of you, too . . . and it's important to me that you know you can bring that. It can be here, while we find a way forward together . . . [additional values engagement]. . . . There is nothing more important to me in here than to find a way to be useful to you—to help you create the life you want; one that is valued and vital . . . and I get that right now it is hard to see how weight restoration is part of that . . . and I wonder if we can talk about what thoughts and feelings that brings up? We know "mad," but what else?

Therapist Barriers to the Therapeutic Alliance

Just as the client brings her thoughts, feelings, and behavioral predispositions that pose challenges to the therapeutic alliance, so does the therapist. Therapists may be fearful of the physical fragility of their clients, particularly when the client herself is indifferent or resistant to change. They may experience an urgency "to do something" that may be further intensified by distressed family and friends. Therapists may also have strong emotional responses to clients' lack of engagement or active opposition to treatment. They may be put off by visual body scanning or judgments that clients express. Body-related judgments may be particularly disturbing if they activate the therapist's own body concerns and contribute to a gulf between the therapist and client. The therapist should be mindful and aware of his or her ongoing experience and how this might interfere with being present and value-guided with the client. Additional tools for assessing therapist barriers are provided in Chapter 11.

Looking Ahead

In Chapter 3, we provide an in-depth description of an ACT-based assessment and case formulation, which directly informs treatment. We describe how to conduct a functional assessment of AN, and how to expand assessment to the six core process or functional domains. We provide a case formulation and treatment planning form (Form 3.1) and dimensional rating scales for the six core process domains (Form 3.2) at the end of Chapter 3. The functional assessment is not just a treatment planning exercise. It is also an important intervention, providing a vehicle to explore the workability of AN behaviors and potentially pave the way for something new.

CHAPTER 3

ACT Case Formulation, Assessment, and Treatment Planning

with **Lisa K. Honeycutt** and **Ashley A. Moskovich**

The central feature of an ACT case formulation is the functional assessment. The functional assessment specifies the contingencies maintaining AN (i.e., how AN is helpful to the individual and/or functions to provide emotional relief, despite physical and psychological harm). Initially, the functional assessment focuses on food restriction, driven exercise, and other maladaptive eating and weight control behaviors. However, it quickly expands to other behaviors that, while topographically dissimilar, are functionally equivalent to the core features of AN. This may include, for example, performing "perfectly" in relationships, school, or work, which, along with eating and weight control, may decrease anxiety, guilt, or shame.

The therapist builds upon this initial functional assessment a more thorough case formulation by viewing the client's struggle through the lens of the six core ACT processes: Acceptance, Defusion, Present-Moment Awareness, Self-as-Context, Values, and Committed Action. This more detailed assessment aids in treatment planning (e.g., identifying specific targets for Acceptance or Defusion) and allows the therapist to track client strengths, weaknesses, and progress in specific skill domains (e.g., capacity for Present-Moment Awareness).

Lisa K. Honeycutt holds a dual licensure as a Licensed Professional Counselor and a Licensed Marriage and Family Therapist in the state of North Carolina. She has served as Clinical Research Coordinator in the Department of Psychiatry and Behavioral Sciences at the Duke University Medical Center since 2009. Ms. Honeycutt also serves as a counselor in the ACT at Duke program and the Duke Center for Eating Disorders and as a medical family therapist in the Healthy Lifestyles program in the Department of Pediatrics at Duke University Medical Center.

Ashley A. Moskovich, PhD, is a medical instructor in the Department of Psychiatry and Behavioral Sciences at the Duke University School of Medicine. She completed her predoctoral internship at the UCLA Semel Institute for Neuroscience and Human Behavior and earned her PhD in clinical psychology from Duke University. Dr. Moskovich completed a postdoctoral fellowship at Duke University Medical Center before joining the Duke faculty in 2017. She is a licensed psychologist with expertise in acceptance and commitment therapy and the treatment of eating disorders.

Antecedents–Behaviors–Consequences (ABCs) and Intervening at the Level of Context

Before discussing AN case formulation, it may be useful to briefly describe behavior analytic or contextual approaches to understanding and intervening on behavior problems.

Behavior analysis applies learning theory to the study of human behavior. Analyses specify the context in which behaviors emerge (e.g., antecedents, consequences) for the goal of predication and influence of behavior.

Historically, behavior analysis focused on behavior and environmental factors that could be directly observed and modified. Clinical applications were limited and focused on problems among individuals with autism and intellectual disabilities, and in classroom settings and group homes (where operant learning principles such as reinforcement could easily be applied). In conducting functional assessments in this setting, behavior analysts would directly observe the individual in his or her environment and identify antecedent and consequent conditions that could be modified to decrease problem behavior and/or increase a desirable alternative response. For example, imagine a child who acts out during math class. Careful observation might determine that the child's acting-out behavior is reliably *preceded by* a performance demand (e.g., when the students are asked to complete math problems at the board or a timed activity; the antecedent) and *followed by* the teacher removing the child from the classroom (a powerful short-term consequence). This consequence maintains the child's behavior, despite the notes sent home to his or her parents, or other more delayed negative outcomes (see Figure 3.1). The child's tendency to act out might be modified by altering antecedent and consequent conditions. For example, the teacher might reduce the demand to the child's skills level a priori, notify the child of the upcoming demand (at 10, 5, and 2 minutes prior), and not allow acting out to result in escape from the task altogether. Engagement in the task might also be incentivized with stickers or something else that the child finds reinforcing.

In this example, a "performance demand" is an external stimulus and only one element of the antecedent conditions. There are also the child's internal experiences that co-occur with this demand. This might include, for example, the thought "I'm stupid," a queasy stomach, and anxiety (see Figure 3.2). In dealing with this issue, second-wave CBT diverges from the core tenets of contextual behavioral science, taking a more mechanistic approach and formulating these thoughts and feelings themselves as the cause of the child's behavior (and thus a target for change themselves). The idea is that by helping the child shift from "I am stupid" to more rational, realistic, or positive thinking (e.g., "It is challenging, but with continued effort, I can learn"), the child will no longer need to escape the situation.

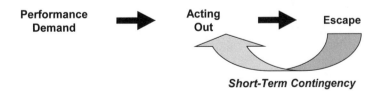

FIGURE 3.1. Observable situational factors influencing "acting out."

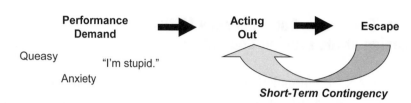

FIGURE 3.2. Additional internal factors influencing "acting out" (which may or may not be observed publicly).

ACT, in contrast, retains the contextual frame when considering these internal events. Rather than change the thoughts and feelings themselves, ACT aims to change *the context* in which thoughts and feelings are situated to facilitate more effective behavior. This includes the context of *literality* (which reinforces treating words like the literal events they represent) and the context of *experiential control* (see Figure 3.3). It is only when "I am stupid" is experienced literally that it has emotional power, and only in a context in which emotional control is good that escape is necessary (see Hayes et al., 2001, for a more extensive discussion). ACT increases the child's behavioral options by creating a situation in which thoughts can be experienced directly, as mental activity, and feelings may be permitted. Environmental factors might also be changed (e.g., adding a warning for a performance demand) to support new behavioral responses.

Functional Assessment

Initial Behavioral Targets

Among individuals with AN, initial targets for intervention are behaviors that maintain dangerously low weight (e.g., excessive caloric restriction). This is followed by eating and weight control behaviors that limit life vitality (e.g., refusal to eat out) (see Table 3.1) and behaviors that have a different form but serve a similar purpose or function as AN. This might include,

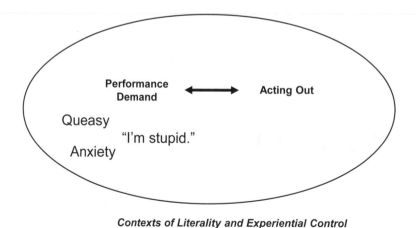

FIGURE 3.3. Contexts that support "acting out" in the presence of thoughts and feelings.

TABLE 3.1. Eating Disorder Behavioral Targets for Individuals with AN

- Restricting intake (overall calories, food types, time of day)
- Exercising excessively; until injury or to the exclusion of other life activities
- Purging (self-induced vomiting, laxatives, diuretics, medication misuse)
- Taking appetite suppressants
- Chewing and spitting
- Picking/nibbling (rather than sitting down to a meal)
- Body checking ("pinching" fat, weighing excessively)
- Avoidance of body information (avoiding mirrors, weighing, trying on clothes)
- Avoidance of body exposure (hiding body under layers of clothing, avoiding communal changing rooms or swimming)
- Cutting food into small pieces, arranging food
- Focusing on fatness or fat talk
- Evaluating nutritional content, counting calories, and so forth
- Making food unappetizing (creating strange concoctions, imagining maggots, etc.)
- Meal planning
- Refusing to buy a bigger clothing size, refusing to get rid of clothes from a lower weight

for example, achievement striving in other domains, such as academics (see Table 3.4 on page 54). The therapist should be aware that some behaviors observed among individuals with AN (e.g., prolonging meals or cutting food into small pieces) are the result of starvation rather than a functional operant. These behaviors may remit without direct intervention as nutrition improves. Additional information about the impact of starvation can be found in Chapter 5 and may be useful to review when initiating treatment.

Contingencies Maintaining AN Behavior

After initial target behaviors are identified, the therapist specifies how these behaviors change the individual's internal experience from less to more preferred, and therefore are reinforced. While somewhat idiosyncratic, thoughts and feelings that AN may attenuate include (1) feeling uncertain, overwhelmed, or a lack of control and (2) feeling like a bad or imperfect person, unlikable, undeserving, or a disappointment or failure. We provide tools for identifying the contingencies maintaining AN behavior in the next major section of this chapter.

Contingencies *Not* Currently Exerting Stimulus Control

Functional assessment also requires identifying the *undesirable* consequences of AN that are not currently exerting stimulus control. These consequences might simply be ignored or denied by the client in order to preserve or protect AN. Consequences might also be severely delayed (such as the effects of prolonged starvation) or only become apparent as the client's nutrition improves and she gains clarity about her personal values (e.g., absence of close relationships). The undesirable consequences of AN are explored over time, in a manner sensitive to the client's stage of change (see Chapter 6).

Functional Assessment Tools

Functional assessment begins in the clinical interview and is aided by a historical timeline of the onset of behaviors and periods of exacerbation or remittance. Functional relationships might also be elucidated by chain analyses, daily experience cards, and observation of in-session behavior. Each of these assessment tools is described below.

The Clinical Interview

The clinical interview situates AN in the client's life and specifies the conditions under which maladaptive eating and weight control have emerged. This information helps the therapist generate hypotheses about the possible functions of AN or related behaviors. During the clinical interview, close attention is paid to transitions in the client's life (e.g., starting a new school or a new job, ending participation in a sport) and events that threatened the individual's competency, social status, or sense of personal control (e.g., getting a "B" on an exam or a negative performance review). These events are common triggers for increased preoccupation with eating and weight and/or rigid attempts to gain emotional and behavioral control (see Table 3.2).

In addition to providing life context, the clinical interview also provides specific information about client strengths and weaknesses that are important in treatment planning. Client

TABLE 3.2. Categories of Potentially Relevant Events in the History of AN Development

Event	Examples
Experiences of feeling ugly or not good enough	• Not being asked out while others around you are • Mention of weight gain at a family reunion
Experience of uncertainty or lack or control	• Transitions (e.g., changing schools or jobs, moving, divorce)
Events that suggested that the individual was "out of control"	• A choice that led to a bad outcome • Onset of intense emotions • Sexual feelings
Events that suggested unlikability or signaled rejection	• Loss of a relationship • Not getting into a sorority • No one to sit with at lunch
Events that threatened competency	• Receiving a "C" on an assignment • Negative feedback from a boss
Events that threatened identity	• Ending participation in a sport or activity • Child moving out of the home • Job loss
Other "shaming" incidents	• Body exposure at doctor's appointment • Sexual activity • Someone mentioning an error, public criticism
New information or rules about food or the body (that differed from what the individual was doing or suggested that she was wrong)	• Nutrition class • Change in group norms

strengths may include the ability to flexibly take perspective or have rich self-knowledge (e.g., awareness of thoughts, feelings and interests outside of AN, clarity about personal values). Weaknesses may include the inverse of these strengths or other skills deficits that may increase vulnerability to AN (e.g., long-standing difficulty making or maintaining friendships).

We provide a script for introducing the clinical interview and outline the key areas for inquiry below. It is neither possible (nor ideal) to cover all of these areas in this depth in the initial interview, and some areas may be skipped altogether.

IN PRACTICE

Therapist Script

"Before we get into our work, I would like to get some more information, to situate your struggle with eating or weight in the broader context of your life. . . . I wonder if you'd be willing to tell me more about how you find yourself here and what led up to this point . . . and times when things have been easier or harder.

"You are also more than your struggle, more than your eating and body concerns . . . and so I also want to know you . . . what you care about [other than eating and weight] . . . the things that have been important or mattered most to you . . . what you have wished for in all of this . . ."

Presenting Issue

- When did the individual first begin to worry about her body, food, or eating? Worry may predate significant caloric restriction/weight loss. (The therapist might also identify when the individual became preoccupied with gaining control over herself or her behavior. If there was a clear onset of preoccupation with emotional and behavioral control, this will also inform the functional assessment.)
- When did the individual first begin restricting calories or food types ("dieting")? What was the time course to AN?
- Periods of exacerbation and relative remission, including significant fluctuations in weight (e.g., highest and lowest weight for current height)
- Events coinciding with changes in eating and weight preoccupation
- Current weight and height
- Detailed information about current food intake and weight control behavior; include a 24-hour dietary recall, with specific probing of quantities (e.g., do not assume that "eating a sandwich" means the entire sandwich with two pieces of bread, meat, and cheese)
- The client's current living situation (does the client live alone, with a spouse, etc.?)
- Conditions of the household (who works, etc.)
- Quality of the relationships of members of the household

Family History

- Where did the individual grow up?
- What were the conditions of family life (members of the family, occupations, etc.)?

- Transitions of childhood that may have coincided with eating and weight preoccupation; examples include:
  - Moving to a new neighborhood or town
  - Changing schools
  - Marriage or divorce or other changes in family structure (e.g., family member leaving for college)
  - Death of a family member
- Family-of-origin patterns/attitudes
  - Closeness of relationships
  - Patterns of communication
  - Management of conflict
  - Attitudes about food, exercise, and body weight/shape
- Traumatic events in childhood
- Family mental health issues

Social

- Current social context
  - Breadth of social support network (e.g., one vs. several friends)
  - Depth of relationships (level of intimacy)
  - Frequency of utilization of social support or social engagement

Assessment of the client's social support system may be aided by the "Social Support Bullseye" exercise. In this activity, the client's name is placed in the center of a bullseye, with each "ring" representing degree of closeness. The rings are populated with the names of individuals in the client's social network. For example, the center ring should include only individuals who are closest to the client, who know her "hopes and fears." The furthest ring may include only minor acquaintances (see Figure 3.4). This exercise provides not only a visual depiction of the individual's current social support network, but it is also intervention and allows for concrete committed actions in the social domain. For example, the client might identify individuals whom she would like to "bring closer" through initiation of plans, disclosure, and other behaviors that build intimacy.

- Social developmental milestones
  - Interest in other children
  - Transitioning from parallel to interactive play
  - Separating from caregiver (to attend school, sleep in own room, attend sleepovers, etc.)
- History of friendship and intimacy/dating
  - Did she interact with peers as a child (rather than gravitating to people who are much older or much younger)? Did she have a best friend?
  - Has she participated in dating or romantic relationships (if developmentally appropriate)?
  - Were there major changes in friendships or intimate relationships that might coincide with changes in eating or weight preoccupation?

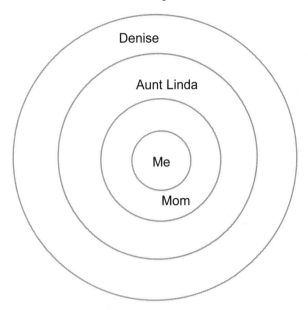

FIGURE 3.4. "Social Support Bullseye" exercise that provides a graphical representation of the client's social context (social support system).

- Social skills; examples include:
  - Ability to join in
  - Ability to initiate interactions or plans
  - Ability to self-disclose and form close relationships (not just acquaintances)
  - Ability to participate in unstructured social activities
  - Ability to maintain boundaries

Academic/Occupational Functioning and Participation in Sports or Other Extracurricular Activities

- Current academic and occupational pursuits
- Past academic or employment history (e.g., types of jobs, stability of employment)
- Participation in sports and other extracurricular activities
  - Competitive versus noncompetitive, team versus individual sport
  - Activities in which body size is relevant (e.g., gymnastics, dance, flyer for cheerleading team, jockeying)
  - Activities that may or may not be supported/valued by family and peer groups
- Sense of personal meaning in pursuits
- Start and end times that might have coincided with changes in eating and weight preoccupation
- Skills in managing activities
  - Ability to not overextend (not take on more than is necessary, expected, or healthy)
  - Ability to take breaks
  - Ability to receive feedback/tolerate mistakes

Medical History

- Illnesses, injuries, and surgeries, particularly those that resulted in weight loss or inability to exercise or that impacted sense of personal control or identity
- Chronic medical conditions
  - Onset of the condition
  - Experience of diagnosis
  - Impact of the condition on body weight or management of the timing and content of food intake or exercise (e.g., as in type 1 diabetes)
  - Relationship to the condition and management behaviors (e.g., accepting vs. rejecting)
- Medical complications associated with disordered eating or maladaptive weight control (e.g., history of an esophageal tear)

Mental Health History

- History of inpatient, residential, and outpatient treatment
- History of suicidal ideation and/or self-harm
- Psychotropic medications
- Reactions of other people to client's mental health issues, particularly if reinforcing

Developmental History

- Pregnancy or early feeding or gastrointestinal problems
- Developmental milestones other than social (walking, talking, toilet training, puberty, verbal vs. performance abilities—e.g., early reading)
- Other:
  - Need for order, structure, or routine and reactions to changes in daily schedule
  - Ability to communicate needs or ask for help
  - Ability to act independently
  - Reaction to pubertal development

Timeline Activity

Supplementing the clinical interview with the creation of a historical timeline may make it easier to see the time sequence of events and highlight antecedent and consequent conditions. It might also be easier to probe specific experiences in the client's life that may be relevant to understanding the function of AN (e.g., loss of a best friend). In creating a timeline, the therapist may use disposable whiteboard paper or several sheets of paper taped together. Key events from the clinical interview are placed on the timeline, and the therapist probes to deepen understanding of corresponding thoughts, feelings, and reactions to various situations. Gaps in the client's history are filled in. This includes gaps between major events (i.e., what was happening in the client's life at those times), as well as gaps in knowledge of the client's experience of her life events.

The timeline can begin anywhere; however, useful starting points include the following:

- When the client first became concerned about eating or her body
- When the client first attempted to deliberately change how her body looked through diet, exercise, or other means
- When friends or family first became concerned about the client's weight loss
- When treatment was initiated

A script for introducing the timeline activity is provided below. Figures 3.5 and 3.6 provide illustrations of historical timelines.

IN PRACTICE

Therapist Script (Introducing the Timeline Activity)

"I am starting to get a sense of how things have been for you, and I am wondering if we could lay this out in a timeline . . . fill in some gaps and dig in a bit deeper . . . into the moments before, during, and after things got better or worse [or your focus on eating and weight intensified]. I want to get a better sense of your experience in those moments, including the thoughts and feelings you were having. If I were to ask you what kind of

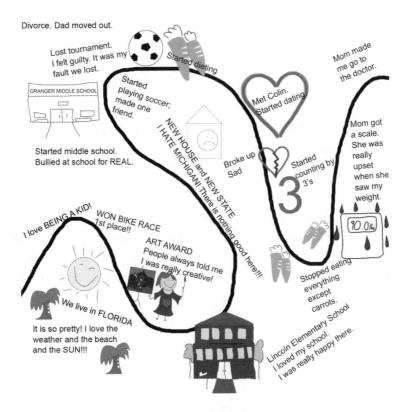

FIGURE 3.5. One example of an adolescent timeline to probe events corresponding with onset or remittance of behaviors.

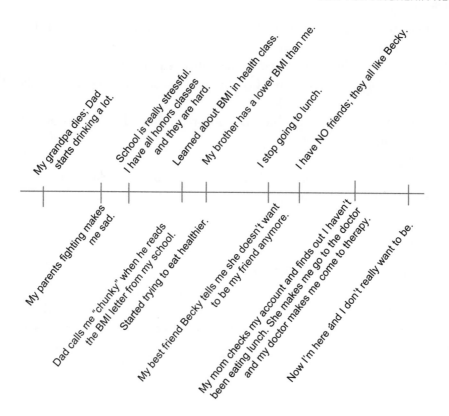

FIGURE 3.6. Another example of an adolescent timeline to probe events corresponding with onset or remittance of behaviors.

fabric is on this chair, you might say leather, but it would be different to describe the richness and variations of the color as they are experienced to your eye or how the fabric feels to your skin. I am hoping we can do that—that you can help me experience your experience . . . get it more from the inside out . . . so I could almost know what it was like to be you in these moments."

Information from the clinical interview and historical timeline is used to generate hypotheses about the psychological function of AN (i.e., how AN was helpful or seemed to improve the client's situation), as illustrated in the dialogue below. We outline common functions of AN along two dimensions for easy recognition in client narratives (see Table 3.3).

Dialogue

THERAPIST: You said you moved around that time. What was that like for you?

CLIENT: OK, I guess.

THERAPIST: What do you remember thinking or feeling about the change?

CLIENT: I remember hating that I had to change schools. I didn't know where to sit in class or at lunch. Everyone knew each other.

THERAPIST: What was that like for you?

CLIENT: (*Describes.*)

THERAPIST: (*Summarizes thoughts/feelings.*) You seem sad; does that bring up sadness talking about it now?

CLIENT: I don't know. I shouldn't be upset. It was 2 years ago . . . and I am in math Olympiad and AP classes now. My other school didn't have the same kinds of opportunities.

THERAPIST: Changing schools is hard.

CLIENT: It shouldn't be.

THERAPIST: Your mind gives you some kind of rule of what things can/should be hard . . . when it is acceptable to be upset.

    (*pause*) So let me see if I got this . . . In the eighth grade you changed schools . . . and while you were happy to have a sense of challenge in the classroom, you weren't sure about your place . . . you felt out of place, maybe even alone . . . ? And you started focusing on your eating around then . . .

CLIENT: Yeah.

THERAPIST: How did things change when you started doing that?

CLIENT: Well, I started spending a lot of time before and after class writing out my meals—what I had eaten or planned to eat. It didn't matter that I didn't have anyone to talk to anymore . . .

THERAPIST: It took your mind off things and gave you something to do while other kids were socializing? . . . In that way, it made things better. And how has it been since then?

TABLE 3.3. Psychological Functions of AN

Positive (what it gave)	Negative (what it took away)
Internal	
• Increased feelings of *safety* or *security* • Made things feel more *predictable* or *controlled* • Made her *feel better about her decisions* (more confident) • Provided a sense of *mastery* or *pride* (i.e., helped the individual feel interesting, special, achieving, excelling, moral/good)	• Decreased *ambiguity* or *uncertainty* • Decreased feeling of being *overwhelmed* or *out of control* • Attenuated feelings of *ineffectiveness* or *low self-worth* (e.g., feeling that one is not good at things, mediocre, uninteresting, or unlikable) • Attenuated feelings of *self-loathing* or *self-disgust*, *guilt*, or *shame* (e.g., feeling wasteful or like a "waste of space") • Reduced fear of *judgment* or *rejection*
External	
• Resulted in *compliments, attention,* or *adoration* from others • Increased *caretaking* from others	• Reduced *uncomfortable sexual attention* • Reduced *weight-related teasing* or *judgment from others* • Decreased *isolation* • Reduced *expectations* or *responsibility*

Chain Analyses

Chain analyses are also helpful in identifying the context in which AN behaviors emerge and are maintained. Chain analyses are conducted in session and have the advantage of being more proximal than a timeline (e.g., centering on an event in the past week). They are also discrete, isolated to a single incident (rather than multiple incidents or a broader pattern of behavior). These features may make it easier for clients to identify relevant thoughts or feelings. In conducting a chain analysis, the therapist starts with a recent time when the client skipped a meal, purged, or engaged in another maladaptive eating or weight control behavior. It might also include times when the client was particularly consumed by eating disorder thoughts. The therapist helps the client identify "links" in the chain to the behavior. This includes environmental/situational factors, as well as thoughts, feelings, body sensations, urges, memories, and so forth. In identifying antecedents, it is important to go beyond the most proximal antecedent (which is often more directly related to body weight and shape; e.g., trying on clothing) to the event that sensitized the individual to the eating disorder cue in the first place (e.g., a rejection experience).

The therapist also goes *forward* in time to identify the consequences of engaging in AN behaviors, for example, emotional relief, or undesirable outcomes, if available (e.g., subsequent increase in guilt after purging). Figure 3.7 provides an example of a chain analysis. Relevant dialogue follows.

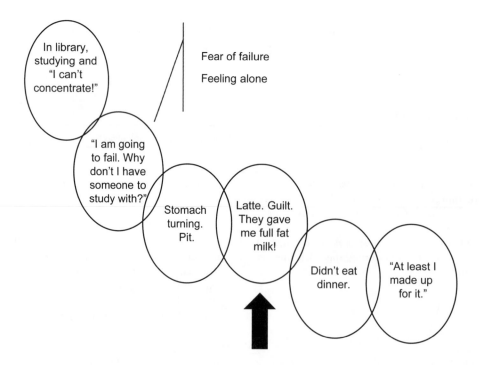

FIGURE 3.7. Sample chain analysis. The presenting concern (identified by the client) and the beginning of the chain analysis is marked with an arrow. Additional links were identified with the therapist. These include earlier antecedents (external and internal), responses, and consequences.

IN PRACTICE

Dialogue

THERAPIST: You said that you restricted dinner.

CLIENT: Yeah, I had a latte at the coffee shop on campus. It was too much. I just felt so bloated . . . and disgusting . . . so I skipped dinner.

THERAPIST: Is it OK if we take a look at how your day unfolded?

CLIENT: OK . . .

THERAPIST: Tell me what was going on before that. Where were you and what were you doing?

CLIENT: I was working in the library—studying for a chemistry test. I was distracted by these two girls talking though. I couldn't focus.

THERAPIST: You were studying and feeling distracted. Did you worry that you wouldn't do well on the test?

CLIENT: Yeah, I started getting anxious about it.

THERAPIST: So you felt anxious. How did you know you were anxious? What did you feel in your body?

CLIENT: Butterflies . . . my stomach was turning. . . . I also felt this sinking feeling. Like a pit.

THERAPIST: You could feel turning and sinking in your gut. . . . Anything else?

CLIENT: I just kept thinking why was I studying alone. . . . What is wrong with me?

THERAPIST: So you were anxious about the exam, but also feeling badly about yourself . . .

CLIENT: Yes. . . . They gave me regular milk in my latte though. That was really upsetting.

THERAPIST: I have no doubt that was upsetting to you (*softly, pause*). . . . I also wonder if the latte was harder to cope with because you were feeling bad about yourself more generally . . . because you were alone? And I am wondering if this comes up for you at other times . . . ?

Daily Experience Cards

Daily experience cards may be used between sessions to identify thoughts, feelings, and situational factors associated with AN behaviors. Daily experience cards have the advantage of decreasing reliance on retrospective recall. Recording closer in time to the actual event, the client may be better able to access detailed information about the conditions under which the behavior emerged (i.e., thoughts, feelings, situational factors that preceded or followed a refused meal, excessive exercise, purging, etc.). Daily experience (or diary) cards, Handouts 7.1 and 7.2, are described in more depth in Chapter 7. They are available at the end of the chapter and can be downloaded and printed for use in your work with clients (see the box at the end of the table of contents).

In-Session Behavior

The client's behavior in session provides some of the richest information about the emotional antecedents of AN (and other functionally equivalent behaviors). The key is for the therapist to be a keen observer and to notice conditions associated with shifts in the client's attention toward eating and weight. For example, the therapist might observe when the client abruptly changes topics to eating and the necessity of weight gain or when she becomes preoccupied with how her stomach feels (as illustrated in the dialogue below). The therapist can mark these changes and ask (privately or publicly with the client), "What was happening right before that?"

- What were the situational factors (e.g., topic of conversation)?
- What was the client likely experiencing immediately prior to the change (i.e., thoughts, feelings, body sensations)?

IN PRACTICE

Dialogue

The client is describing when she first starting restricting her eating.

CLIENT: I think I was 15 [years old] and after we moved, it just wasn't possible to do volleyball.

THERAPIST: That sounds like it was really hard—to lose this thing that was so important to you at the time. (*long pause*)

CLIENT: I don't even know why I am doing this and why I am here. I have already added more food than I wanted to. My body is disgusting . . .

THERAPIST: I am wondering what happened for you there. . . . You were talking about volleyball, and then it shifted. . . . You started talking about why you are here, and if you need to be, and I am wondering, what were you feeling right before that . . . before you turned your attention to eating and weight?

Challenges and Opportunities in the Functional Assessment

Lack of Clear Episodes for Analysis

Some AN behaviors are fairly discrete, such as an episode of purging or intense exercise. Other behaviors are less so. For example, dietary restraint may occur as a continuous behavior, with little variability. Thus, it may be difficult to isolate the episode or pinpoint the factors that preceded it. This can pose a challenge in functional assessment. There are several possible solutions. First, the absence of behavior (eating) when it is supposed to occur (at a mealtime) is an event for analysis. Second, *relative* increases in restriction urges or eating or body preoccupation, may be the target behavior for analysis (we elaborate this point with the "Eating Disorder Volume" metaphor, introduced in Chapter 7). Finally, the target behavior may be expanded to hours or days. For example, it might be possible to identify factors that discriminate a "high-restriction day" from a day in which food intake was relatively more consistent.

Lack of Clear Onset of AN

For some clients, the onset of AN is experienced as a gradual development of their identity, without a clear "onset" per se. This is particularly common among adolescents. In this case, the therapist can inquire more deeply about factors that influenced the client's ideas of who she was or what she should care about, as illustrated in the following dialogue.

IN PRACTICE

Dialogue

THERAPIST: I wonder if we could take a look at what was going on when you changed your eating?

CLIENT: I don't really know when you are talking about. My mom said something to me in December, but I was eating salads way before that. I just want to be healthy. Being healthy is important to me. It is who I am.

THERAPIST: Tell me more about that moment you decided that you cared about health, that this was important to you . . .

CLIENT: I guess I learned about nutrition in the seventh grade. . . . We learned all about what to eat/not eat. . . . I guess it just became "my thing."

THERAPIST: So it was kind of like your identity, "Kate was healthy or the nutrition guru."

CLIENT: Yeah, all my friends were dating, talking about boys. I just didn't care about that stuff.

THERAPIST: What was it like to have your friends caring about boys when you weren't into it?

Limited Emotional Awareness

Limited emotional awareness is common among clients with AN and may interfere with their ability to identify emotional antecedents. For example, clients might only be aware of somatic experiences, without associating this with an emotion (e.g., they might report only that they "feel fat" or that their "stomach hurts" when experiencing anxiety or report "fatigue" when experiencing sadness). They may simply repeatedly respond "I don't know" to any question about how they feel. Limited emotional awareness may be compounded by a lack of willingness to acknowledge feelings, which they may view as a personal weakness. This may delay understanding of how AN helps the client cope. Case formulation may need to be updated as clients' emotional awareness and willingness increase and emotional antecedents become known.

Using "Response Prevention" to Identify Feelings

A client with AN may be so skilled at controlling internal experience that she has not felt vulnerable emotions in a long time. As a result, she may now have limited awareness of the thoughts/feelings that are distressing to her. These experiences might remain inaccessible as long as extreme caloric restriction, list making, planning, conforming, or other rigid control behaviors are at high strength. Thus, it may be necessary to temporarily block avoidant behaviors and observe what thoughts and feelings emerge. This work is done with the client's informed consent and in a valued context. The following dialogue illustrates the process of obtaining informed consent and introducing this strategy to gain access to feelings.

IN PRACTICE

Dialogue

THERAPIST: What feelings do you think you were managing in that moment?

CLIENT: I don't know.

THERAPIST: I notice that comes up for you a lot. . . . Is this familiar to you . . . this experience of not knowing how you are feeling?

CLIENT: Yes. . . . It's just been like this for so long . . . I don't know why I do it [AN] anymore . . .

THERAPIST: It seems gaining access to these things might require letting go of the strategies that you have developed to keep feelings at bay . . . so that we can see what is in there: What thoughts and feelings show up. Just for a moment . . . like in a moment when you feel compelled to restrict a meal or make a list . . . that you resist and, instead, pause and check in . . . see what is there. Would you be willing to do that? [Purposely uses *willing* rather than *want*. The client is unlikely to *want* to do this, but she might be *willing* to.] (*long pause*) I would not ask you to do this if I didn't think that it could be helpful to you in some way (although admittedly very hard in the moment). And by "helpful," I mean helpful in having the kind of life you would choose.

CLIENT: I'm not sure . . .

THERAPIST: You can think about it and let me know. . . . In anything we do, know that you are the driver. You are the one saying if and when you are willing, and how much. Also know that you can always pick the strategy back up. You are not committing to letting go of it indefinitely, just long enough to learn what feelings it might be protecting you from.

Additional Therapeutic Purposes of the Functional Assessment

In addition to identifying factors maintaining AN (or related behavior), the functional assessment serves a number of other important therapeutic purposes. First, gathering detailed information about the client's experience is an opportunity to connect with the client, to know what thoughts and feelings are painful to her, and to learn her personal narratives or fused beliefs (e.g., "People expect me to be perfect"). Sometimes, it is also an opportunity to learn about the client's values or what the client finds personally meaningful. Second, the functional assessment is an opportunity for skills building. Throughout the assessment, clients are asked numerous questions about their thoughts and feelings. This builds skills in noticing and describing internal experiences (e.g., labeling emotions). The client may also gain skills in flexible perspective taking as she takes her own perspective at different times and places (how she feels now, how she felt last month, how she felt 2 years ago, etc.) and describes her experience from these various vantage points. Finally, the functional assessment lays the groundwork for creative hopelessness and contacting the futility of avoidance and control (the topic of Chapter 6).

Functional Classes of Behavior

The initial functional analysis focused on food restriction or other AN behaviors that maintain dangerously low weight. However, the broader aim of treatment is to shift the entire system of avoidance and control. This requires identifying other behaviors in which the individual engages that serve a similar purpose as the core features of AN and similarly limits life vitality or causes psychological harm. This might include, for example, achievement striving in other domains to feel worthy or planning/list making that decreases uncertainty in a manner similar to dietary rules. Behaviors that serve a similar purpose as AN can be identified in several ways:

- *Examining psychiatric comorbidities*, which describe co-occurring behaviors that may serve a similar purpose as AN.
- *Identifying behaviors that are rigid or situationally insensitive*. For example, the client may describe that she *always, must, or has to* engage in a behavior or that she rarely deviates from particular patterns of activity (e.g., always doing things for other people, always apologizing). If these behaviors *always, must, or have to* be done, they are likely driven by avoidance and control.
- *Asking the client* what behaviors (other than AN) produce similar changes in her experience. For example, a client might describe how exercising attenuates feelings of being undeserving (by making her feel as though she has earned or deserves her food). The client might be asked, "Do you do other things to feel deserving or worthy? For example, is working long hours also something that makes you feel that way?"

Table 3.4 lists some of the most common behaviors observed among individuals with AN that may serve a purpose similar to restrictive eating and weight control. In some cases, functionally equivalent behaviors may be opposite to one another. For example, a client might appease people sometimes and lash out at other times. Both behaviors could function as escape from interpersonal rejection, even though they are formally polar opposites.

TABLE 3.4. Behaviors Common among Individuals with AN That May Serve the Same or Similar Purposes as Restrictive Eating and Weight Control

- Working long hours
- Not taking breaks
- People pleasing (always doing for others; trying to predict their needs)
- Avoiding conflict (passivity, lack of expression of ideas or hurts)
- Mimicking other people (deciding action based on what others are doing)
- Not initiating or avoiding unstructured social interactions
- Staying "busy," avoiding "nonproductive" activities
- Only spending time with individuals who are much older or much younger
- List making
- Planning (including anticipating problems and solving them in advance)
- Being compliant
- Excessive morality (following the letter, not the spirit, of the law)
- Overscheduling
- Focusing on achievement and clear markers of success
- Extremely measured decision making
- Seeking advice or reassurance from others
- Gathering information excessively
- Extreme responsibility
- Always putting others' needs first
- Perfectionistic persistence (persisting despite diminishing returns)
- Excessive frugality (needing to not need anything)
- Inhibiting expression of thoughts, opinions, feelings
- Berating oneself for minor transgressions
- Overapologizing
- Prefacing everything before speaking
- Downplaying strengths or rejecting compliments
- Comparing oneself to other people
- Being "the best"

Behaviors more common among AN–binge/purge subtype

- Cutting or other self-harm behaviors
- Substance use
- Sexual engagement
- Taking on more than one can do
- Procrastination
- Impulsive decision making
- Sleeping in, avoiding responsibilities

The System That Has Trapped the Client

The functional assessment culminates with the articulation of the "system that has trapped the client," that is, how her behavior improves her immediate situation (by attenuating painful or unwanted internal experience) but ultimately causes physical and psychological harm or has costs for her personal values (see Figure 3.8). At this stage, the goal is not to press strongly on the undesirable consequences or costs of the client's behaviors. The therapist's insistence on the negative consequences or attempt to get the client to contact consequences too early (before the therapist is clear about all that AN does for the individual) may diminish rapport. This does not mean that the therapist should ignore evidence of negative consequences when they are available (e.g., if the client mentions missing out on time with

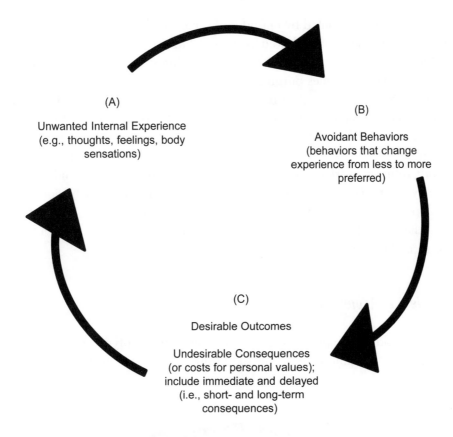

(A)

Unwanted Internal Experience
(e.g., thoughts, feelings, body
sensations)

(B)

Avoidant Behaviors
(behaviors that change
experience from less to more
preferred)

(C)

Desirable Outcomes

Undesirable Consequences
(or costs for personal values);
include immediate and delayed
(i.e., short- and long-term
consequences)

FIGURE 3.8. The system that has trapped the client (Antecedents–Behaviors–Consequences).

friends because of exercise routines) or that information about the medical consequences of
low weight should be withheld, but rather that these things should be observed in a matter-
of-fact or compassionately curious manner. Making experiential contact with the costs of
current behavior patterns is the focus of Chapter 6. Case examples and Figure 3.9 illustrate
the initial case formulation.

Case Example 3.1 (Adult)

Jane, a 33-year-old European American female presenting with AN, reports a long history
of eating disorder symptoms beginning in high school and one prior hospitalization for low
weight when she was 17. Symptoms have been in remission until this past year, when they
reemerged in the context of a job promotion. Jane describes significant anxiety with this
transition, which increased substantially after her first performance review. From her perspective, the review was "OK" but far from her usual "exceeds expectations." She describes
feeling like a "failure" following her review and developing intense worry of being fired.
Within several weeks of the review, Jane began restricting her food intake to 750 calories a day and exercising excessively, which resulted in significant weight loss. She reports
that watching her weight decline gives her feelings of success and control. Her regimented

eating is occasionally punctuated by episodes of subjective binge eating (i.e., feeling out of control when she eats more than allowed by her strict dietary rules). She describes compensating for these episodes that she labels as "eating failures" by further reducing her daily caloric allotment and sometimes purging. Jane adheres to a rigid work schedule, devoting 70 hours a week to work and neglecting time with friends, pleasurable activities, and self-care (including sleep). She describes that she "needs" this time in order to be successful. She describes excessive list making and checking and rewriting reports numerous times to prevent mistakes at work. She also works hard to appear knowledgeable and in control while at work, refusing to ask for any help, criticizing the work of others, and blaming other people for any errors. Despite the negative impact this collection of behaviors has had on her friendships, relationships with colleagues at work, and her health, Jane is terrified of making any changes out of tremendous fear that she may lose her job and be a failure. The initial case formulation is summarized in Figure 3.9.

Case Example 3.2 (Adolescent)

Julie is a 15-year-old female presenting with AN–restrictive subtype. About 8 months ago, Julie's health class did a unit on nutrition and healthy weight. She began tracking her food

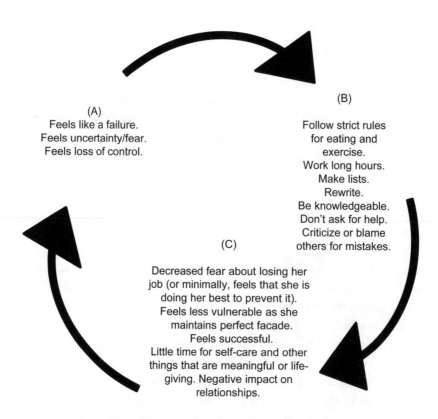

FIGURE 3.9. Functional assessment for Jane (Case Example 3.1).

intake and calories as part of an assignment for the class. Julie initially began cutting back on the amount of "junk food" she was eating and lost a little weight. This was followed by lots of compliments from peers; this was really nice because she had been struggling with her friendships since transitioning to middle school and felt like she no longer fit in with friends, who were now focusing on boys and less on school or sports. Soon, cutting out junk food turned into a diet, then to severe restriction. She currently restricts herself to 900 calories a day, with exactly 300 calories at each meal. She limits her eating to packaged foods that have nutrition labels on them (e.g., oatmeal, yogurt) so that she can be sure she does not exceed her calorie limit. She also weighs herself daily and keeps detailed diaries of her food intake and weight. A similar rigid approach is observed in her schoolwork. Described as a "perfectionist" by her parents, Julie studies relentlessly and gets upset if she receives anything less than a perfect score on tests or assignments—often isolating herself in her room and reviewing the material for hours if she does not achieve 100%. She reports that she feels like she has to punish herself for making a mistake and make sure she does not do it again, describing significant fears of embarrassment and failure. A constant theme for Julie is a fear that others will not like her or that she will let them down. She has devised many systems to ensure these things do not happen. In this case, anxiety and fear of disappointing others and making mistakes are key antecedents. Excessive tracking of calories and food restriction, and the punitive way in which she engages with her schoolwork, reduce risk of these events and allow her to avoid embarrassment and feelings of failure. However, these benefits come at a severe cost to her well-being.

Refining the Functional Assessment

The functional assessment begins when treatment is initiated; however, it is continually refined as new information emerges or the contingencies supporting behavior change. For example, the therapist might have the initial formulation that fear of rejection is keeping an individual locked in eating and exercise routines and not pursuing relationships. Over time, it might become clear that the client *also* fears success in connecting to others or that there are relevant skills deficits (e.g., deficits in her ability to accurately read another person's interest in friendship). Updating the case formulation with this information allows for more effective intervention.

Challenges to Identifying Functional Classes of Behavior among Individuals with AN

The Impact of Undernourishment

Some behaviors that appear to be operant (i.e., maintained by contingencies) are actually the result of severe undernourishment. This includes, for example, taking inordinate amounts of time to complete a meal, cutting food into small pieces, or even excessive movement. This distinction is important, as it may be unnecessary to target these behaviors directly. The behaviors will remit spontaneously as the individual eats with greater regularity and weight improves. Knowledge of the impact of starvation on behavior can help therapists avoid formulating starvation behaviors as operant and increase credibility and rapport with clients.

Fat Talk

Fat talk includes statements such as:

> "I am fat."
> "I like that I can see my bones."
> "I don't understand why I can't be under 100 pounds."
> "My thighs are disgusting."
> "She is thinner than I am."

In most cases, "fat talk" is formulated as experiential avoidance: avoidance of other, more painful thoughts or feelings or of the deeper emotional experience (e.g., feeling unworthy). This formulation differs from second-wave CBT, which views the content of these cognitions as central to AN etiology. This difference in formulation has direct implications for treatment. Rather than engage these cognitions at the content level (e.g., targeting the individual's biased perspective on her body weight), ACT helps clients with AN observe the thought "I am fat" as a thought or a product of the mind that emerges in times of stress or emotional pain, with little to no therapeutic attention to the truth or accuracy of the thought (workability is the metric; see Chapter 9).

Desirable Behavior

Individuals with AN may be highly accommodating, responsible, and hardworking. While these behaviors are often desirable, they often also function as emotional control, and individuals with AN engage them in a manner that is highly rigid and self-depriving (e.g., studying for hours when additional preparation is unnecessary and despite fatigue). Paradoxically, this means that treatment goals might include minor acts of rebellion, and decreased people pleasing or excessive compliance may indicate improvement.

Case Formulation and Treatment Planning Form

A case formulation form (Form 3.1) is provided at the end of this chapter; you can download and print a copy from the publisher's website and use it in your work with clients (see the box at the end of the table of contents). The form outlines the basic functional assessment of avoided events and avoidant repertoires (targets for acceptance) and provides prompts to consider cognitive fusion maintaining ineffective behaviors (discussed in depth in Chapter 9), degree of undernourishment, strength of external supports (e.g., parents or family), and the client's commitment to change. Completing the form is useful for treatment planning. An example of a completed form is provided next with Case Example 3.3 on page 61 (Figure 3.10).

1. **Identify AN behaviors.** Include overt (e.g., food restriction) as well as covert behaviors (e.g., calorie counting). Be specific (e.g., eliminates all fat from diet, does not eat snacks, limits food intake to 400 calories a day, exercises 2 hours a day).

Diet is limited to four to five safe foods. Avoids all meat, dairy, bread, and desserts. Does not consume snacks between meals (>8 hours between meals at times). Will not eat anything prepared by another person or eat at restaurants. Runs >9–10 miles/day.

2. **Identify how the client's behavior is helpful.** Include **unwanted internal experiences** that AN eliminates (e.g., feelings of failure) and **desired internal experiences** that AN provides (e.g., mastery). (These are contingencies maintaining AN.)

Reduces insecurities/provides her with positive feelings about herself. (She feels accomplished in her goals and increasingly fast run time; these accomplishments are particularly important to her because of her feeling of failing in social situations.)

Decreases loneliness/provides her with a distraction. (She stays busy with meal planning and preparation and exercise, gives her something to do, she does not feel as lonely as she would otherwise.)

Decreases anxiety/fear. (She feels comfortable/safe and has a "reason" to avoid social situations.)

3. **Identify other behaviors that produce similar changes in the client's internal experience.** Include these behaviors as treatment targets if they are rigid, situationally insensitive, or diminish life vitality. Examples include not expressing opinions, compliance, working long hours, imposing rigid daily structure or planning, counting or other rituals. (These are behaviors that are functionally equivalent to AN.)

Does not express her thoughts/feelings, even with safe people (compliance or quiet defiance).

Overrelies on family for social interactions.

Avoids school or other places where her peers are likely to be.

4. **Identify cognitive fusion that is maintaining problem behaviors despite physical or psychological harm.** Include rules or strongly held beliefs about how one "should be" or the implications of having feelings or making mistakes. Also include painful or evocative self-relevant thoughts (e.g., "I am unlikable").

I must run X miles/day, not eat X, etc.
People don't like me/People do not want to interact with me.
I am unlikable, uninteresting/boring.
I am too quiet.
Feelings are weak and stupid.
I am a burden to my family.

(continued)

FIGURE 3.10. A completed ACT for AN Case Formulation and Treatment Planning form for Jennifer (Case Example 3.3).

5. **Identify undesirable consequences of AN or other problematic behaviors** (e.g., lost time due to overexercise, lack of meaningful relationships). Include what the client has lost, as well as things that she has not had the opportunity for. (These are consequences of AN that are not currently exerting stimulus control but, if contacted, would maintain more adaptive repertoires of behavior.)

She does not have relationships with her peers or with individuals outside her family.

Intimacy in family relationships is limited due to a lack of disclosure.

There are lots of places that she cannot go because they involve feared social engagement (e.g., college campus). This has limited life engagement, exploration, and overall vitality.

She has not been able to travel or try new things, despite a desire for "adventure."

---

6. **Assess degree of undernourishment and strength of external supports.** What percentage of ideal body weight is the client (based on the client's age, sex, and weight history)? Should there be limits or conditions to outpatient treatment? To what extent should other people in the client's natural environment be brought into treatment?

    What are the family resources (i.e., parents, siblings, and extended family) that can provide emotional or instrumental support? What is the client's willingness to involve the family, and the family's ability to communicate effectively around AN, food/eating, or set and follow a plan? What are the primary barriers?

85% of ideal body weight

Jennifer's parents have been mostly "hands off" and have limited information due to Jennifer's lack of communication/disclosure.

Jennifer reports fear of burdening her family members.

Parents report fear of "making things worse" by being more involved.

---

7. **Assess commitment to change.** How committed is the client to treatment? Are there aspects of living with AN that the client does not like that might be leveraged to engage the client in treatment (e.g., occasional binge eating due to nutritional depletion)? Are there other outside contingencies compelling change (e.g., is the individual mandated for treatment to continue playing on a sports team, etc.)?

Jennifer is motivated and coming to treatment on her own. She is experiencing more boredom and burden with AN. Although she is ambivalent re: facing fears, she is willing to work toward weight restoration and social engagement.

Other members of the treatment team:

Physician: *Dr. XXXX (seeing every 2 weeks)*

Nutritionist: *XXXXX, RD, Appointment scheduled for next week (XX/XX/XXXX)*

Psychiatrist: *None*

Other: *None*

Initial behavior change goal and plan (e.g., eat dinner with a support person present, mark other meals with some food intake, add a snack or nutritional supplement to daily intake):

Discuss with client the importance of providing psychoeducation for the family and the need to involve her parents more if her weight trajectory does not improve over the next 3–4 weeks.

Family meals in the evening (conforming to vegan for now), food intake every 2.5–3 hours (snacks between meals ~200–300 kcal), activity limited to 10 minutes of walking/every other day.

FIGURE 3.10. *(continued)*

Case Example 3.3

Jennifer is a 19-year-old female who presented with restrictive eating and overexercise. She lives with her biological parents. She identifies as "vegan" and her diet is limited to four or five "safe" foods. Jennifer withdrew from public school as a sophomore in high school due to increasing social anxiety. She is currently completing college coursework online and rarely interacts with individuals outside her immediate family. Jennifer reports her anxiety began when she was out of school frequently for medical reasons and increased when her peers began to comment on her quietness. She describes fears of being uninteresting and unlikable. She feels comfortable at home and prefers the structure and routine of a rigid eating and exercise schedule (which consumes most of her time). She spends some time with her older sister (whom she identifies as her best friend) but does not disclose feelings to her for fear of being a burden and her belief that emotions are weak or stupid. Jennifer has been training for half-marathons and feels good about her increasingly fast run times. However, she also feels burdened by the obligation to run at least 9–10 miles a day and reports increasing discontent with the narrowness of her life and interactions. Jennifer is aware of her recent feelings of boredom and, somewhat surprisingly, fantasizes about leaving the country or moving to a big city. She is also experiencing increasing fatigue as her caloric intake decreases and her running increases.

AN through the Lens of the Six Core ACT Processes (or Functional Domains)

Viewing the client's struggle through the lens of each of the six core ACT processes (or functional domains) helps with treatment planning. This more advanced case formuation helps the therapist know which therapeutic process to engage when and how to leverage client strengths in treatment. It also identifies opportunities for honing skills in each of the six process domains to improve client functioning.

We describe AN through the lens of Acceptance, Defusion, Self-as-Context, Present-Moment Awareness, Values, and Committed Action (summarized in Figure 3.11 on the next page) and provide guidance on identifying key targets and assessing capabilities for individual clients in each process domain.

Acceptance (Experiential Avoidance)

Viewed through the lens of acceptance, individuals with AN can be described as having an experience phobia, in that they are fearful of feelings (emotions, drives, or urges) and of experiencing life in a way that is not predictable or well controlled. Aversion is to both positive as well as negative affect, which might feel equally compelling or out of control. Those with AN may specifically fear needing or wanting "too much," being self-centered, and being judged or rejected by other people. Fears are managed by imposing structure ("rules") to maintain emotional and behavioral control and prevent mistakes.

Deficits in Present-Moment Awareness
Attention narrowed to the body and other threat cues (e.g., rejecting facial expression); difficulty being "in the moment" or engaging in play; excessive attention to past wrongs and planning to avoid future mistakes

For case formulation: Is the client's attention on the moment or in some other time/place? Are they able to flexibly attend to internal and external events as they occur?

Experiential Avoidance
Attempts to avoid or suppress feelings and other experiences that feel uncertain or out of control; avoidance of ambiguous situations, imperfection, failure, making mistakes, guilt and shame, and the possibility of being rejected or judged

For case formulation: What are the client's unwanted internal experiences (avoided events) and avoidant behaviors?

Deficits in Valuing
Adoption of external systems of control and rigid definitions of what is "good" or "right" and will please others; limited awareness of what is personally meaningful or brings true joy

For case formulation: Is there evidence of true mattering (caring about something in a genuine way, rather only "shoulds" or "oughts")? What are the client's barriers to authoring personal values?

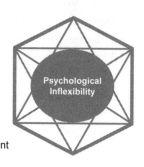

Cognitive Fusion
Overreliance on structure and rules; frequent comparison/evaluation of themselves and their performance, using concrete markers like body weight/shape; fusion with thoughts like "People won't like me" or "Perfection is expected"; feelings and meeting needs are judged as "weak" or "selfish"

For case formulation: What mental activity is the client fused with (e.g., "I am fat," "I need too much," or "People won't like me"; rules for diet and social interaction)?

Deficits in Self-Awareness
Self and self-worth is based on things that are observable to other people (body, achievements); self-knowledge (e.g., personal preferences) is limited; difficulty differentiating their perspective from others' or showing self-compassion

For case formulation: What are the client's self-narratives, self-knowledge, and ability for perspective taking?

Deficits in Committed Action
Action is overscheduled and overcommitted; goals are persistently pursued despite diminishing returns; lack of spontaneity and experimentation with different strategies

For case formulation: What is the focus and the quality of the client's actions? What are the client's barriers to making commitments or taking action?

FIGURE 3.11. AN viewed through the lens of each of the six core ACT processes. Copyright © Rhonda M. Merwin, Nancy L. Zucker, and Kelly G. Wilson. Reprinted by permission.

Identifying Targets for Acceptance

The therapist identifies the specific internal experiences (i.e., thoughts, feelings, and body sensations) that the client avoids with AN or other rigid control behaviors. These internal experiences are targets for acceptance (or willingness) interventions. Table 3.5 summarizes common targets for acceptance work among individuals with AN.

Assessing the Client's Capacity for Acceptance

The client's capacity for acceptance is reflected in the range of acceptable internal experiences (i.e., whether some feelings are permitted or permitted in some contexts). The

TABLE 3.5. Common Targets for Acceptance in AN

Target	Description
Anxiety	Fear of making a mistake, being rejected or judged
Guilt	Feeling of doing something wrong, upsetting or burdening others
Shame	Feeling of being a bad person, not meeting expectations or failing
Uncertainty	Feeling unsure in daily decisions and in new situations, transitions, and change
Lack of control	Feeling limited influence over a situation, other people (their reactions, etc.), or one's body
Overwhelmed	Feeling unable to cope with situations or meet demands
Positive affect	Feeling of being satisfied or enjoying things, having pleasure, or being comfortable or relaxed
Biological drives	Feeling a drive or urge for food, sex, rest, and so forth.[a]

[a]A lack of distress regarding biological drives may not be indicative of high levels of acceptance. Rather, drives may be muted as a biological adaptation to starvation (and thus less distressing). Distress will be revealed as the client restores weight and the body awakens. While clients may experience aversion to the drive/urge to eat, they may find hunger appetitive (desirable) because it signals self-discipline and self-restraint. Similarly, the urge to rest may be aversive, while fatigue or soreness (after exertion) may be appetitive.

therapist may also rate the client's capacity for acceptance using a dimensional scale (see Figure 3.12), which can be useful in treatment planning and observing change over time.

Defusion (Cognitive Fusion)

Viewed through the lens of defusion, AN may be described as overattachment to structure and external systems of control ("rules"). Rules not only occur in the domain of eating and

Capacity for Acceptance

Constantly suppresses feelings or avoids activities that may generate strong feelings (positive or negative).	−3 −2 −1 0 1 2 3	Consistently allows feelings to be present; approaches activities that have emotional valence.
Always judges, rejects or denies feelings.	−3 −2 −1 0 1 2 3	Validates and respects feelings and what they communicate (if anything).
Persistently imposes rules or structure; avoids unplanned activities; avoids or limits decision making by eliminating choices.	−3 −2 −1 0 1 2 3	Allows uncertainty or imprecision; engages in activities with less structure and planning; actively makes choices even when feeling uncertain.
Never takes interpersonal risks (e.g., avoids eye contact, does not express opinions, does not self-disclose).	−3 −2 −1 0 1 2 3	Engages in behaviors that feel interpersonally risky.

FIGURE 3.12. Dimensional ratings of the client's capacity for acceptance.

weight, but also across domains of living (e.g., how to behave in social interactions). Individuals with AN may engage in *near constant* comparison and evaluation, with continual scrutiny of themselves and their performance using concrete markers of success (e.g., body weight, grades, job evaluations). Some individuals with AN may also be attached to harsh self-talk (e.g., "You don't need that, you fat pig"), which they view as motivating excellence or deserved. The directly available functions of meeting one's needs for food, rest, or support (e.g., the experience of being adequately nourished or rested) are dominated by verbal functions (i.e., self-indulgence).

Identifying Targets for Defusion

The therapist identifies cognitive fusion that contributes to the client's problems (see Table 3.6). Defusion strategies decrease attachment to the content of this mental activity (when this mental activity does not serve the individual and her values) and increase the client's capacity to use direct experience in decision making.

Assessing the Client's Capacity for Defusion

The client's capacity for defusion is reflected in her ability to recognize thoughts as mental activity (rather than the events they represent), and to discriminate when listening to thoughts is useful and when it is not. The therapist may rate the client's capacity for defusion using a dimensional scale (see Figure 3.13 on page 66), which can be useful in treatment planning and observing change over time.

Present-Moment Awareness

Individuals with AN are rarely in the present moment. Instead, their minds are running backward and forward in time, assessing whether they made a mistake in the past and how to be better in the future. When attention is focused on current experience, it is often narrowly deployed to the body (e.g., feelings in the gut) or other threat cues (e.g., the bodies of other people, signals that they said or did something wrong). Individuals with AN may have extreme difficulty engaging in "play" or other activities that are non–goal directed and may be spontaneous or unplanned.

Identifying the Client's Difficulties in Present-Moment Awareness

The therapist identifies areas of narrow and rigid or distracted attention. These areas provide opportunities to build the client's capacity for flexible attention to events as they unfold in the moment (see Table 3.7 on page 66). The ability to flexibly attend allows the client to situate events in their broader context, and thus better understand their meaning. It also expands the stimuli that are available to guide behavior (e.g., the client may be aware of an inviting face, in addition to the discomfort they are experiencing in their gut).

TABLE 3.6. Common Targets for Defusion in AN

Target	Examples
Self-management rules	• Eat less than 400 calories a day. • Don't stop running until you have doubled your distance from yesterday. • Always defer to the other person's needs. • Don't burden others. • Work is priority.
Harsh self-talk to compel compliance with rules	• "You are weak. Get up." • "You are a fat pig. Stop eating." • "Shut up, you don't need that."
Body-related thoughts	• "I am disgusting." • "My thighs [stomach, arms, etc.] are too big." • "I'm ugly."
Thoughts about expectations and the impact of mistakes	• "Perfection is expected or imperfections are intolerable." • "Everything must be earned." • "Mistakes are irreparable." • "I will make a mistake that has devastating consequences."
Thoughts about one's acceptability or basic worth/self-judgments	• "I'm not worth anything." • "I'm unlikable." • "I'm a failed person." • "I'm too much; I'm a burden." • "I'm bad or wrong (e.g., weak, selfish, lazy, needy, or greedy)." • "I'm undeserving, or I deserve to be punished."
Thoughts about feelings and their implications	• "Feelings can't be trusted." • "Feelings lead to behavior that is out of bounds." • "Feelings cause mistakes." • "Feelings are a weakness or a personal failure."
Verbally ascribed functions of meeting physical and emotional needs that dominate over other available functions	• Meeting needs (to eat, sleep/rest, get support) is greedy, indulgent, selfish, lazy, needy, and so forth.

Assessing the Client's Capacity for Present-Moment Awareness

The individual's capacity for present-moment awareness can be assessed on a continuum and tracked between sessions and/or within a session. This includes the ability to maintain flexible and focused attention in the present moment and to broaden awareness beyond a threat cue, situating it in its broader context (see Figure 3.14 on page 67).

Self-as-Context

Individuals with AN may be described as having a weak self-as-verbal process (or *knowing self*), with limited awareness of their feelings or personal preferences. Self-as-content

Capacity for Defusion

Always follows self-imposed rules despite unworkability or negative consequences.	−3 −2 −1 0 1 2 3	Deviates from rules when doing so would be effective or value-guided.
Never makes a distinction between thoughts about events and the events themselves (e.g., the thought "I am a bad person" is treated as the literal event rather than a judgment that one makes about oneself).	−3 −2 −1 0 1 2 3	Consistently recognizes thoughts as mental activity and discriminates from direct experience.
Speech is dominated by eating disorder content, judgments, and reasons for not eating; is repetitive or rote; lacks voice prosody.	−3 −2 −1 0 1 2 3	Speech is varied in content and delivery; is animated in emotional tone.
Contacts only negative verbal-evaluative functions of food, eating, or meeting needs (e.g., greed).	−3 −2 −1 0 1 2 3	Experiences the direct benefits of eating, sleeping, or seeking support. Other functions of food or eating exert influence over behavior (e.g., increased energy, texture, taste, interest, social value).

FIGURE 3.13. Dimensional ratings of the client's capacity for defusion.

TABLE 3.7. Common Areas of Narrow or Rigid Attention

Area	Description/examples
Past mistakes	• Something she did and said that was "wrong" • Including minor perceived transgressions, such as eating the wrong thing, saying the wrong thing in a meeting or class, or expressing an opinion
Daily decisions	• What to eat or what to wear • What to say
The feared distant future	• Failure in a career • Becoming obese
The body	• Weight • A specific part of the body • Internal gut sensations
Evaluation/feedback	• A negative job review • A less optimal grade
Interpersonal threat cues	• Signals of conflict or displeasure from others (e.g., an ambiguous facial expression, an individual having a different viewpoint) • Challenges to social status (e.g., a thinner individual)

Capacity for Present-Moment Awareness

Is always ruminating about the past or worrying about the future.	−3	−2	−1	0	1	2	3	Is able to be in the here-and-now.
Is constantly vigilant about how the body looks or feels.	−3	−2	−1	0	1	2	3	Flexibly attends to the body; is able to also notice other people or the situation.
Is constantly scanning the environment for threat (e.g., reactions of other people, negative feedback).	−3	−2	−1	0	1	2	3	Is able to rest attention on the current task or something that is interesting or meaningful.
Does not easily disengage from a stimulus that has captured attention (e.g., ambiguous social cue).	−3	−2	−1	0	1	2	3	Is able to broaden attention in the presence of a perceived threat cue.
Must always be doing something productive.	−3	−2	−1	0	1	2	3	Is able to engage in non-goal-directed activity.

FIGURE 3.14. Dimensional ratings of the client's capacity for present-moment awareness.

(or the *conceptualized self*) is narrowly defined by AN and their outward appearance (i.e., how they look to others). Individuals with AN may also have deficits in flexible perspective taking. They may have difficulty taking their own perspective at another time or place or differentiating their thoughts/feelings from the experiences of another person. As a result, they have difficulty with self-compassion and may view the world as full of judgment, harsh, and unsafe.

Identifying the Client's Difficulties in the Self-as-Context Domain

The therapist identifies the client's overattachment to self-content. This includes overidentification with the eating disorder or other self-narratives. The therapist also identifies areas of impoverished content or limited self-knowledge (see Table 3.8 on the next page).

Assessing the Client's Capacity to Deviate from Self-Narratives, Use Self-Knowledge, and Engage in Flexible Perspective Taking

The client's capacities in self-as-context domains can be assessed using dimensional ratings (Figure 3.15 on the next page). Capacities may be tracked between and within sessions.

Values

Viewed through the lens of values, individuals with AN may be described as having little awareness of what brings meaning, vitality, or true joy. Instead, values are based on perceived societal definitions of what is "good" and "right" or will meet expectations/please others. Fear of failure, or of making mistakes, prevents deeper exploration of personal meaning. Avoidance

TABLE 3.8. Common Areas of Overattachment and of Impoverished Content in AN

Area	Examples/description
Common areas of overattachment (or overidentification)	
Eating and weight control/eating disorder identity	• "I am anorexic [an eating disorder patient, a vegan]." • "I only eat 'clean'."
Outward appearance (i.e., what other people "see" rather than who they sense themselves to be)	• One's body • Achievements, accolades
Narratives of persistence	• "I don't give up."
Narratives of being flawed (see also defusion)	• "I'm [bad, failed, inadequate, etc.]."
Common areas of impoverished content/deficits in self-knowledge	
Limited awareness of personal opinions or preferences	• Referencing or reporting what she perceives to be others' opinions or desires, when asked her own
Limited knowledge of one's emotions	• Reporting feeling "fat" or "upset" rather than using more specific emotion language

Capacity for Self-ing

Never deviates from self-narratives.	−3 −2 −1 0 1 2 3	Is able to behave in ways that contradict self-narratives when doing so would be effective or value-guided.
Defines self narrowly by achievements or measurable outcomes.	−3 −2 −1 0 1 2 3	Possesses rich and varied self-content.
Never uses personal preferences and opinions in making decisions (in domains other than eating); conforms and complies.	−3 −2 −1 0 1 2 3	Takes personal preferences and opinions into account when making decisions.
Is consistently unaware of ongoing emotional experience (beyond being fat or upset).	−3 −2 −1 0 1 2 3	Has ongoing awareness of his or her feelings; labels emotions.
Is unable to take a different perspective (of oneself at another time or place, or the perspective of another person); perspective is experienced as static and universal.	−3 −2 −1 0 1 2 3	Is able to flexibly take perspective; appreciating the impact of situational factors on behavior and allowing for empathy and compassion (for self and other people).

FIGURE 3.15. Dimensional ratings of the client's capacities in the self-as-context domain.

of emotions might also make it extremely difficult for clients to know what they desire or what is important to them. If AN emerged early, a lack of values clarity may reflect halted or delayed individuation or identity formation. Values may also be confused by years of AN and its demands.

Identifying the Client's Difficulties in Values Clarity and Potential Valued Directions

The therapist identifies issues limiting values clarity or authorship in AN (summarized in Table 3.9) and notes potential valued directions. The therapist may formulate hypotheses regarding personal meaning based on the client's life history (e.g., things that the individual cared about before AN).

Assessing the Client's Capacity for Valuing

The client's clarity about personal values and the extent to which her values are organizing behavior can be assessed on a continuum. Tracking capabilities within and between sessions can aid in treatment planning (see Figure 3.16 on the next page).

Committed Action

Individuals with AN are overcommitted in their actions and persistently pursue a goal, despite high personal costs and diminishing returns. Time is disproportionately allocated to achievement striving and often is overscheduled/overstructured such that commitments do not take into account the person's needs. At times, individuals with AN might reject their overcommitted approach and behave in an impulsive or disinhibited manner. This is more likely among clients with AN with the binge/purge subtype.

TABLE 3.9. Common Difficulties with Values Clarity in AN

Difficulty	Examples/description
Valuing determined by other people or rules	• Adopting parent values • Basing valuing on "shoulds"
Avoidance mistaken for values	• "Valuing" thinness, achievement, perfection, or control because they limit emotional pain
Avoidance of valuing because of the potential for discomfort	• Denying relationship values because relationships are emotionally challenging, or because they feel as though they will fail
Development of values disrupted by eating disorder	• Emergence of AN thwarting the typical process of adolescent identity formation
Decreased awareness of values due to years of struggle	• Less contact with potential sources of meaning due to prolonged underweight (e.g., loss of relationships or job)

Capacity for Valuing

Completely unaware of what she cares about other than AN, perfection, or control.	−3 −2 −1 0 1 2 3	Deeply aware of personal values.
Behavior is primarily motivated by relief from discomfort, "shoulds," etc.	−3 −2 −1 0 1 2 3	Behavior is strongly motivated by personal values/vitality.
Always avoids value domains that are important to her because of fear.	−3 −2 −1 0 1 2 3	Explores values in domains that are important to her.

FIGURE 3.16. Dimensional ratings of the client's capacity for valuing.

Identifying Client Difficulties in Committed Action

The therapist identifies how the client invests her time, and whether action is motivated by avoidance and control or personal values. The therapist also observes *the way in which* the client engages activities, and whether she can deviate from a course of action when helpful. Common difficulties in committed action are outlined in Table 3.10. The therapist might also create a pie chart of hours of energy invested in particular activities (over the course of a day or a week) to aid in this assessment (see Figure 3.17).

Assessing the Client's Capacity for Flexible Committed Action Linked to Values

The therapist assesses the client's capacity for flexible committed action linked to values (Figure 3.18). This includes whether the client is able to adjust behavior (deviating from routines) as needed, "do less," and participate in activities with greater meaning.

Form 3.2 (at the end of this chapter) compiles the assessment scales for the six core process domains (presented earlier) for reproduction and use in treatment planning. The form is also available on the publisher's website for downloading and printing (see the box at the end of the table of contents) and use in your work with clients.

TABLE 3.10. Common Difficulties in Committed Action

Difficulty	Description/examples
Actions are overdevoted to achievement or good behavior	Doing things that are not personally meaningful because they build a vita or look good (e.g., participating in a club or sport in which they do not have interest)
Engaging in actions despite high personal costs or diminishing returns	Spending unnecessary additional time studying or perfecting work
Actions are overscheduled/ overstructured	Following a schedule for the day without "checking in" on needs; inability to accept a spontaneous social invitation)

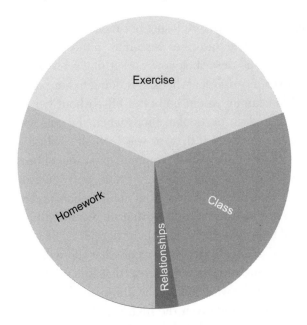

FIGURE 3.17. Allocation of personal time for assessment of committed action.

Case Example 3.4

Abigail is an 18-year-old female presenting for treatment after a brief stay in a residential treatment facility (that she left against medical advice [AMA]) and 5 days of participation in an intensive outpatient program (also AMA). Her current weight is at 85% of her ideal body weight. Abigail rejects her ideal body weight, reporting that her body "wants to be 10 pounds less" and that she is not experiencing hunger. She has been steadily losing weight since her discharge. She provides extensive reasons for the weight loss and tries to adjust her calorie intake by 50 calories/day to stop its progression. Abigail has not menstruated in

Capacity for Committed Action		
Fills all available time with activities based on what she "should" be doing.	−3 −2 −1 0 1 2 3	Engages in activities that take into account personal needs or sources of fulfillment or joy.
Cannot deviate from plans.	−3 −2 −1 0 1 2 3	Is able to behave spontaneously sometimes.
Always persists, even when actions are not improving outcomes or are causing harm.	−3 −2 −1 0 1 2 3	Is able to stop or adjust goals based on feedback.
Never engages in activities that are not goal-driven or do not produce a measurable marker of success.	−3 −2 −1 0 1 2 3	Participates in activities that are personally meaningful even when they do not have a measurable outcome.

FIGURE 3.18. Dimensional ratings of the client's capacity for flexible and effective committed action.

months, which is pleasing to her. Before losing her menses, she worried that she was dirty and that others would know. She describes herself as "a mess" and states that she is trying to get a handle on things. She describes how everything feels out of control and chaotic. Abigail also describes extreme guilt for what she is doing to her parents and sisters, and she sometimes wonders if her family would be better off without her. She is also upset about her decisions in the past and, in particular, times when she was not a good friend (giving examples of when she has put herself first, or was "selfish"). Most of her friends are from treatment, and Abigail describes herself as "unpopular" at school because she is "awkward" or "weird." Crowds make her extremely uncomfortable, and she avoids situations with lots of people when possible. She has withdrawn from public school and has been homeschooled for several years due to anxiety and her report that she would kill herself if she had to stay in public school. Abigail feels like she is "less than" her peers. She describes wanting to see "how far her body can go," although she is not clear what she will do next (once she reaches such a dangerous weight). She reports some sense that this might make her feel special or more accomplished and that she would enjoy the diminished responsibility or expectations. This would be particularly freeing given the high standards she held for herself academically (before AN) and the punitive way in which she engaged in studying.

Abigail describes feeling as though there is no joy in life, in part not only because she feels as though she has to count/calculate everything, but also because there is so much loss and pain; she says that if "this is all there is," she would prefer to die. She denies active plan or intent. She says that she is "anxious all the time," fearing that she is going to "mess up" in some way. Abigail worries that she is "making it up" and that really, deep down, she is just lazy and doesn't want to work hard (at school, etc.). She fears that if she were kinder to herself, then she would never stop eating or move her body. She complains of low energy and that she is "depressed." She is specifically bothered by her difficulty concentrating and her fogginess, which has made it more difficult to do academic tasks. As Abigail experiences more mastery in restrictive eating, she has been experiencing more failure in her school-work. She would like to "feel better" (less fatigue, depression) and may be willing to make behavior changes to help with this (e.g., facing fears regarding eating).

Formulation of the Problem

Abigail manages feelings of guilt, shame, and fear and thoughts about being a bad person (greedy, selfish, lazy, or incompetent) or unlikeable (awkward, ugly) by keeping a tight leash on her behavior; using strict rules, structure, and routine; and trying to improve herself. The weight loss she has experienced, as well as her increased sense of control, has been highly reinforcing of her behavior. Abigail has also experienced decreased expectations for herself (in academics) and less caring about her social struggles. However, the cognitive fog resulting from her low weight has only strengthened her feelings of incompetency and her desire to escape tasks in which she might fail. It has also led to more isolation from her peers and greater fear in engaging with them. Abigail values her family and her relationships with others, but she has not defined what this means deeply (i.e., who she is or wants to be in these relationships). Her behavior sometimes negatively impacts her relationships, and this bothers her.

Acceptance and Defusion

Abigail has a limited capacity to allow anxiety. She is attached to a narrative of herself as a bad, undesirable, or incapable person, which increases her pain and keeps her stuck. Acceptance interventions will help Abigail allow anxious feelings, including the fear of letting go of rigid constraints on her behavior, and take personal, social, and academic risks (e.g., eating more flexibly, interacting with peers). Defusion strategies will help Abigail observe her constant comparison and evaluation as mental activity and hold thoughts such as "I am a mess, selfish, incapable" lightly. This will reduce her overall level of suffering, as well as help her be more in the present moment (aware of her environment and what might be effective for the situation). By being curious about her guilt (and generally her sources of pain), Abigail may be able to define her personal values.

Self-as-Context and Present-Moment Awareness

Abigail will need help connecting to a sense of self that transcends momentary thoughts/feelings (including her categorical judgments of herself) and practicing taking the stance of the observer ("I notice that I am having the thought that 'I am lazy'."). More self-compassion might be possible once she is able to distinguish herself from her thoughts, feelings, and actions and to take her own perspective across time (appreciating the different contextual variables influencing her behavior). It might also be enhanced by practice offering compassion to herself at an earlier place and time. Present-moment interventions will help Abigail stay in the here-and-now rather than spending all of her time in her head, remembering past regrets or worrying about the future. Present-moment interventions will also help her practice broad and flexible attention, rather than hyperfocusing on her body or signals of rejection or incompetency.

Values and Committed Action

Abigail's guilt feelings might inform her personal values in relationships, learning, and other domains. Values will have to be distinguished from rules of what she "should" do and from rigid expressions (e.g., "Valuing relationships is always forsaking myself"). Committed actions will include eating more, and generally breaking self-imposed rules that are overly rigid and nonresponsive to her needs. They will also include practice making decisions that have the potential for mistakes and investing in her relationships. This will mean letting go of other time investments (e.g., obsessional counting of calories and nutritional content) and experimenting with new behaviors. Value-guided behavioral activation might also be used to increase alternative (adaptive) sources of competency and mastery.

Other Elements to Consider in Treatment Planning

- *Weight and external supports.* Abigail will likely need some external support (at least initially) for restoring weight. Her parents have allowed her to leave treatment AMA on more than one occasion, and this may suggest the need for parent psychoeducation about the seriousness of their daughter's low weight and how they can help with warm but firm boundaries around AN. There might also be the need to address psychological barriers for the parents (difficult thoughts and feelings that interfere with persistence in expectations/

boundaries, such as fear of disrupting their relationship with their daughter or causing her more pain). A multidisciplinary team with clear and consistent expectations for eating (e.g., meal plan, exchanges) and weight will also be essential.

• *Motivation for change.* Abigail's motivation for change is low, increasing the importance of parental support during the early stages of treatment. Her aversion to fatigue, cognitive fog, and general depressive feelings might be leveraged to increase willingness to experiment with less punitive self-treatment and improved nutrition. Abigail might also be motivated by her relationship values or values she holds related to learning/academics if she were willing to approach her fears in these domains.

Updating the Case Formulation as Treatment Progresses

As mentioned earlier, it is often necessary to refine the functional assessment throughout treatment. To illustrate, an update from the previous case is provided here.

Later, Abigail's weight improved (to low normal) with the assistance of her parents in treatment and weekly meetings with the nutritionist. She no longer feels fatigued and as suicidal. She has begun to face many of her fears and has started dating and working. She is considering returning to school. This has provided Abigail with alternative sources of mastery. However, as things have improved, the degree of her obsessionality is clearer than it was initially and, no longer focused on eating, is centered more squarely on her relationships. Abigail is constantly concerned about whether she is liked and fears rejection by her boyfriend and friends. She manages these feelings by limitless giving to these relationships. She frequently buys gifts for other people (despite having limited resources) and is always available for favors or unsolicited help. Abigail reports her behavior serves her relationship values; however, the rigidity of their execution suggests that they are also driven by avoidance and control. She is likely avoiding fear (of rejection), guilt (of being a burden to people), and shame (not feeling worthy/worthwhile). Abigail's behavior is maintained by the emotional comfort she experiences in the moment. However, paradoxically, she never really knows if she is liked for who she is, which maintains her obsessional worry. Abigail also feels unfulfilled as her needs are not met. Treatment will necessitate continued practice of disentangling from worry, rumination, and thoughts of low self-worth to come to the present moment and facing her fear of doing less (setting limits) and "being herself" in relationships. Over time, as Abigail has positive experiences in relationships (experiences acceptance for who she is), she may be better able to accept herself as well. Her value of treating people well may be extended to herself (i.e., choosing to treat herself as worthwhile; equal to others, whether or not she feels this way).

Looking Ahead

Reversing starvation and improving weight and nutritional status is an essential element of treatment in AN. In Chapter 4, we describe orienting clients to the goal of weight restoration and preparing them for weight gain and structuring interventions to facilitate increased food intake.

FORM 3.1

ACT for AN Case Formulation and Treatment Planning

This form outlines the core components of the functional assessment of AN behavior and key considerations in treatment planning. It may be useful to complete this form at the beginning of treatment, along with Form 3.2. Both forms may be updated as treatment progresses and new information emerges.

---

1. **Identify AN behaviors.** Include overt (e.g., food restriction) as well as covert behaviors (e.g., calorie counting). Be specific (e.g., eliminates all fat from diet, does not eat snacks, limits food intake to 400 calories a day, exercises 2 hours a day).

---

2. **Identify how the client's behavior is helpful.** Include **unwanted internal experiences** that AN eliminates (e.g., feelings of failure) and **desired internal experiences** that AN provides (e.g., mastery). (These are contingencies maintaining AN.)

---

3. **Identify other behaviors that produce similar changes in the client's internal experience.** Include these behaviors as treatment targets if they are rigid, situationally insensitive, or diminish life vitality. Examples include not expressing opinions, compliance, working long hours, imposing rigid daily structure or planning, counting or other rituals. (These are behaviors that are functionally equivalent to AN.)

(continued)

Note. Copyright © Rhonda M. Merwin, Nancy L. Zucker, and Kelly G. Wilson. Reprinted by permission.

4. **Identify cognitive fusion that is maintaining problem behaviors despite physical or psychological harm.** Include rules or strongly held beliefs about how one "should be" or the implications of having feelings or making mistakes. Also include painful or evocative self-relevant thoughts (e.g., "I am unlikable").

5. **Identify undesirable consequences of AN or other problematic behaviors** (e.g., lost time due to overexercise, lack of meaningful relationships). Include what the client has lost, as well as things that she has not had the opportunity for. (These are consequences of AN that are not currently exerting stimulus control but, if contacted, would maintain more adaptive repertoires of behavior.)

6. **Assess degree of undernourishment and strength of external supports.** What percentage of ideal body weight is the client (based on the client's age, sex, and weight history)? Should there be limits or conditions to outpatient treatment? To what extent should other people in the client's natural environment be brought into treatment?

   What are the family resources (i.e., parents, siblings, and extended family) that can provide emotional or instrumental support? What is the client's willingness to involve the family, and the family's ability to communicate effectively around AN, food/eating, or set and follow a plan? What are the primary barriers?

(continued)

7. **Assess commitment to change.** How committed is the client to treatment? Are there aspects of living with AN the client does not like that might be leveraged to engage the client in treatment (e.g., occasional binge eating due to nutritional depletion)? Are there other outside contingencies compelling change (e.g., is the individual mandated for treatment to continue playing on a sports team, etc.)?

Other members of the treatment team:

Physician:

Nutritionist:

Psychiatrist:

Other:

Initial behavior change goal and plan (e.g., eat dinner with a support person present, mark other meals with some food intake, add a snack or nutritional supplement to daily intake):

FORM 3.2

Key Targets, Strengths, and Weaknesses in Each Core Process Domain

Instructions: For each of the six core ACT processes, list the most salient targets for your client. Next, use the anchors below to estimate your client's current capacities in each domain, ranging from *very weak* (–3) to *very strong* (3). Ratings may be used for case conceptualization and ongoing treatment planning.

Key Targets for Acceptance (i.e., unwanted thoughts/feelings):

Capacity for Acceptance

Constantly suppresses feelings or avoids activities that may generate strong feelings (positive or negative).	–3 –2 –1 0 1 2 3	Consistently allows feelings to be present; approaches activities that have emotional valence.
Always judges, rejects, or denies feelings.	–3 –2 –1 0 1 2 3	Validates and respects feelings and what they communicate (if anything).
Persistently imposes rules or structure; avoids unplanned activities; avoids or limits decision making by eliminating choices.	–3 –2 –1 0 1 2 3	Allows uncertainty or imprecision; engages in activities with less structure and planning; actively makes choices even when feeling uncertain.
Never takes interpersonal risks (e.g., avoids eye contact, does not express opinions, does not self-disclose).	–3 –2 –1 0 1 2 3	Engages in behaviors that feel interpersonally risky.

Note. Copyright © Rhonda M. Merwin, Nancy L. Zucker, and Kelly G. Wilson. Reprinted by permission.

(continued)

Key Targets for Defusion (i.e., unhelpful attachment):

Capacity for Defusion

Always follows self-imposed rules despite unworkability or negative consequences.	−3 −2 −1 0 1 2 3	Deviates from rules when doing so would be effective or value-guided.
Never makes a distinction between thoughts about events and the events themselves (e.g., the thought "I am a bad person" is treated as the literal event rather than a judgment one makes about oneself).	−3 −2 −1 0 1 2 3	Consistently recognizes thoughts as mental activity and discriminates from direct experience.
Speech is dominated by eating disorder content, judgments, and reasons for not eating; is repetitive or rote; lacks voice prosody.	−3 −2 −1 0 1 2 3	Speech is varied in content and delivery; is animated in emotional tone.
Contacts only negative verbal-evaluative functions of food, eating, or meeting needs (e.g., greed).	−3 −2 −1 0 1 2 3	Experiences the direct benefits of eating, sleeping, or seeking support. Other functions of food or eating exert influence over behavior (e.g., increased energy, texture, taste, interest, social value).

(continued)

Key Targets for Present-Moment Awareness (i.e., fixed or distracted attention):

Capacity for Present-Moment Awareness

Is always ruminating about the past or worrying about the future.	−3 −2 −1 0 1 2 3	Is able to be in the here-and-now.
Is constantly vigilant about how the body looks or feels.	−3 −2 −1 0 1 2 3	Flexibly attends to the body; is able to also notice other people or the situation.
Is constantly scanning the environment for threat (e.g., reactions of other people, negative feedback).	−3 −2 −1 0 1 2 3	Is able to rest attention on the current task or something that is interesting or meaningful.
Does not easily disengage from a stimulus that has captured attention (e.g., ambiguous social cue).	−3 −2 −1 0 1 2 3	Is able to broaden attention in the presence of a perceived threat cue.
Must always be doing something productive.	−3 −2 −1 0 1 2 3	Is able to engage in non-goal-directed activity.

(continued)

Key Targets for Areas of Self (e.g., unhelpful self-narratives, impoverished content areas):

Capacity for Self-ing

Never deviates from self-narratives.	−3 −2 −1 0 1 2 3	Is able to behave in ways that contradict self-narratives when doing so would be effective or value-guided.
Defines self narrowly by achievements or measureable outcomes.	−3 −2 −1 0 1 2 3	Possesses rich and varied self-content.
Never uses personal preferences and opinions in making decisions (in domains other than eating); conforms and complies.	−3 −2 −1 0 1 2 3	Takes personal preferences and opinions into account when making decisions.
Is consistently unaware of ongoing emotional experience (beyond being fat or upset).	−3 −2 −1 0 1 2 3	Has ongoing awareness of his or her feelings; labels emotions.
Is unable to take a different perspective (of oneself at another time or place, or the perspective of another person); perspective is experienced as static and universal.	−3 −2 −1 0 1 2 3	Is able to flexibly take perspective; appreciating the impact of situational factors on behavior and allowing for empathy and compassion (for self and other people).

(continued)

Key Targets for Values (e.g., signs of deep caring, barriers to authoring values):

Capacity for Values

Is completely unaware of what is cared about other than AN, perfection, or control.	-3 -2 -1 0 1 2 3	Is deeply aware of personal values.
Behavior is primarily motivated by relief from discomfort, "shoulds," etc.	-3 -2 -1 0 1 2 3	Behavior is strongly motivated by personal values/vitality.
Always avoids value domains that are important to her because of fear.	-3 -2 -1 0 1 2 3	Explores values in domains that are important to her.

(continued)

Key Targets for Committed Action (e.g., areas of over- and underinvolvement):

Capacity for Committed Action

Fills all available time with activities based on what she "should" be doing.	−3 −2 −1 0 1 2 3	Engages in activities that take into account personal needs or sources of fulfillment or joy.
Cannot deviate from plans.	−3 −2 −1 0 1 2 3	Is able to behave spontaneously sometimes.
Always persists, even when actions are not improving outcomes or are causing harm.	−3 −2 −1 0 1 2 3	Is able to stop or adjust goals based on feedback.
Never engages in activities that are not goal-driven or do not produce a measurable marker of success.	−3 −2 −1 0 1 2 3	Participates in activities that are personally meaningful even when they do not have a measurable outcome.

CHAPTER 4

Weight Restoration

Reversing low weight is an essential goal in the treatment of AN. This is because extreme low weight has significant medical consequences, and while some of these problems reverse with renourishment, others are more permanent (e.g., loss of bone density). Treatment also becomes more challenging the longer an individual engages in extreme food restriction. Behavior patterns become more ingrained and starvation impairs cognitive and behavioral flexibility/adaptability (e.g., attention becomes increasingly narrow and fixed on food).

Starvation also alters body functions in a way that maintains inadequate food intake. For example, with prolonged undernourishment, individuals experience delayed gastric emptying and diminished hunger. Restoring weight can interrupt the downward spiral of progressively less food intake and low weight and advance other therapeutic goals by improving the individual's ability to more fully participate in treatment.

Although a higher level of care is relatively common in the course of AN (American Psychiatric Association, 2006; Anderson et al., 2017), the majority of weight restoration often occurs in outpatient treatment. For some individuals with AN treated in an outpatient setting, it may be possible to restore weight with minimal disruption of their daily lives. For others, weight restoration may require a significant change in the client's living situation or activities. This might include returning home from college, family members temporarily moving in, oversight of meals at school, relinquishing activities with high-energy expenditure (e.g., sporting activities), or other concessions.

While the ultimate aim of treatment is for clients to end rigid, rule-based self-regulation, often an early step in this process is to give clients clear directives about when to eat and how much. This may seem counterintuitive given the desire to move clients away from rules; however, these directives are often essential in disrupting AN and beginning the process of weight restoration. Clients will feel safer to eat more with clear guidelines, and this is the priority. A clear message about the importance of halting dangerous weight loss (by eating more) may also paradoxically provide relief by imposing a limit on AN and allowing the individual to relinquish tight control with dignity. Over time, the therapist helps the client approach the fear, guilt, or uncertainty of choosing to eat more sufficiently based on internal cues and personal preferences.

In restoring weight, the clinical focus is on the process of eating with greater regularity, adequacy, and variety, typically in that order. Goals will vary based on the severity of the client's condition. Initial goals for eating with *regularity* might include "marking meals" by eating something three times a day or adding snacks in between meals (eating every 2–3 hours). Increasing the *adequacy* of caloric intake might include replacing diet foods with regular versions, adding nutrition to something already being consumed (e.g., mixing nuts or nut butter into oatmeal or adding cheese to a sandwich or chickpeas to a salad), increasing portion size (e.g., a full serving rather than half a serving), adding a nutritional supplement of 250–350 calories, or replacing a snack with a nutritionally dense shake (shakes may be particularly useful when calorie needs are very high due to increased metabolism during refeeding). Variety is typically the last concern and includes diversifying the foods that are consumed. This might include trying variations of acceptable foods (e.g., eating another variety of bean, if beans are typically consumed) or eating foods considered "off limits" (e.g., desserts). Variety might be addressed earlier, if limited food selection is making it difficult to get sufficient calories and restore weight without excessive bulk.

Weight restoration plans are developed in collaboration with the client and the other members of the treatment team (nutritionist, physician). Target weight gain for outpatient treatment typically varies from 0.5 to 1 pound per week. Ideal body weight is determined by the client's sex, height and individual growth curves, and, potentially, recent weight history and history of menstruation. Setting expectations for weekly weight trajectory and defining weight parameters for continuation in outpatient treatment is important (an issue we return to later in the chapter).

Motivating Increased Food Intake

Values

Ideally, eating and weight restoration are motivated by the client's values (what she cares about most deeply and wants for her life, as illustrated in Dialogue A) or the kind of person she wants to be (e.g., a person who treats herself with kindness, a person who faces fears). However, many clients are compelled to treatment by other people, and thus unlikely to identify a personal value that is served by eating or weight restoration (at least initially). In this case, the therapist may begin with the client's desire to end unwanted oversight (from family, friends, and medical providers) as motivation for change. This desire can be framed as valuing personal autonomy, which has been lost as the weight loss has become more extreme (illustrated in Dialogue B below).

Focusing on reducing unwanted oversight may be helpful in the initial reversal of starvation; however, it is unlikely to sustain long-term health. Rather, it will be necessary for the client to identify something of personal meaning that can encourage sufficient nourishment "when no one is looking." We describe how to facilitate values authorship in Chapter 8.

IN PRACTICE

Dialogue A

THERAPIST: It can be so hard to initiate treatment, yet here you are after years of dealing with this. I am wondering, why now? What is important about facing this fear and changing your eating?

CLIENT: I know if I don't, then I'm going to have to leave nursing school. I've wanted to be a nurse for as long as I can remember . . .

THERAPIST: So facing the fear of eating . . . this is about being able to do the work that you care about—that is important to you. I wonder if you could tell me more about nursing and what it means to you . . . most deeply . . . what it would mean to you to bring your whole self to that work. . . . We are going to have to be really clear about this—and to have it accessible to you when it is most hard to persist in eating. You'll need to be able to remind yourself why you are doing something that feels so difficult or overwhelming at times . . .

Dialogue B

CLIENT: I have no interest in gaining weight. This whole thing is stupid. I just want people to leave me alone.

THERAPIST: I hear you. This is really hard—and annoying! I also hear that it is important to you to be self-determining—to have other people not telling you what to do. That has been one consequence of AN. It has caused other people to step in.

CLIENT: It's really none of their business.

THERAPIST: It certainly is frustrating to have people acting as though they know what you need. I wonder if we can work toward you getting your freedom back . . .

Logical Consequences

Logical consequences can also be used to create a context that supports eating. This approach is not meant to be punitive; rather, it is to increase client contact with the consequences of behavior. The body has an incredible capacity to adapt to conditions, including conditions of prolonged nutritional deprivation. Thus, AN is a situation of degraded and delayed contingencies—too miniscule and too far off in time to influence behavior. By instituting logical consequences, it might be possible for behavior to be shaped more adaptively sooner.

Logical consequences are consequences that are not naturally occurring (i.e., they are imposed), but they logically follow the behavior. For example, it is logical that if we cannot nourish our bodies sufficiently, then we need to conserve energy. Thus, a logical consequence for insufficient food intake is the removal of activities that require energy expenditure (e.g., participation in sports, dance, or exercise at the gym). Logical consequences may be centered on daily activities (i.e., the ability to eat a meal, snack, or supplement determines daily activity participation) or a pattern of behavior over days or weeks (i.e., following a meal plan or a positive weight trajectory allows continued participation in an activity). An inability to nourish oneself sufficiently over a period of time might also have a logical consequence of a change in the frequency of therapy appointments or level of care. This consequence is logical in that the lack of improved intake is a signal that "something is not working" and needs to change. Therapists can work with the physician on the treatment team to reinforce limits, or, in the case of younger clients, can work with parents who implement contingencies at home.

Additional information about developing behavior change plans can be found in Chapter 5 and is relevant to working with clients individually, as well as with the family.

Therapist Support

Therapist support for weight restoration might include in-session meal exposures, the use of coaching calls at difficult mealtimes, or postmeal check-ins to increase accountability for eating. If the therapist is providing additional support outside of sessions, the parameters of this support need to be clearly specified, as well as a plan for transitioning to less-frequent contact.

Treating Denial of Low Weight Functionally

Denial of low weight or the seriousness or gravity of low weight is common in AN. It is most pronounced among clients who are severely undernourished and compelled to treatment by other people. It might sound like the following:

"My weight is not too low; other people just have a problem with it."
"People are lying to me about my weight. It's not that bad."
"I am not losing weight anymore; it's fine."
"The medical problems of low weight do not apply to me (I know that they happen to some people, but not me)."
"I feel better than I have ever felt; how could this be a problem?"

It might also have a more subtle presentation of a continual internal debate about whether the client really needs to gain weight (or not). Among patients who are improving, denial of low weight might reemerge in times of stress, when there is a strong need for AN behaviors to cope.

It may be tempting for therapists to address denial by providing psychoeducation about undernourishment or the medical indicators of the client's nutritional status. Whereas this is fine from the perspective of expanding the client's current context with information, there are two problems with *over*relying on psychoeducation. First, despite obvious undernourishment, individuals with AN might have normal laboratory results due to the body's ability to adapt to conditions (although this adaptation does not prevent long-term consequences). Injury might also only reveal itself as the individual starts to eat with greater regularity and the body begins to repair. Second, information that contradicts the individual's beliefs is likely to be rationalized or ignored. This is because denial is not an information deficit; rather, it is a behavior motivated by fear. Thus, it may be more effective (and ACT consistent) to respond to denial functionally, as a way to protect AN, as illustrated in the dialogue below.

IN PRACTICE

Dialogue

CLIENT: I don't know what everyone's problem is. I am huge!

THERAPIST: Eating more is really scary. . . . Let's see if we can get a sense of all the things your mind says to you about it. So one thing it says is "Everyone is wrong, you are huge, keep doing what you are doing" . . . what else? (*elicits content*) In this way, then, your mind tries to protect you from this scary thing . . . from changing your eating . . .

CLIENT: (*Fidgets.*)

THERAPIST: It must be hard to feel so afraid. Like jumping off the high dive . . . and into water that is unfamiliar to you. You can't see the bottom, and you can't be sure whether it is safe.

CLIENT: Yes . . . and there are all these people ushering me to the edge. But they aren't the one that has to jump.

THERAPIST: You are absolutely right. You are the one that is doing the hard work. I want you to know that I am here, and we can put in place as much or as little support as is useful (during meals, etc.) . . .

"I'm Not Hungry" as a Reason Not to Eat

During weight restoration, "I am not hungry" might emerge as a reason to not eat. This expression is likely under complex stimulus control, with both biological and psychological constituents. For example, hunger might simply be diminished as individuals eat more frequently and consume larger quantities of food to restore weight, particularly if energy expenditure is low. Decreased hunger might also be the result of biological adaptations to starvation, including slowed gastric emptying or hypometabolism. Denial of hunger might also be functional and reflect the client's fear or uncertainty of eating more. In any case, the therapist may validate how hard it is to eat when not hungry (or when less hungry). Typically, the client should be encouraged to continue with prescribed eating, following nutritional recommendations for total calories and macronutrient distribution. As weight is restored, the client may begin to practice appetite awareness and more intuitive eating.

Sometimes clients report the opposite problem, indicating that they are hungry between meals or snacks. Clients may be encouraged to deviate from their prescribed meal plan and eat when hungry, given that this likely signals increased metabolism and a need to consume more energy. Hunger should stabilize as clients continue to eat with regularity. If clients continue to struggle with the urge to overconsume food, the therapist may need to address psychological factors (e.g., difficulty finding the "middle ground" between rigid overcontrol and limitless eating, or the trauma of starvation, discussed later in the chapter).

Weight Monitoring

Weight monitoring is necessary in the treatment of AN, particularly in the early stages of treatment, when nutritional plans might need to be adjusted fairly frequently due to changes in metabolism. The therapist can conduct weight checks (e.g., at the beginning of weekly sessions), or if it is more therapeutically appropriate, another member of the treatment team, such as the nutritionist or the physician, can be responsible for gathering and communicating this information to the other providers. In using weight-related information, the therapist models being flexible and effective rather than rigid and rule-governed. Weight *trends*, rather than individual weight data points, are observed and situated in the broader context of the individual and her behavior. However, the therapist should also be cognizant that being too flexible or dismissive of weight data may be a disservice to the client.

Weight checks might be blinded or nonblinded to the client. Nonblinded weights are used in FBT (Lock & Le Grange, 2015); however, the impact of this specific element of treatment has not been studied, and the effects might be different for adolescents who have the support of their parents than for independent adults. In the absence of data to guide this decision, it is made on an individual basis.

Some clients have a strong preference for whether they are blinded to their weight. The therapist should consider factors that might influence client preference in treatment planning. This may be determined by not only asking the client about her motivations, but also by observing behavior before or after weighing or after receiving weight-related information. For example, the therapist might observe that the client restricts food prior to a medical appointment (when she expects to be weighed) or evidences positive affect after hearing she has lost weight. This suggests that having the client see her weight is reinforcing restriction and is thus counterproductive. Blind weighing during acute weight restoration will help the client restore weight more efficiently. Future therapeutic goals may include helping the client see and accept her weight *without* working for weight loss. For other clients, not knowing their weight may impede progress. Allowing nonblinded weights may help the client engage in weight restoration because they feel safer and more trusting of the treatment providers. In this case, later therapeutic goals will include the client gradually facing the discomfort of not knowing her weight (e.g., increasing the time between weighing). Observations (and hypotheses about how seeing or not seeing one's weight is functioning for the client) should be discussed openly with the client, and a plan should be devised that is sensitive to the client's preference *and* therapeutic needs.

Although the process of weight monitoring is best decided collaboratively, occasionally the therapist may take greater ownership of this decision and "prescribe" blind weighing, particularly for severely undernourished clients. Clients might be discouraged from weighing themselves at home in between appointments. The script below illustrates how a therapist might introduce weight checks to a client. In Script B, the therapist discusses changing the plan for weight checks as therapy progresses.

IN PRACTICE

Therapist Script A

"You might remember that we planned to do a weight check today. . . . This will give us a sense of how things are going and where we might need to make changes. The important thing will be trends rather than individual data points (we actually expect weight to fluctuate in a range). . . . Trends will tell us if we need to adjust our plan . . . If you are willing, I suggest that we start with blind weights. We can discuss whether it would be helpful to do nonblinded weights in the future as the situation improves. (*pauses*) I know that this is a scary thing, and you are not completely comfortable with this idea . . . and if I did not insist that we do this, I would be doing a disservice to you [abandoning you to the eating disorder]. It is essential that we know whether we are being helpful to you, whether outpatient is enough . . ."

Therapist Script B (with the "Closed-Closet" Metaphor)

"In the past, we have been doing blinded weights, mostly because you felt as though that helped you not get entangled with thoughts and feelings about your body. And I think that was great insight on your part, as you have been able to just focus on doing what you need to do (in terms of eating). I am wondering how you are feeling about seeing your weight today, and working through it together? (*pause*) Imagine that we have a closet where we shove all the stuff that we don't want to look at. If there is something that we really don't want to see, we may never open that closet or even go into that room. We might even start to avoid that side of the house! Not only does that limit our space to live, but also our mind can tell stories about what's behind the door. . . . This would be about opening the door, letting the light shine in . . . seeing it for what it is (not for what our mind says it is). . . . I imagine what we will find is some discomfort, maybe some hard memories . . ."

Preparing Clients for the AN Extinction Burst

All animals (including humans) prefer aversives that they can predict to those that they cannot. Predicting discomfort that clients might experience as they begin to eat more and restore weight can increase their capacity to allow these experiences and persist in effective behavior. It is often particularly helpful to prepare clients for the temporary increase in the intensity and frequency of their AN thoughts and feelings, as illustrated in the script that follows. This may be thought of as an *extinction burst,* as behavior that was reinforced in the past is not any longer. The script below may not be appropriate for all clients. Clients who are overly identified with AN early in treatment may be put off by the externalizing language.

IN PRACTICE

Therapist Script

"As you do this work [of restoring weight] [i.e., stop restricting, stop punishing yourself, stop requiring that you 'earn' meals], we can expect AN to get really loud. It may yell and shout at you . . . try to convince you to not eat. It may call you names. Those are the moments we need to prepare for together."

Body Experience during Weight Restoration

Clients with AN may experience changes in their body during weight restoration that they may not understand. These changes might perpetuate feelings of fatness or fears of being indulgent or out of control. Open and honest communication about what to expect when the body is restoring weight can help clients persist in behavior change. It can also increase trust in the therapist and the treatment team. The depth of discussion will require clinical judgment. Time should be taken to process the client's response and appreciate her fear or discomfort. Some clients may not be able to integrate or use all of the information in the early stages of treatment. This content may be presented again in smaller segments. It can also be presented more in metaphor, which provides the opportunity to begin to recontextualize the body and the body experience. The therapist script that follows describes changes that might occur as the client renourishes her body. The dialogues illustrate using metaphor to recontextualize the client's experience of her body and persist in weight restoration.

IN PRACTICE

Therapist Script (Psychoeducation about the Body during Renourishment)
"The body responds to starvation by slowing basal metabolic rate (i.e., the amount of energy that the body requires at rest in order to carry out normal physiological processes) and maintaining only the most essential processes (those that are necessary for survival). This is why you have stopped menstruating. This is a biological adaptation that helps humans survive during a famine. Burning energy more slowly, your body can conserve its resources and make the most out of what it is given. If the body continues to be depleted, it will begin to feed on itself, using your muscle, including your heart, as an energy source. You may have noticed some loss of muscle in your own body. It is when this is no longer sustainable that people die. The gastrointestinal system also slows down during starvation, resulting in delayed gastric emptying. This may create a sense of fullness, even when you have eaten very little. You can see how the hypometabolic state leads people to eat less—the body is burning more slowly so you need fewer and fewer calories to maintain dangerously low weight as your body fights for survival, and because of delayed emptying, you feel full. The good news is that as you start to eat again, your basal metabolic rate will increase—you will start to use energy more quickly.

"As your basal metabolic rate increases, you might become hypermetabolic. This is your body 'revving' back up. It might produce intense feelings of hunger and a strong drive to eat. It is important to respond to hunger cues as your body is working to repair itself, and this requires a good deal of energy. This is biology, not you losing control. We will have to help you keep up with your metabolism during this period. This may require levels of energy consumption that you are not used to (even before AN) or that are intensely scary to you. But it is important to know this now: The meal plan that you have is a starting point that we will have to adjust to meet your body's requirements.

"As your gastrointestinal system becomes more active, you may also notice other things that are uncomfortable. For example, you may have some bloating and abdominal pain. Most of these feelings are normal and just mean your body is functioning again. Bloating or distension is not weight, but gas or fluids. The other thing that happens is that, initially, weight may be restored disproportionately to your midsection (and sometimes the face). This is a physiological consequence of starvation (e.g., elevated cortisol levels). It also helps protect the vital organs when the body is depleted. With continued weight restoration, the weight will redistribute and things will 'even out' . . . ."

Dialogue A (with the "Swamp" Metaphor)

CLIENT: I hate my body . . . all it does is bloat and hurt . . . I don't want to do this anymore.

THERAPIST: That sounds so uncomfortable . . . and I am not sure that there is anything that can be done right now. It's like being on a journey and you run into a swamp and it is deep and thick, and you feel like you are just dragging your legs through it. One option is to turn back and head the other direction. And you have done that before. Many times, in fact. Sometimes that is the best option, to see if there is another path. In this case, there is only one path . . . the only way is through. If you turn back, you will continually find yourself here . . . and have to start again . . .

Dialogue B (with the "Body Protector" Metaphor)

CLIENT: I just don't know if I can tolerate it . . . it is awful. And my stomach looks fat.

THERAPIST: Your body has been working hard to adapt to these (impoverished) conditions. It has slowed everything down and is conserving energy. This was to protect you and preserve your life. As you have started to fuel it, it is revving up; things are starting to move again (that's why you are experiencing some bloating) and the body is prioritizing your midsection to protect your most vital organs. . . . I know this is hard . . . and if you continue to give your body what it needs, it will settle down. It won't need to protect your organs because you are. I wonder if you would be willing to give it a little while—keep putting one foot in front of the next . . . for now . . . and see if things improve.

The Trauma of Starvation

Starvation, although self-imposed, is traumatic. The mind and body remember the massively depleted state and fear that it will happen again. As an adaptive mechanism, individuals might be driven to overconsume food, even after weight is restored. Individuals might also have psychological barriers to setting *any* limits on eating (e.g., balancing meals) because it will remind them of past restriction. For some clients, this will develop into patterns of binge eating and, potentially, maladaptive weight control strategies to compensate. While some overeating is expected, normal, and likely time-limited, it is important to monitor this behavior and potentially intervene to help clients reestablish healthy guidelines for eating. A script for discussing the loss of control individuals might feel and how to approach healthy limits is provided below.

IN PRACTICE

Therapist Script

"It makes sense that your body is pushing so hard for food. It has experienced a significant trauma, and it is afraid that it will be faced with another period of life-threatening deprivation. Psychologically, you have experienced a trauma as well. You can remember so clearly what it felt like to be starved. I can hear that you are scared that any limit, even a moderate, lightly held limit, will return you to that state. We will work on approaching this together . . . and slowly introduce healthy, flexible limits (guidelines, really). Our ultimate goal is that you have the *freedom to choose* when you eat and when you don't, and how much based on your needs and preferences—and not on fear."

What If the Client Refuses to Work on Weight Restoration?

It is not possible to work with a dead client or a client who does not have her emotional and cognitive faculties because she is starved. There is also considerable evidence that some AN behaviors (as well as some of the rigidity that characterizes AN) will remit as a result of renourishment. Thus, improving nutritional status is a clear goal of AN treatment, and client refusal to consider weight restoration places the therapist in a professional and ethical dilemma. Our strategy for dealing with this has been to be very up-front with our values as therapists and what we can and cannot sign on for, and for how long.

Luckily this is rare. Most often, the issue is finding the "yes" (the place where the client is willing to work). Sometimes this means accepting smaller changes than we would like. Typically, the client's goal is not to die. Most often, the client wants something for her life (and thinness is viewed as a prerequisite). It is our job to create some curiosity about whether there is another way that does not threaten her well-being and is life-enhancing.

Sometimes, when faced with a chronic client, the decision might be made to relinquish the expectation of weight restoration and take a more palliative care approach. However, this is an ongoing debate that depends on the therapist's own willingness to enter into this type of therapeutic contract with a client or refer her to another provider.

Looking Ahead

The amount of time spent in therapy is miniscule relative to the hours clients spend outside the therapy room. Most behavior takes place in the natural environment surrounded by parents, partners, and family members. In Chapter 5, we describe how to work with loved ones to support the individual with AN. The content is also useful for work with individual clients.

CHAPTER 5

Working with Parents, Partners, or Other Family Members of Individuals with Anorexia Nervosa

with **Lisa K. Honeycutt** and **Ashley A. Moskovich**

Historically, families of individuals with AN were purposefully excluded from the treatment. This was based on the unfounded assumption that AN is a reflection of an individual's need for autonomy and personal control that has been stymied by the parents or family (e.g., Bruch, 1962, 1982). Since that time, there has been clear empirical evidence that including families is efficacious for children and adolescents, particularly when the diagnosis of AN occurs shortly after onset (American Psychiatric Association, 2006; Le Grange et al., 2010). This is sensible given that most meals and snacks occur outside of the therapy room, and often with various members of the biological or nuclear family. Engaging families in treatment can also minimize accommodation or reinforcement of maladaptive behaviors and improve family dynamics or interactions that might be strained by the presence of AN (e.g., Ciao, Accurso, Fitzsimmons-Craft, Lock, & Le Grange, 2015).

The way in which family members are included in treatment is highly variable. Family members may participate only in an initial consultation or in multiple meetings throughout treatment. In the case of adolescents with AN, family members might be included for some portion of *every* session. Family members may also be seen with the client (in a conjoint session) or separately. Whether to conduct conjoint or separated sessions is determined by clinical judgment and is informed by the strength of the therapeutic alliance and the level of expressed emotion in the family (Eisler et al., 2000). If the therapeutic alliance is weak, the therapist might avoid meeting frequently with family members in the absence of the client. Greater levels of critical communication or low warmth within the family might suggest meeting with the client and family members separately (Eisler et al., 2000).

In working with family members, therapists have the following therapeutic goals:

- Provide a frame for understanding AN, and specifically how AN functions as a maladaptive coping strategy.
- Provide psychoeducation about the impact of starvation on behavior.
- Help the family separate their loved one from AN.
- Encourage family members to avoid entanglement with AN or accommodation of AN behavior.
- Determine how the family can help facilitate weight restoration.

Helping Families Understand AN

Family members often need help understanding the behavior they are observing in their loved one. It can be confusing to see her narrow so much in focus, to become completely preoccupied with food and eating, and to increasingly withdraw from other activities. It can also be difficult to synthesize discrepancies in her performance: how she may be high functioning in domains such as schoolwork, yet not able to meet her basic needs. In fact, this incongruity may lead some parents to question the severity of the problem given that the child's performance remains superior in many areas. Families often want to understand what caused AN and parents, in particular, may report guilt and a sense of responsibility for their child's condition.

It may be useful to orient families to a *diathesis–stress model* (that individuals have some degree of biological predisposition that combines with a confluence of environmental factors or learning), but to emphasize that, ultimately, etiology cannot be fully known and to shift focus to the present moment, or "Given that this is where we find ourselves, what do we do now?" When families are stuck asking "Why did this happen?", this indicates the need for acceptance of the current situation, defusion (of stories of blame), and practice coming to the here-and-now. In Dialogue A, the therapist is responding to family members' repeated questioning of why their loved one is struggling with AN. In Dialogue B, the therapist provides a frame for understanding the broader class of behavior that the family is observing in the individual with AN and a general strategy for addressing this behavior to improve her health and well-being.

IN PRACTICE

Dialogue A (with the "Rearview Mirror" Metaphor)

FAMILY MEMBER: I wish someone could just tell me why, why is this happening!?

THERAPIST: I hear you . . . This is so confusing and you just wish you could make sense of it all. I also wonder if trying to make sense of it (asking "Why?") is actually keeping you stuck a bit. . . . (*pause*) These things are complex . . . often a confluence of factors, and cannot fully be known. I wonder what it would be like to look forward, rather than back. . . . It's hard to drive when our gaze is fixed on the rearview mirror. When we are driving we need to look ahead of the car, not behind it . . . [This metaphor can be elaborated and returned to when attention is unduly focused on the past, quickly bringing therapeutic attention to the present.]

Dialogue B (with the "Poured from the Same Vessel" Metaphor)

FAMILY MEMBER: I just don't understand. She is making all A's and has always done everything so well. She is so hardworking and responsible—this is not like her. We have never had to worry about her. . . . Her brother, that is a different story. But not Kate. Did I tell you? She even has early admission to Stanford . . .

THERAPIST: I know it doesn't seem to make sense—how she can perform so well and at the same time cannot feed herself. The problem is that this drive to perform or be "good" and AN are poured from the same vessel. This drive has led her to neglect her needs, even her most basic need to eat.

The other thing I want to speak to is that I see how proud you are of her and what she has done—and that her ability to motivate and do is something you appreciate about her (and that she has appreciated about herself). We don't want to squash her drive, we just want to help her harness it—so that she can have it, instead of it having her. As it stands now, it threatens her life. This might seem strange, but we will actually be working to reinforce *doing* less . . . to teach her to be *kinder and less demanding* of herself. Often, this shift results in similar performance outcomes but with less personal cost, although not always.

AN as Maladaptive Coping

It might also be useful to describe to families how AN functions for the individual. In the simplest terms, AN can be formulated as a maladaptive coping strategy—a way of managing emotional distress by redirecting attention to areas of life that are less distressing or provide a sense of mastery or pride. Describing AN in this way can sometimes help families appreciate how difficult it would be to relinquish AN, which has served a clear purpose in the individual's life. Maslow's (1943) hierarchy of needs has intuitive appeal for describing how, by focusing on food, the individual turns away from other aspects of life that might feel more challenging (e.g., socializing). If the therapist has permission to share details of the personal struggle of the client, it is possible to specify what the individual is "turning away from" (i.e., what is hard for her). This is illustrated in Script A. Script B provides an alternative metaphor serving the same purpose.

The therapist might also describe how AN functions to simplify life by providing rules for behavior. The advantage to this description is that rather than put undue emphasis on food and eating, it allows for a broader description of the individual's chosen strategy of self-regulation and how it is helpful in a sense. This is illustrated in Therapist Script C.

IN PRACTICE

Therapist Script A (Maslow's Hierarchy of Needs)

"Have you heard of Maslow's hierarchy of needs? [*Draws pyramid.*] Humans have all kinds of needs. At the most basic level, we need food, water, and shelter to survive. If these basic needs are met, then we can attend to our social or self-esteem needs, to things higher up on the pyramid. AN takes us back to this bottom rung—directs all of our attention to food and eating—and allows these other things to recede into the background. In turning toward eating and weight, we can turn away from the more complicated or upsetting aspects of experience—areas in which we may feel as though we have failed or will fail—or other areas over which we have less control. It feels kind of nice . . . not to worry so much about X or Y and let life just be about the next meal . . .'"

Therapist Script B (with the "Magic Cloak" Metaphor)

"Imagine that your [family member] has been working hard, living her life, and no matter what, she still finds herself feeling anxious and worried. One day, while she is out walking, she uncovers a magic cloak. Skeptical at first, she looks at it and reads the card that's attached, and it says, 'Wear me and all your worries will fade away.' She puts it on, the cloak itself vanishes, but she has never felt more alive. The cloak gives her confidence and takes away many of her worries, fears, and doubts. People start to notice that something about her is different. She gets compliments and feels good about herself for the first time. Imagine what a relief this would be. . . . You can see why she wouldn't want to give it up and might be upset that people are asking her to."

Therapist Script C (Rules Simplify Life)

"Have you ever had the experience of going to a new restaurant and find that it has a huge menu, and you are overwhelmed with all the possible choices? While this might cause you to pause for a moment, for [your family member], this is incapacitating. The possibility of making a wrong choice feels quite significant. By applying rules (e.g., no meat or dairy), she limits her options to a more manageable set of choices. Now imagine that this is her experience all the time, not just at meals or new restaurants. The choices in her life feel overwhelming—and rules, well, rules help winnow it down a bit, make it more manageable. . . . She is no longer frozen in fear that she will make a wrong choice (make a mistake) . . ."

The Impact of Starvation on Behavior

Providing psychoeducation regarding the impact of undernourishment on behavior to help family members appreciate that some aspects of their loved one's behavior, which may be frustrating or upsetting (e.g., increased rigidity or obsessionality), are the natural by-product of starvation. Much of what we know about the impact of starvation on behavior comes from the Ancel Keys study from the 1940s (Keys, Brožek, Henschel, Mickelsen, & Taylor, 1950). In this study, conscientious objectors from World War II agreed to participate in a study as an alternative to going to war. The aim of the study was to understand how best to refeed prisoners of war who were dying upon refeeding. Psychologically healthy men were observed for 3 months, then their typical caloric intake was reduced by 50% over the course of 6 months. The men lost approximately 25% of their original body weight. They continued to be observed as they became renourished. This study indicated that starvation could induce some of the behaviors observed among individuals with AN among healthy men. For example, the men became preoccupied with food and eating and lost interest in other things (e.g., social interactions). Food dominated their conversations, and many of the men became interested in nutrition and cooking when they had not shown an interest in these things before. They began creating strange food concoctions and cutting their food into small pieces to make the meals last longer. They even demonstrated increased concern about body weight and shape and, when additional food was available, binge eating, followed by self-reproach. This study suggests that many of the behaviors that family members observe, and may be upset or frustrated by, are induced by starvation. Some of these behaviors may be contained, if they are really problematic, with contingencies (e.g., time limits on meal length), although many will simply remit as a consequence of renourishment.

Family members might also be reminded that starvation is a state of physical threat. Thus, the individual with AN might be more vigilant and reactive when undernourished than she typically is. This does not mean that all behavior (e.g., lashing out at a loved one over a meal) can be excused; rather, the family can validate the client's experience, while also establishing a limit for what is acceptable behavior (e.g., "I understand that this has upset you, and it is also not OK to talk to me like that"). Some of the cognitive narrowing and rigidity/obsessiveness might also be attributed to a starved brain.

The medical consequences of starvation are also important for family members to know. The medical consequences include more acute manifestations of undernourishment (e.g., hypothermia) and potential long-term consequences for growth velocity or bone density. It is important to emphasize that swift renourishment can mitigate many of these.

Separating the Individual from AN

Externalizing language is used in many therapeutic traditions as a way to help the individual see her problems as separate and distinct from herself. When externalizing AN, it is objectified as a collection of thoughts, feelings, and actions. *Externalization* defuses the individual from her thoughts and feelings and discriminates between problematic behavior and a problematic person. When the individual is not conflated with her thoughts, feelings, or actions, family members may be better able to love and support her, while also creating a context for behavior change. Sometimes families find it useful to give AN a name to more clearly discriminate their loved one from her difficult thoughts, feelings, or behavior patterns. This strategy is illustrated in the dialogue below.

IN PRACTICE

Dialogue

FAMILY MEMBER: She was horrible last night. You wouldn't believe the things that she said to her father! He just left dinner, and they didn't speak the rest of the night. I just don't know how much longer we can do this.

THERAPIST: What happened next?

FAMILY MEMBER: Well, she went to her room and I assume was on her phone.

THERAPIST: It sounds like AN has been really strong the last several days, and it feels as though it is tearing your family apart a bit (*pause to acknowledge the emotion that is present*). It can be challenging in these moments to remember that [your family member] is in there (she is). I wonder if we can find a way to stand with her, the part of her that you can sense with your heart, at these times. Validating how hard this is, while setting warm but firm boundaries around AN . . . so that she knows (deeply) that you won't lose her to this, no matter how horrible AN is.

Not Getting Entangled with AN

At some point during the course of AN, family members will find themselves locked in a debate about nutrition or what the individual has or has not eaten, or unhelpful conversations about body weight or shape. At these times, it might be more useful for family members to respond to the emotional rather than the literal content of their loved one's communication. If family members are attending sessions regularly, it is also possible to teach them to identify possible antecedents to the momentary exacerbation of AN (e.g., a negative work evaluation or a low grade on an exam) and help their loved one practice approach-based coping in the moment. The following dialogue illustrates how the therapist can coach the family to validate the emotion (rather than behavior) and see eating disorder thoughts/feelings functionally rather than getting hooked by their content.

IN PRACTICE

Dialogue

FAMILY MEMBER: Last night, she got so mad at me for using olive oil. I always use olive oil in this recipe . . . and then when we were leaving, she asked me several times if she looked fat. I thought that she looked great . . . a lot healthier than she has before, and I told her that. I think that upset her more. What am I supposed to do when she asks me this over and over? Like last week, she said she was too fat to go to my work dinner . . . and of course, that's ridiculous.

THERAPIST: I would encourage you step out of the eating disorder content as much as possible and instead speak to her emotions: "I'm sorry that today has felt hard . . . or that you are feeling badly, or that you are feeling sad or anxious or [ ]."

If she seems open to it and you are aware, you might suggest something that is upsetting her: "It sounds like you might be worried about the impression you are going to make tomorrow. . . . Do you want to talk about it?"

Remember that when [your loved one] is really consumed by eating disorder thoughts, this is a signal that she is experiencing painful emotions. Sometimes the thing that is deeply upsetting to her will be unrelated to food and eating, for example, a conflict with a friend or at work that made her feel badly about herself. However, her emotion will seem to be about a meal or tight clothes because these things capture her attention. Of course, these things might be upsetting in and of themselves, but their emotional impact comes from this other deeper pain.

Ultimately, the goal is for her to begin to see eating disorder thoughts and feelings as a *signal* that something is wrong and identify what that is—what emotional distress she is managing by focusing on eating or her body. You can help her do this, if she will allow it, but it would need to be done in a validating, compassionately curious manner.

I would also encourage you to avoid making comments about appearance (positive or negative) or answering questions about whether she looks healthy or sick. These are often emotionally loaded and unhelpful—things like "healthy" may be distorted by AN to mean "fat" or "failure." I don't want you to walk on eggshells, but these kinds of conversations are often unfruitful. If you are faced with a lot of questions, rather than respond to content, I would encourage you to respond to the process of what is happening and provide support: "I am wondering why you are asking this, if there is something bothering you that you would like to talk about. . . . I am here for you."

Accommodation of Maladaptive Behavior

In the OCD literature, illness accommodation is recognized as a barrier to effective exposure-based treatment (Storch et al., 2007). *Illness accommodation* refers to families accommodating to the rituals of the individual with OCD and, while well intentioned, this functions to maintain the individual's fear and avoidance behavior. Families of individuals with AN face a similar situation regarding how much they should accommodate the individual with AN. Examples of accommodation might include choosing restaurants with only clearly labeled nutrition information and safe foods and preparing foods in particular ways (e.g., without butter or oils). Overall, AN should not rule the family; at the same time, the family might have to adjust some to support their loved one. Families should be advised to "meet her where she is at," such that the challenge is not so great that she is unable to cope, but they are also not conceding to AN. When accommodations are made, they should be to increase food intake (prioritizing quantity and sufficient energy over food variety, etc.). The dialogue that follows coaches the parents on setting flexible boundaries.

IN PRACTICE

Dialogue

PARENT: I told her we were going to Magianno's and she said, "I can't eat there! I will just wait until after the game," and I didn't know what to do. That would be well after dinner.

THERAPIST: I think this is probably a place for flexible boundaries; not eating is not an option, but where she eats might be. It might sound something like this: "I would rather you eat at the place that everyone else has agreed on; however, I know it is hard for you to go out to eat unexpectedly. I am willing to go to [alternative location] on the way to the football game, which has some of the foods that are on your current meal plan; however, not eating before the game is not an option."

PARENT: We used to love to go to out for Italian food or to cook these Italian meals together. . . . It reminds me of when I was a kid, and my grandmother. . . . Now she refuses almost everything . . .

THERAPIST: I know this feels like such a loss. . . . It sounds like you have fond memories of mealtimes together. Right now, sufficient calories are so important—we just have to prioritize that. However, we should also think about how you can reclaim some part of that. It will probably look like meeting her where she is and encouraging her to challenge the eating disorder and take a step forward. I am imagining, for example, making the pasta that you enjoyed together, but with the sauce on the side. Maybe the full dish is beyond her reach at the moment, but perhaps she would have half a serving of the pasta, along with other "safe" foods to make a full meal . . .

Emotional and Instrumental Support

Family members often have questions about how best to help their loved one with AN. Family members can provide emotional or instrumental support, or a combination of the two (as outlined in Table 5.1). *Emotional support* refers to being present and offering support at times of greater stress or difficulty. This might include family members simply being present, physical contact (e.g., hand-holding, a hug), or a verbal expression of empathy or understanding. *Instrumental support* includes actions that directly facilitate effective behavior or block ineffective behavior. Individuals with AN may have specific ideas about how their family can be helpful, and plans are developed in collaboration with the client. Plans should be developed a priori, not at mealtime, when urges to restrict will be strong and it will be harder to accept help.

Reluctance to Include Others

Some adult clients might be reluctant to include family members in their treatment. Sometimes this is because of difficult family history (e.g., trauma or estrangement). Other times, it is because of the toll AN has taken on family relationships, or it is a direct effort to protect AN. For adults who are extremely undernourished, having *someone* in their external

TABLE 5.1. Examples of Emotional and Instrumental Support

Emotional support	Instrumental support
• Being present at meals or snacks. • Calling or texting before or after a meal. • Accompanying individuals to medical appointments. • Setting aside special time together outside of eating or meals.	• Helping the individual with grocery shopping. • Tracking food intake. • Establishing methods of accountability for following meal plans. • Preparing meals that provide a mix of "safe" and "unsafe" foods. • Engaging the individual 30 minutes after eating to prevent vomiting. • Engaging in alternative activities with the individual during typical exercise times. • Maintaining contingencies for eating and weight restoration.

environment who is knowledgeable about the situation (including meal plans and the goal of gaining weight) may be a contingency for outpatient treatment. This can help minimize the expansion of unhealthy behavior. It does not have to be a family member, but could be another person who can provide support. The dialogue that follows introduces the idea of including support people to a client and uses perspective taking to increase willingness.

IN PRACTICE

Dialogue

CLIENT: I don't want my family to know. . . . I don't want to worry them.

THERAPIST: I know this is a scary thing—to think about talking with your family. It is a powerful thing to "out" the eating disorder. It is a major act of willingness, and it has to be your choice.

CLIENT: I don't know.

THERAPIST: One thing we do know is that "doing it alone" hasn't been working. . . . AN is too strong . . . and if things keep going as they are, you will be too medically compromised for outpatient treatment.

CLIENT: Yes . . . I know that is true . . . I just worry about being a burden.

THERAPIST: This thought is something that comes up for you quite a lot. . . . And I also wonder, what is it like for you to sit on the sidelines when someone you love is suffering . . . do you know this place? What do you imagine this is like for them . . . to know something is wrong but not know what, or how to help?

The Role of Family Members in Weight Restoration

Beginning in the 1980s, several studies testing the Maudsley model of FBT for adolescent AN were published. This model empowered parents to assume temporary control over their child's eating in order to restore weight and it outperformed individual adolescent treatment, particularly in amelioration of physical manifestations of AN. Thus, it was concluded that direct family involvement in meals is helpful for *adolescents* with AN, and this became the standard of care.

Parents assuming temporary control over meals (determining food type and quantity for their child) may be equally beneficial for *dependent, young adult children,* although there are logistical challenges if children are not living at home. Young adults may need to return home from college, or parents may choose to live temporarily in a dorm or apartment to help their child finish out a semester. When choosing to intervene in this way, the family should consider whether the risk of continued low weight outweighs the cost of temporarily disrupting their child's developmental trajectory. The role of family members in weight restoration of *fully independent adults* is less clear; however, as previously mentioned, having someone at least aware of the client's situation often helps in minimizing expansion of unhealthy behavior. Simply eating with another person may be beneficial, increasing accountability for food intake. These additional supports may be systematically reduced as the individual's eating and weight improve.

Some clients have family members who are unable to participate effectively in weight restoration for a variety of reasons. In this case, *family* might include other people who are close to the individual, or the therapist may provide additional support to help the client restore weight. Therapist support for weight restoration might include more frequent in-session meals, the use of coaching calls at difficult mealtimes, or postmeal check-ins to increase accountability for eating. If the therapist is providing additional support outside of sessions, the parameters of this support need to be clearly specified. Plans for providing additional support for weight restoration are developed collaboratively with the client. The outcome of these plans should be monitored and plans should be adjusted if they are not helping the individual eat more and restore weight. Clients might have ideas about what is and is not working to help them eat more. These ideas can be tested as hypotheses, as illustrated in the dialogue on page 111.

Additional Information for Working with Parents of Adolescents and Dependent Adults with AN

Caring for someone with AN is extremely challenging (Treasure et al., 2001; Whitney et al., 2005). Many parents benefit from additional therapeutic support to address AN behavior and cope with having a child who is starving. To truly appreciate the experience of parents, consider the following narrative:

"Prior to your child's recent dramatic weight loss, your daughter had been a remarkably easy child to parent. She was a diligent, conscientious, and serious young girl who was very respectful of authority, completed her homework without prompting, and always strove to be the best at everything. In fact, she often *was* the best at everything. However, her acquisition of status was often at great personal expense. Your daughter always worked excessively hard, sacrificing sleep or leisure so that she could achieve the often untenably high standards she established for herself. She had difficulty saying no, for fear of missing out on a chance to achieve something. As a result, even in grade school, she seemed constantly overly stressed, as she always had too many activities to accomplish in seemingly too little time. Yet you hesitated to cancel or limit any activities, as she always excelled in them and professed to enjoy them. What was sneaking under the radar was the fact that there was a dangerous cost to your daughter's relentless striving: her health. Indeed, coupled with this need to achieve was a toxic perfectionism. You watched with horror the consequences your daughter would impose on herself when she made a mistake. It seemed like she was a harsh, cruel dictator, who would articulate a verbal diatribe of self-loathing, make herself work even exceedingly harder than before, and further restrict any form of leisure or luxury. How does one parent a child such as this? It always seemed as if your child was doing the parenting task for you, but in a much more stern and harmful way than you ever would. You had the ironic task of trying to set limits on a child who was doing too much of a good thing.

"With the onset of this phase of 'healthy eating,' you watched with distress as the same method of discipline unfolded. Your child set up untenable expectations about her new attempts to eat healthier and, at first, it didn't seem too terrible. After all, who could complain about an adolescent striving to eat more fruits and vegetables? However, as with all things your daughter attempted, she just couldn't stop and do things 'good enough.' Everything always had to be 'better.' For your daughter, 'better' implied the establishment of harsher expectations and more stringent standards for her diet. Any dietary transgression your daughter committed (according to her harsh rule book), was met with extreme agitation and self-loathing. You had even witnessed your daughter do self-injurious things when she ate something she 'shouldn't.' As time passed, this quest for healthier eating morphed into severe dietary restriction, and the weight loss began. Of course, you would suggest that your child eat. You would even make her meals and sometimes get so desperate that you would have outbursts of rage condemning all the harm she was causing herself and how challenging it was to be her mother. In fact, this was perhaps the first time in your history of parenting your daughter that you ever lost your temper with her. Of course, when you did succeed in getting your child to eat, the results were horrible. The pattern of self-loathing you had witnessed was as powerful as it had ever been. Yet now she blamed you for being the cause. The result, of course, was not only no improvement of eating but the beginning of a seemingly increased emotional distance between the two of you."

It is easy to see how impossible this would feel. Parents are stuck choosing between two types of harm: the harm of their child not eating and the emotional berating that ensues when she does. They may fear that they are making things worse by stepping in, or that they will permanently damage their relationship with their child if they insist that she eat.

Although eating disorder behaviors are unique in some ways, behavioral principles may be applied in a similar fashion as with other child behavior problems. We outline key elements of behavior management plans below, and describe their application to AN, beginning with preparing the child and family for parent involvement.

Behavior Management Plans

The key elements of behavior management plans are:

- Identifying specific behavior change goals
- Using contingencies
  - Providing logical consequences
- Clearly communicating expectations
- Maintaining consistency
  - Avoiding intermittent reinforcement
  - Expecting an extinction burst
- Monitoring the outcome
- Modifying the plan

Providing a Frame for Parental Involvement

If parents have been relatively hands-off, it can be useful to provide the client and parents with a frame for parental involvement. The key message is this: Even though the child is chronologically old enough to feed herself, at present, she is struggling to perform actions that would be expected of someone her age (i.e., nourish herself sufficiently). Parents can protect their child by temporarily reverting to an earlier stage of development (and assuming greater responsibility for regulating their child's food intake). This frame is illustrated in the scripts that follow. Script A is directed to the client, and Script B, to the parent or caregiver.

IN PRACTICE

Therapist Script A (to the Client)

"Do you remember when you were learning to do something for the first time, like tie your shoe? You probably first watched a parent many times. You then tried and struggled, and your parent probably let you try for a bit and then stepped in if you needed it. This is the dance of parenting: Leaning in and stepping back as needed to help our kids master new skills. Now tying your shoe doesn't have major implications. If your shoe isn't tied, you might trip, but that is probably all. Eating is another story. Your parents have stepped in because they fear for your life. I know this feels yucky right now—you want to make your own decisions. Our job will be to help them know that it is safe to step back—and for it really to be [safe]."

Therapist Script B (to the Parent/Caregiver)

"I know that this is scary to see your daughter like this, and it's hard to know what to do. At this point, we need to think developmental rather than chronological age. Developmentally, she is much younger, and she is going to need you to do more of the daily management (of her eating and meal planning, preparation, and serving). Over time, as she gains strength, you will pass responsibility back to her. This is similar to when she was learning to walk or ride a bike: When it was clear that she needed your help, you leaned in and offered more support, and when it looked as though she could do it on her own, you stepped back to let her try it (stepping in again if needed). This is the dance of parenting . . ."

Identifying Specific Behavior Change Goals

The overarching goal is to stop acute weight loss and begin to reverse life-threatening starvation. This is accomplished by increasing caloric intake and reducing excessive exercise or other maladaptive weight control behaviors, such as self-induced vomiting. Later, attention shifts to increasing food variety and helping the client develop her own capacity to adaptively regulate her eating (using hunger/satiety and personal preferences, rather than rigid rules).

Specific behavior change goals are typically identified in conjoint sessions that include the parents, as well as the adolescent or young adult. Goals are informed by assessment and feedback from other members of the multidisciplinary team (nutritionist, physician). These individuals provide dietary recommendations and input regarding the rate of weight restoration and target weight range.

Strategies to increase calorie intake could include "marking" mealtimes that had previously been skipped with some eating, adding snacks, adding to meals that are typical eaten, or adding nutritional supplements (or some combination of these things). Strategies should be specific and measurable (e.g., +200 to 250 kcal/day) and adjusted to meet the individual's dynamic energy needs (e.g., change in metabolic rate, activity level). See also Chapter 4.

In identifying behavior change goals, it is important to work with the adolescent's preferences whenever possible (e.g., some adolescents find it easier to eliminate exercise than to increase food intake). Providing choices is also helpful to allow the individual to experience some sense of personal control. For example: "We need to add something to your meal plan. Would you like to add to your lunch or dinner? We could add a piece of fruit or a caloric beverage. Do you prefer either of these options or have another idea?" Flexibility without compromising health is key at this stage. For example, if the child reports increased guilt with consuming a greater number of food items, the plan might include mixing nutritionally dense foods (e.g., seeds, nuts, protein powder, dried fruit) into foods that are already consumed (e.g., oatmeal) or creating dense shakes that are experienced as one food item. Guilt regarding the number of food items can be addressed later, after the initial threat of undernourishment is mitigated. Some elements of behavior change plans are likely to be non-negotiable. For example, in order to reduce self-induced vomiting, it might be necessary to establish house rules of no bathroom use for 60 minutes after a meal (however, what happens during those minutes, i.e., who stays with the individual and whether they engage in an activity together, would be the client's choice).

Contingency Management: Using Logical Consequences

The immediate emotional benefits of AN are often more powerful than the long-term negative consequences of low weight. In order to disrupt current patterns of restriction, there will need to be something to compete with these benefits. Ultimately, this will be the individual's deeply meaningful personal values. However, for some young people, defining personal values may take time. In some ways, this is developmentally expected; however, this delay is also a function of undernourishment, which narrows attention to food and suppresses feelings (including felt sense of meaning). In the interim, parents can increase eating or decrease maladaptive weight control through the use of logical consequences.

Logical consequences can be used when the natural consequence for a behavior is too delayed or incremental to impact behavior. These consequences, rather than being arbitrary or general, logically follow from the behavior. For example, the logical consequence for breaking something in the house is using one's own money to replace the item. Similarly, the logical consequence for being unable to nourish oneself with food might be a nutritional supplement. An inability to consume any nourishment might lead to rest and energy conservation. Thus, rather than going to school, seeing friends, or even engaging in homework (all of which require sufficient nutrition), the adolescent would be expected to rest and regain strength to try again at the next meal.

For logical consequences to be effective, they need to be reasonable (not exaggerated), time-limited, and implemented in a warm but firm manner. It is also important that the young person always have the opportunity to reengage the healthy behavior (i.e., it is never too late to decide to rejoin a meal or complete a snack or nutritional supplement). Each moment is a new moment for effective action. Past conflict or behaviors are in the past. For example, if a child is asked to rest in bed rather than attend school due to refusing breakfast, but comes back to the table to complete her meal or completes an acceptable alternative (e.g., supplement), she may be taken to school late. The behavioral principle of *shaping*, or reinforcing successive approximations toward the desired behavior, should also be kept in mind. Expectations for the adolescent's behavior increase as she meets challenges, but not in a manner that punishes progress.

Clearly Communicating Expectations and Contingencies

Whenever new limits are put in place, children need to be informed, such that expectations for behavior are clear and consequences are predictable. Parents may want help in planning these conversations with their children. It might also be useful to role-play conversations or to facilitate these discussions in a conjoint session. Key points for parents to communicate to the child include (1) the need for increased support: "We are stepping in more to help manage your eating or exercise (or restore your energy balance)"; (2) the strength of the relationship: "This is because we love you and want you to be healthy"; (3) confidence in the plan: "We have a specific plan that we are going to follow to help restore your health"; and (4) the collaborative nature of changes: "Your feedback is valuable and will be included in the plan when it is coming from you (or a value-guided place) and not AN." These conversations are also a nice opportunity for parents to model for their child the willingness to experience difficult emotions, be genuine, and try and fail. In the therapist script that follows, the therapist is modeling how the parents can communicate clear expectations to their child in a warm and supportive manner.

IN PRACTICE

Therapist Script

"It might sound something like this:

"'Your dad and I love you so much. There is nothing more important to us than you and your health. This time has been difficult and we have been unsure what to do . . . how to be helpful to you. And, rather than leaning in, we have been leaning back, hoping things would get better. We want to stand with you, and stand for you more strongly against the eating disorder.

"'We are going to be stepping in more, making and serving meals based on your meal plan from the nutritionist. What we need to figure out together is what we are going to do if AN is so strong that you are unable to eat the meal with us. We need to decide what alternatives we have to get your nutritional needs met (for example, supplements or shakes that might be easier to consume) and if you are not able to do that [consume a supplement], how we can conserve your energy.

"'One thing that your dad and I have decided is that days that you are unable to get adequate nutrition, we absolutely can't let you go to dance class. That wouldn't be safe, and we care too much about you to put you in harm's way . . .'"

Consistency

Behavior change plans need to be implemented consistently to prevent intermittent reinforcement of unwanted behavior. Intermittent reinforcement occurs when behavior contingencies are inconsistently implemented and behavior is permitted *some* of the time.

The result of intermitted reinforcement is that it is difficult to extinguish behavior because *sometimes* it results in the desired outcome (in this case, the outcome of not eating). Consistency in implementation also refers to activity between parents (i.e., that both parents implement the plan similarly).

Every parent can reach a level of exhaustion that might result in inconsistent implementation of a behavior change plan. This can be minimized by a parental tag team (i.e., one parent taking turns with the other) or bringing in other social supports (a grandparent or other family member who can take over when the parents need a break). Parents might also use reverse "time-out" (i.e., the parent removing him- or herself from the situation temporarily) and practice self-care to conserve emotional resources. We describe parental self-care in greater depth on pages 117–118.

Consistent implementation does not mean that the parent is rigid or harsh. Rather, the parent takes into account other factors of the situation and implements consequences in a manner that is warm but firm. In the script below, the therapist is modeling this approach for a parent.

IN PRACTICE

Therapist Script

"It might sound something like this:

"'Because you haven't eaten dinner, I just can't take you to dance. I know that dance is important to you, but you wouldn't have the physical resources that you need and it would not be safe or responsible to take you. You still have the option of the Ensure [nutritional supplement], and because we got home late today, you can complete it in the car if you prefer. I know today has been hard, and if you want to talk, I am here . . .'"

Extinction Bursts

As parents begin to set limits on AN, there is likely to be an *extinction burst* (i.e., a temporary increase in the frequency or intensity of unwanted behavior). For parents this will seem as though the situation is getting worse. Their child may be more upset or confrontational at mealtimes, refuse food more vehemently, and so forth. Educating parents about extinction bursts can help them persist through this temporary exacerbation with the warm and consistent implementation of the plan, as illustrated in the script on the next page.

Parents are encouraged to use an *authoritative* parenting style to set boundaries around the eating disorder. This parenting style is characterized by clear limits for behavior, combined with high warmth, and is associated with better overall mental health outcomes for children (e.g., better interpersonal adjustment, higher self-esteem). It is differentiated from *authoritarian* parenting, which demands obedience based on parental authority and focuses on compliance and punishment, and *permissive* and *neglectful* parenting, which have no limits.

In the case of an adolescent with AN, parents might also need to set boundaries on other forms of punitive self-control (doing "good or right" to the neglect of her needs) because without them, she will keep working or giving, to her own detriment.

IN PRACTICE

Therapist Script

"It is likely that as you start to put limits on AN, it will get louder and more insistent. This is an extinction burst, and it can scare parents. You might worry that you are making things worse, but this is a natural, normal thing that happens when we put limits on behavior that weren't there before. The most important thing is for you to stay warm and consistent at these times. If you are finding it difficult in the moment, I would encourage you to take a break (implement a reverse time-out or use the parental tag team; see p. 108)."

There is an interesting parallel to draw here. The parents are not the only ones enduring an extinction burst. Rather, the adolescent is also coping with an extinction burst of AN. As she has begun to challenge AN (at her parents' urging or of her own accord), it has become louder and more insistent inside her head. AN has begun to make threats about what will happen if she eats ("You are going to be obese, you fat pig") and what this means about her ("I thought you were better than this—why are you so lazy? Why do you give up so easily?"). If parents are aware of this, they will better understand their child's behavior, which may seem obstinate, and empathize with how hard this is for her too. The script below uses metaphor to help parents appreciate their child's experience and persist.

IN PRACTICE

Therapist Script (with the "Temper Tantrum" Metaphor)

"Can you think of a time when you have seen a child having a really big, loud temper tantrum? Imagine a little toddler running around playing in the park and Mom says, 'It's time to leave,' and suddenly that cute little blonde figure turns into a raging ball of fury. Her little fists pound the air; she screams, 'No, no, no,' and throws herself on the ground, refusing to move another inch. So imagine that very experience going on inside your daughter's head—except the child is AN. When you begin to insist on adequate intake and refuse to give in, AN will have a temper tantrum. It will kick and scream, and call her names, and as a result, your daughter will fight back against you more aggressively. You might actually notice yourself thinking, 'This is not my child,' and in some ways you are right. In those moments it can be helpful to remind yourself that this is AN having a temper tantrum in her head (and this is impacting her behavior). We should anticipate what this may look and sound like and prepare for it together . . ."

Monitoring Outcome

In monitoring the outcome of behavior change plans, it may be tempting for parents to equate success with the absence of negative emotions or conflict. The problem is that difficulty and hard feelings are part and parcel of change. If it feels easy, it may mean that the eating disorder is not sufficiently challenged. For example, the adolescent might have traded restriction for overexercise, or she might have reached a milestone (e.g., allowing more calories) and need to move on to something more challenging (e.g., increasing variety in food selection).

If adolescents are not experiencing difficult feelings, it might also be because they plan to return to restriction ("I have to eat now, but I can lose weight later"). While it is important to be mindful of this, it might not require direct intervention. Rather, attachment to this belief may simply allow the adolescent to eat more now. It may not persist as she contacts reinforcement inherent in nourishing her body and engaging more fully in life. The plan to return to restriction can be reassessed later in treatment. The dialogue below illustrates how the therapist might coach the parent on defining success behaviorally, rather than by the presence or absence of emotions.

IN PRACTICE

Dialogue

PARENT: This week was horrible. I think my daughter was possessed by a demon. Before every dinner she would scream and cry in her room in protest. We had to remind her several times this week that she wouldn't be able to go to school the next day if she didn't eat dinner. On Wednesday, she flat out refused to eat dinner, so we had to keep her home from school the next day.

THERAPIST: What happened Thursday night?

PARENT: She came down to eat dinner but was really upset at us.

THERAPIST: This sounds really hard . . . and it sounds like you encountered a dinnertime extinction burst. . . . While painful, this is a good sign.

PARENT: Ugh.

THERAPIST: I know . . . and it is really wonderful that you were able to consistently implement your plan even when AN was pushing back really hard. (*pause*) This is so important—to show AN that you are not going to back down, that you are going to do whatever you need to do to be there for your daughter.

One thing we can think more about is how you and she can connect at other times—times that are completely separate from eating. These will be replenishing moments for you and for her. (This also functions as differential reinforcement of non–eating disorder behavior.)

Modifying the Plan

It will be necessary to modify the plan. Some things work well, while other things do not, and some things that were working before will stop being effective. New information will also emerge. Common reasons that plans might not be working include:

- *Insufficient oversight.* Eating disorder behaviors are not being monitored effectively. The plan may then be tweaked to incorporate additional monitoring support at home, at relatives' or friends' homes, or at school.

- *Opposition to oversight.* Oversight is increasing oppositional behavior in a way that is counterproductive. Removing oversight could function as a positive contingency; that is, the adolescent could "rise to the occasion" (and increase food consumption) to prove that oversight is not needed.

• *Contingency is not meaningful or it is no longer meaningful.* Consequences are ineffective in changing behavior. For example, going to school may have initially encouraged eating. However, as school has become more difficult (academically or socially), it is no longer a motivator and may even be functioning to increase food refusal. The contingencies for food refusal need to be changed.

• *Behavior change exceeds the child's capacity.* The parents, therapist, or adolescent have not accurately assessed the adolescent's capacity to go against AN and its demands. It will be necessary to assess which elements of the plan exceed adolescent capacity and adjust goals accordingly. Adolescents might also need additional emotional or instrumental support.

Whenever possible, the adolescent's ideas about what needs to be changed should be used in modifying behavior management plans. However, suggestions might be approached as hypotheses and tested to see whether they result in the desired outcome (more adequate nutrition), as illustrated in the dialogue below. In some cases, what the child believes will help is actually what will increase comfort or quiet AN (but not necessarily increase food intake).

IN PRACTICE

Dialogue

CLIENT: My dad just stares at me. I can't stand it. I could eat better if he wasn't sitting right there.

THERAPIST: It makes you feel like you are being scrutinized . . .

CLIENT: Yes! Why can't he go do something? I really think it would help me.

THERAPIST: Why don't we try that out? How far away do you think your dad needs to be— out of the room or just not over your shoulder?

CLIENT: Out of the room!

THERAPIST: OK, we'll need to figure out how your parents can still monitor things, but generally, you would like your dad to back off. Let's come up with something that we can try for a week or two. If it helps you make progress in your eating, then we'll keep it in place. If not, we'll have to try something else. Either way, you and I can work on allowing that feeling [of being scrutinized] while staying effective. Sound good? Let's get your parents in here and see what they think and finalize a plan.

Stepping Back

Just as parents need a strategy for entry, they need a strategy for exit. Determining when to reduce supports or oversight is challenging. Parents may be cautioned against stepping back too early, after only days or weeks of increased food intake. Complying with meal plans may simply be a "honeymoon" phase, and while parents deeply want the ordeal to be over and their child to be OK, pulling back too soon may result in a resurgence of eating disorder behavior.

At the other end of the continuum is fear of letting go of oversight. AN is traumatic for parents and family members who witnessed their loved one deprive herself and waste away. A natural outgrowth of this trauma is family members overreaching or micromanaging, or communicating anxiety or distrusting the adolescent's ability to make self-care decisions. Fearing that their child will return to an undernourished state, parents may overreact to normal restraint (e.g., the child forgoing an extra serving of something) or to weight gain that happens quickly or exceeds the child's premorbid weight. A trauma frame can help parents understand their own emotional reactions and inhibit unhelpful responses. This requires that parents recognize in the moment how they are feeling and that this feeling comes from a deep fear for their child's health and well-being, which was threatened but may no longer be. A script for discussing this issue with parents is provided below.

IN PRACTICE

Therapist Script

"You all have been through a lot. Your daughter's life has been threatened. And your response is a very normal one. Like any other trauma, there is vigilance to signs of danger. If we have been caught in a storm, it is only natural to attend to every dark cloud.

"On the flip side, sometimes it can be tempting to turn away (and deny that there are clouds because they are too painful to see). We are going to be mindful of this as well, and see if together we can find a place to live in between—not over- or underresponding out of fear."

The Desire for Certainty

In early meetings with parents, as well as throughout treatment, parents have a lot of questions and want to be certain that what they are doing is "right." It can be easy to allow Q&A or psychoeducation to fill all the therapeutic time. However, excessive questions are often driven by parental anxiety (or a desire to reduce uncertainty). Providing a lot of rules for eating disorder management is problematic in that it might decrease parents' sensitivity to what is needed in the moment.

While parents are given guidelines (based on behavioral principles) and a specific plan is identified, this plan should not be overspecified verbally, and the family should be encouraged to stay open to their experience and what they might learn. A flexible, trial-and-error approach is encouraged. The mantra is: Try things, check in with how it is working, and make changes or modify your approach to enhance outcomes. In taking this approach, parents are also modeling flexibility for their children and determining the workability of our actions based on their effectiveness, rather than rigid rules of what is "good," "right," or "safe." This will be immensely helpful for their children, who are likely to be rule-based and adverse to experimentation. The dialogue below provides an example of how the therapist might respond to parents who are struggling with uncertainty about how best to help their child. In addition to discriminating rules from guidelines, the therapist also puts uncertainty/anxiety in a frame of coordination with the parents' values to enhance willingness (i.e., parents may allow themselves to feel uncertain or anxious for their child).

IN PRACTICE

Dialogue

The parent has asked multiple nuanced questions, looking for rules about how to respond to his or her child in different situations.

THERAPIST: I know this must be so scary to see your daughter like this and you feel uncertain about what to do. I'm hesitant to provide hard rules. If you go into situations with your daughter with rules, rather than guidelines, it will be harder for you to adjust to the demands of the situation. One thing we will also talk more about is "making room" for this feeling of uncertainty. . . . I think it will be here for a while . . . this is often more like a marathon than a sprint.

PARENT: But how do I know this is the right thing to do?

THERAPIST: I know this is so hard. I wish there was an absolute answer that I could give to you.

Instead, we will have to take general guidelines: what we know about behavior and about AN, and experiment to find what works. This can be unsettling. It will feel uncertain and you may worry that you are doing it wrong.

Our job will be to help you have those thoughts and feelings without them having you (without getting overly hooked by them, which will make it hard for you to help your daughter).

In some ways, you are doing exactly what your daughter is doing, facing something that is so hard and unknown . . . and practicing an open, flexible approach. In this way, you are modeling life skills for her. It could be very powerful for her to see you willing to experiment and find what works.

Parental Inflexibility

Parents of children with AN will experience a lot of painful emotions: intense fear for their child's life and sorrow or grief for what they have lost. Because of the legacy of parental blame in the history of AN, they might also be experiencing guilt for their child's condition. For some parents, their child's struggle will be personally familiar and resemble their own difficulties with food or eating, now or in the past.

Parents might also be dealing with behaviors (other than AN) they have never witnessed before in their child. For example, their child who has been compliant and kind may suddenly be overtly oppositional or cruel, even as the parent is working hard to support her (e.g., "You just want me to be fat, like you!"). These new behaviors can evoke feelings of anger or sadness and make it extremely challenging for parents to respond effectively at mealtimes or to access their full range of parenting tools. Instead, they might find themselves pleading or yelling at their child (different manifestations of the same desperation for change), or being caught up in needless battles that take attention away from the primary task of renourishment. The challenge for the therapist is to help parents discriminate when their actions are workable (and when they are not), to observe their thoughts and feelings (without getting hooked by them), and to stay effective and value-guided in the moment. The dialogues and script that follow illustrate how this can be facilitated in session through metaphor and practice. Dialogue A focuses on allowing emotion (without being overtaken by it). Dialogue B focuses on taking the power out of the child's hurtful words toward her parents (using a defusion exercise). The final therapist script uses a metaphor to illustrate the unworkability of the parent's response to facilitate willingness to try something new.

IN PRACTICE

Dialogue A (with the "Riding Emotion Waves" Metaphor)

PARENT: I was just so fed up; I couldn't believe that she wouldn't just eat her lunch!

THERAPIST: So what did you do?

PARENT: Well, I just kept saying to her that she had to do it. . . . I also said some things that were not good . . . like that it is exhausting being her mother and I didn't understand why she was doing this to me . . .

THERAPIST: Can you contact the feeling that you were experiencing—the frustration but also what is under that?

PARENT: (*Tearful.*)

THERAPIST: I wonder what it would be like to allow that feeling to be here, to maybe watch it (and frustration) rising and falling like waves.

You can be taken by it, you know, we all can . . . lose our grounding, feet swept from under us—swept away by the tide. There is another option though. . . . We can bury our feet more deeply in the sand . . . grounded in what we want to "be about" in that moment (our values) and breathe through the experience . . .

Right now, can you feel your breath? There is this sort of rise and fall—can you breathe that emotion like that?—inhale, exhale.

Riding the waves of breath, allowing the rise and fall of emotions . . .

Not gritting your teeth, but softening your face, allowing it to be what it is. And in this moment, imagine that you say exactly what you would want to say to your daughter in that moment . . . maybe even say it out loud now.

Dialogue B (with the "I Hate You" Song)

THERAPIST: As your daughter lets go of restriction, thoughts and feelings will come up that will be hard for her. She may feel a lot of fear, guilt, or shame. She may say, "I hate you" or "You are ruining my life!" Your job (as her parent) is just to validate that this is hard for her or that she feels upset with you. You don't need to engage these comments any more deeply than that.

PARENT: Are you kidding? These are awful things to say to your parent! She was never like this before. I have had to leave work every day for lunch, and the medical appointments, nutrition . . . and . . . we used to be so close . . .

THERAPIST: I am wondering if we can do something together. . . . Right now those words are so powerful, they hook you—grab you by the gut . . .

Now, this is going to be a little playful, is that OK? First, let's write some of these things she says in these moments on this card: "I hate you" . . . "You are ruining my life."

PARENT: How about "You are the worst mom in the world"? . . . once she said, "I wish I wasn't your daughter."

THERAPIST: (*Pauses to honor and allow the emotions that this brings up for the parent.*) I know it is so hard to hear her say those things. It also probably means that AN is being challenged . . . and that she is practicing speaking up (which she doesn't always do, even when it would serve her) . . . (*pause*) So this is our sheet music. We are going to put her words to music, and sing a song together. Now we need a tune. Can you think of a familiar song that we can use?

PARENT: "You Are My Sunshine"?

THERAPIST: Perfect, OK—let's sing! (*Sing words to the tune of "You Are My Sunshine"; some light laughter.*) What happened there?

PARENT: Well, I started laughing—that wasn't expected!

THERAPIST: Yeah, for a moment these were just words . . .

Therapist Script (with the "Slow Computer" Metaphor, Assessing the Workability of Pressing Harder)

"Have you ever had to work on a really old computer? You know how slow they can be? Ahhhh, it's *so* frustrating. I need to get work done! I have very important things to do. So, if I run into a problem, or something gets slow, I just keep clicking and clicking and clicking on the same button over and over again trying to get it to just *do* what I want it to do! And then what happens? Before too long, it freezes up. Now it isn't doing anything. The process takes even longer; it becomes even slower and sometimes I have to start all over again.

"It's kind of like that. . . . You sort of press harder and it overwhelms her capabilities . . . she shuts down more. . . . Now, I totally get why you are pressing, and the question is, is it working?"

The Parental Instinct to Protect Children from Pain (Including Painful Feelings)

Some parents vehemently maintain that protecting their children from feeling bad, and making them happy, is their number one priority. This is based in the broader assumption that painful emotions, in and of themselves, are harmful, and parents want to protect their children from harm. While this comes from a place of love and caring, it may also have unintended consequences that actually contradict what the parents want for their child. In the case of AN, this might manifest as feeding the child the food and the meals she requests (e.g., low calorie, insufficient). In other circumstances, it might manifest as intervening with peers or teachers when there is the potential for any conflict, correcting assignments, or making decisions for the child rather than allowing her to decide on her own and potentially make a mistake.

Although it is with valued intentions, protecting the child in this way also prevents her from learning and unintentionally communicates that perhaps she cannot navigate difficult situations (or tolerate internal distress, mistakes, or failure). In this way, the parents' strategy of protecting the child from harm in the short term is at odds with their value of protecting the child from harm in the long run. While the child feels protected, cared for, and loved, she is also learning that the (external and internal) world is dangerous, and perhaps that she is hopelessly dependent on her parents to keep her safe. While seeming counterintuitive to the parents, the way to protect the child from harm is to help her to repeatedly approach challenging situations and build resilience and adaptability in the face of threat. Unpacking issues surrounding protecting a child from harm is an essential component of work with parents, and it may necessitate detoxifying internal discomfort and helping parents to appreciate short-term versus long-term expressions of their values, illustrated in the dialogue below.

IN PRACTICE

Dialogue

THERAPIST: It's been really hard for you to keep your daughter from dance on days that she has not eaten enough. . . . One of the things we want to think about is whether we should change the plan. We want to choose something that you are willing to do, so that contingencies have meaning and can be effective.

I also wonder if we can dig into what is happening there a bit more . . . what thoughts and feelings are showing up for you?

PARENT: I really just want Becky to be happy. Dance makes her happy. Is that wrong, to want her to be happy?

THERAPIST: Of course not; there is nothing wrong with wanting your daughter to be happy! (*shared pause*) I just wonder if there are other values that this might conflict with . . . or that you see as equally important . . .

Like, kids don't really like going to the doctor, and you could say, "It's OK, you don't have to go," but what would that mean for the broader value of protecting her or teaching her about doing things that are hard for the sake of her health? . . .

PARENT: Yes, I can see that . . . (*pauses reflectively*) but it's so difficult to see her feeling bad . . .

THERAPIST: We also might want to consider what feelings are hardest to allow your daughter to have, and what it brings up for you . . . and whether it might be valuable to allow her to have those feelings, to be able to navigate these hard places . . .

Caregiver Burden and Self-Care

Helping a child with AN restore health is a marathon, not a sprint. Parents are better equipped for this challenge if they are taking care of themselves. They have more physical and emotional reserves, and they are better able to be consistent and value-guided. In caring for themselves, they are also modeling something quite important for their child (i.e., that it is important to respond to one's physical and emotional needs). The therapist script below uses an "Oxygen Mask" metaphor to illustrate this to parents. This is followed by a list of sample self-care activities.

Parents may find it challenging to commit to self-care. Self-care activities may seem frivolous or a waste of time, especially when their child is suffering. Parental willingness to engage in self-care is increased by putting self-care in a frame of coordination with parents' deeply held personal values. It might also be helpful to work with parents on acceptance and defusion of thoughts and feelings (e.g., guilt) that might make it difficult to follow through with self-care commitments. These ideas are illustrated in the final dialogue.

IN PRACTICE

Therapist Script (with the "Oxygen Mask" Metaphor)

"When you are flying on an airplane, you receive some really specific instructions about self-care. The flight attendant tells you, 'If the cabin loses pressure, oxygen masks will drop down, secure your mask before securing your child's.' I realize that this goes against our instincts as parents, yet isn't it the case that if we pass out, we can't be there to help our child? We must be conscious and aware, breathing and able-bodied (*pause*). This [self-care] is your oxygen mask. Caring for yourself, you are better able to care for your child . . . and that is your number one priority (*pause*). In engaging in self-care, you are also modeling something really important—something with which your child struggles. It may be helpful for her to see you taking time for yourself, too."

Sample self-care activities include the following:

- Prioritize 7–8 hours of sleep.
- Have a date night/take time alone with my partner.
- Enjoy leisure activities (e.g., reading, watching a movie).
- Have mindful moments (e.g., savor a cup of coffee in the morning).
- Engage in physical activity (e.g., evening walk, yoga).
- Engage in a hobby.
- Have an afternoon vacation.
- Cook a favorite food.
- Enjoy a sunset.
- Call a friend to talk about the situation.
- Call a friend to *not talk* about the situation.
- Take a bath.

- Get a manicure or a massage.
- Watch a favorite TV program.
- Start a garden.
- Write in a journal.
- Create something.

IN PRACTICE

Dialogue

PARENT: I know I was supposed to take some time for myself this weekend, but really, it just wasn't feasible to do. Things were hectic as usual. Jaimie was having a hard day emotionally, and my son wanted to spend time with his friends. So I, of course, was running around taking him back and forth to activities. By the time I'd get home and even have the opportunity to think about doing something for myself, it was time for Jaimie's next meal . . .

THERAPIST: It is so very clear to me how much you care about your children—you work so hard to take care of your daughter's needs and also let your son know that he is important, too.

PARENT: I'm really scared for her . . .

THERAPIST: (*Is aware of the parent's exhaustion.*) I know . . . and you feel like the thing to do is to pour more and more of yourself into her care. It's also essential that you maintain your life support. . . . to protect against physical and emotional exhaustion. This is more like a marathon than a sprint. You have to be able to make the long haul . . .

PARENT: I just don't know, I just feel awful if I do anything that is unnecessary . . . anything for me.

THERAPIST: It sounds like guilt is keeping you from doing the thing that would be effective. . . . I wonder if you could hold guilt lightly and orient to what your experience tells you about the effectiveness of not attending to your needs.

We also know that one of the things that Jaimie struggles with most is taking care of herself . . . skipping meals, staying up late to study, putting everyone else's needs above her own. . . . What a gift it would be for you to model self-care for her. You have this wonderful opportunity to show her this. . . . It will be hard . . . and it could be exactly what you both need . . .

Looking Ahead

The focus in Chapter 6 is on creating a context for change. This is sometimes referred to as *creative hopelessness* in ACT. For individuals with AN, this includes first appreciating what AN does for the individual, and later, separating the individual from AN and increasing contact with contingencies not currently exerting stimulus control (undesirable consequences of AN and costs of behaviors for personal values).

CHAPTER 6

Creating a Context for Change

You and I are infinite choice makers.
—DEEPAK CHOPRA

Among individuals with AN, action is dictated by rigid, punitive rules for behavior to the neglect of the individual and her needs. While following rigid rules might make the individual feel better about herself or her situation, it ultimately results in a state of extreme physical and emotional deprivation. The way out of AN is *into experience*—that is, allowing oneself to experience signals arising from the body, unmuted by starvation, and using this information to care for oneself, not only physically but also emotionally. This includes eating when hungry and seeking support when sad. It also includes allowing life experiences that are meaningful, even if they are not "productive," predictable, or well controlled.

Individuals with AN may have limited motivation to relinquish rigid rules, which have not only provided relief from psychological discomfort, but have also led to conventional measures of success (including extreme thinness) and have produced feelings of mastery and pride. In order for individuals with AN to consider change, they must make experiential contact with the ways in which rigid control is *not working*, and ultimately limits life vitality. Through guided exploration, clients may begin to notice that nothing is ever enough, and that they have become more entrenched in increasingly severe attempts to feel better (i.e., restricting from 1,000 to 800 to 500 calories). As clients open up to experience, they might also begin to notice that their behavior has other unintended consequences, including costs for deeply held personal values.

Clinical Goals

We describe nine clinical goals in this chapter. The first several goals focus on appreciating how rigid self-regulation *has* been helpful to the individual and loosening attachment to AN through externalization and other strategies. This preliminary work allows for a more honest assessment of the undesirable consequences (or costs) of AN or using rigid rules to maintain emotional and behavioral control. Making experiential contact with the costs of AN is iterative and elaborates as individuals gain clarity about their personal values. For each clinical goal, we provide illustrative therapist scripts and dialogues that situate the scripts in the context of a therapeutic encounter.

CLINICAL GOAL 1: *Appreciate the Immense Emotional Benefits of AN*

It is essential that the therapist have a deep appreciation for the emotional benefits of AN and convey this appreciation to the client. Acknowledging how AN is helpful increases trust in the relationship and client willingness to consider change.

The therapist names the positive feelings associated with AN, as well as the emotional discomfort that AN functions to alleviate. Emotional discomfort that AN behaviors alleviate typically fall into one of two categories. The first category includes feeling uncertain, overwhelmed, or out of control. These feelings are alleviated by the structure imposed by AN and via starvation-induced reduction of somatic–affective variation. The other cluster includes feeling like a bad or defective person (e.g., unlikable, needy, selfish, and/or a failure or disappointment). AN behaviors alleviate these feelings by giving clients a way to be a "better" person. Scripts A–C provide illustrations of therapist responses that focus on the positive experiences that AN "gives" the individual. Scripts D–F provide illustrations of therapist responses that focus on what AN "takes away." We include several examples to illustrate how these responses are personalized to the client's unique experiences. Scripts are followed by sample dialogue. Additional interventions that may be used to meet this clinical goal may be found in Chapter 5 (e.g., the "Magic Cloak" metaphor, p. 97; Maslow's hierarchy of needs, pp. 96–97).

IN PRACTICE

Therapist Script A

"It sounds like it felt good to watch your weight go down: like you were taking control of the situation. That's a nice feeling . . ."

"It seems like it is a basic human need, too . . . to feel effective or masterful . . . in charge of yourself or your life."

Therapist Script B

"AN made you feel like you are good at something . . . [restricting your eating] was something you could do well, and it was something that set you apart from other people. . . . It made you feel special in a sense. I can get why that would mean something (deeply) to you . . . (*pause*) so often you have felt mediocre, like you are not as good as other people . . ."

Therapist Script C

"It seems that AN, with all of its rules, has provided a sense of safety and security in your decisions. Like, what you 'should do' feels clear . . ."

"It seems like that would be such a relief . . . not to have to question everything or worry so much about making mistakes."

Therapist Script D

"It seems that AN has taken away that feeling of being overwhelmed by daily life. What a wonderful gift . . ."

"Feeling overwhelmed is painful [scary, etc.] . . ."

Therapist Script E

"It sounds like you've had this feeling for a long time . . . the feeling of being too much—too emotional, too needy. It sounds like AN has been one way to take up less space . . . (*pause*) and it has worked to take these feelings away to some extent . . ."

"It makes sense that you would appreciate AN for this . . . that you wouldn't want to let it go."

Therapist Script F

"It seems AN directs all of your attention to food and eating and, when it does, it turns your attention *away from* other things that are upsetting to you. You don't have to worry so much about whether you are liked by other people, or whether you are worthy of their time and attention; you can let life just be about the next meal . . . (*gentle*) what a relief."

Dialogue

The therapist is gathering information about AN onset.

THERAPIST: Tell me more about what was going on before your attention turned to food and your body.

CLIENT: I was playing volleyball, but I couldn't take the pressure of being on a team . . . everyone was counting on me and it was too much . . . so I dropped out. I thought I would still be friends with the other girls on the team, but we stopped talking once I didn't see them at practice. I thought that we were really close . . . (*trails off*). I didn't expect that to happen. Then I got a "C" on a quiz . . . and didn't make the honor roll. . . . Everything was going wrong.

THERAPIST: That sounds really hard, to feel like you had lost your place in the group . . . lost your friends . . . like you were failing at things . . . (*long pause*). And then what happened?

CLIENT: Well, I started focusing on my eating. I thought that if I lost weight, then I would feel better . . .

THERAPIST: How did it work?

CLIENT: I did start to feel better. . . . People started giving me compliments, and that was nice. Even though I wasn't spending any more time with friends really, I didn't really care as much . . .

THERAPIST: AN took away the pain . . . of feeling alone . . . and like you were failing at things. . . . And it gave you something too . . . something to focus on and succeed at . . .

CLIENT: For sure.

CLINICAL GOAL 2: *Validate the Fear of Losing the Emotional Benefits of AN*

For individuals with AN, normalizing weight means losing a sense of safety or security or choosing to return to a time of extreme emotional discomfort (when they were experiencing profound shame or low self-worth). Clients might feel as though they cannot cope with their emotions or with life without AN. These fears are appreciated as elements of the client's experience, as illustrated in the therapist scripts that follow.

IN PRACTICE

Therapist Script A

"It must be upsetting to think about letting go of AN. . . . Even if AN is oppressive at times, it also feels comfortable and safe. . . ."

Therapist Script B

"I hear you. . . . Thinking about letting go of AN . . . and beginning to restore weight . . . feels like choosing to return to a time when you were profoundly unhappy. And no matter how painful life is now, that seems worse . . ."

Therapist Script C

"It sounds like AN has been such an important part of your identity . . . of who you are . . . it may even feel like *all of you*. It makes sense that it would feel incredibly scary to think about letting it go . . . (*pause, gentle*). Of course."

CLINICAL GOAL 3: *Appreciate How Rigid, Punitive Self-Regulation Has Been Helpful*

AN is part of a broader behavioral repertoire of rigid rule following and punitive self-control (to the neglect of one's needs). This self-depriving approach to managing oneself, however costly, has also paid off. It has resulted in an impressive list of achievements (academically and professionally), admiration, and praise. Forsaking oneself (and one's needs) for others has also solidified the individual's place in relationships, even if it has not generated true intimacy. The therapist aims to appreciate what punitive self-regulation has meant to the individual and how difficult it would be to consider change, as illustrated in the scripts below.

IN PRACTICE

Therapist Script A

"Your ability to push yourself has been helpful. It has allowed you to excel in soccer and positioned you for an Ivy League college. I get why it would feel scary to consider a less punitive approach . . . one that is kinder and more responsive to your needs . . . (*pause*) like maybe you wouldn't achieve these things anymore, and then how would you know you were worthwhile, or a valuable human being . . ."

Therapist Script B

"You have spent your entire life oriented to other people and *their* needs. . . . And it has helped you approach social situations, by providing you with a role or clarity about what you should be doing: You are the caretaker.

"I can imagine it feels incredibly risky to think about taking up more space yourself (i.e., doing less for others [at times] and taking yourself, your feelings, and your needs into account) . . . like, maybe you wouldn't be liked or valued by other people anymore . . . "

CLINICAL GOAL 4: *Invite Curiosity about Whether Rigid Self-Regulation Is Optimal in All Situations*

The therapist invites the client to consider whether a rigid, punitive approach to managing themselves and their behavior is optimal in all situations. At this stage of treatment, this should only be a gentle curiosity. Over time, the therapist will invite a more extensive exploration of how rigid rules and excessive goal striving may decrease effectiveness or limit life vitality. Illustrative scripts and dialogues are provided below. Script A includes the "Neglected or Abused Child" metaphor, which might be evoked throughout treatment.

IN PRACTICE

Therapist Script A (with the "Neglected or Abused Child" Metaphor)

"It occurs to me that this is like the situation of a neglected child. Imagine that you are the parent and your job is to take care of a child's needs. This requires that you observe the child's signals and respond: identifying feelings of hunger or fatigue and creating conditions for the child to eat or rest.

"This is essentially your position. You are *your* parent or caretaker. By ignoring signals of your needs, you create a situation of neglect. Like a neglected child who goes hungry, tired, or alone . . .

"Sometimes it is more of an abusive situation: The parent (or caretaker) who not only neglects the child's needs, but also berates her for having them: calling her weak or out of control when she feels hungry, tired, or sad [rather than feeding her, putting her to bed, or providing her with comfort] . . . "

(*If the client has reported corresponding mood symptoms*) "It seems like this would be a hard [painful] way to live. . . . Like, I can't imagine *not* feeling [awful] when being treated this way . . . "

[In an alternative version of this metaphor, the therapist orients the client to the four parenting styles identified in the parenting literature (authoritative, authoritarian, permissive, neglectful; Baumrind, 1991). The therapist helps the client identify her (self-)parenting style and explore its potential implications.]

Therapist Script B (with the "Emergency Situation" Metaphor)

"Have you heard stories of emergency situations where mothers lift cars to save their children or other heroic feats? When in an emergency situation, humans have an incredible capacity to override signals, including pain. They run with broken bones, and so forth. This is adaptive in emergency situations. We need to be able to override any feeling that might stop us, and just get the job done. If there is a burning building, we shouldn't stop to eat or take a nap. We should just get out of there! Your capacity to have a laser focus on a goal and *push, push, push* is adaptive if there is an emergency. I wonder, though, as a way of life, does it take a toll . . . ?"

Dialogue (with the "Shoe Store" metaphor)

CLIENT: I have always been the kind of person that just gets things done. No matter what.

THERAPIST: Being hard on yourself has worked so well for you (*pause*). . . . I also wonder whether there is another way of being that, if you could access it, would be useful or life-giving? I don't know, but it could be . . . ? Imagine going into a shoe store and it only has one type of shoe. It's a running shoe and it has all the latest and greatest features. You buy it. And then you go back the next month and it's the same thing. The store only has this shoe . . . and don't get me wrong, the shoe is great. It's comfortable and it really gets you places. But what if it is the only shoe you have? Running is the only thing you can do. . . . You don't have any other options . . . all you can do is run. (*pause*). What if you *could* run, but you didn't *have to* . . . what if you had a choice? (*pause*) When we have choices or *the freedom to choose* . . . we can do what works for the situation . . . or what enhances our lives.

CLIENT: (*Looks concerned.*)

THERAPIST: We don't want to take away your ability to push yourself and drive toward a goal. It can be a useful thing. The question is whether something else might be useful, too (another way of being), if you had access to it.

   We don't have to answer this question now, just something for us to think about.

CLINICAL GOAL 5: *Acknowledge Clients' Fear in Experimenting with a Less Rigid Approach*

Experimenting with a less rigid approach to life is risky. Clients will be afraid to break or flex rules or allow themselves to feel and have needs. The therapist reflects this fear, as illustrated in the therapist scripts and dialogue that follow.

IN PRACTICE

Therapist Script A

"I imagine that it is overwhelming to think about life that is not bound by strict rules and routines . . ."

Therapist Script B

"It seems like it would be scary to try another approach—one that is gentler to yourself— that takes your needs into account. You have been doing things this way for so long . . . maybe forever."

Therapist Script C

"I hear you. . . . This brings up the fear that this will make you self-indulgent or lazy. I wonder if we can just hold that for now. That it feels scary and your mind has stories about what it means to treat yourself differently, with more compassion, or to not doggedly pursue goals and expect so much from yourself all the time . . .

Dialogue

CLIENT: Eating more now just feels like I am giving up.

THERAPIST: You've never quit anything. . . . Not even when it's been in your best interest. And beginning to respond to yourself and your needs feels like that . . . I see why this would be scary to you . . . it feels as though it *means something* about you . . . or your integrity as a person.

Loosening Attachment to AN

We now turn to loosening attachment to AN, which prepares the client to more fully consider the workability of current behavior patterns for deeply held personal values. Loosening attachment to AN can be divided into two clinical goals. Clinical Goal 6, encouraging a separation between AN and the person, and Clinical Goal 7, helping the client contact the less desirable aspects of living with AN.

CLINICAL GOAL 6: *Encourage a Separation between AN and the Person*

The therapist may encourage a separation between the client and AN using externalizing language, common in other therapeutic traditions. This way of speaking treats AN as a functional entity (a collection of eating- and body-related thoughts, feelings, and behaviors) that is separate and distinct from the individual. Observations may be made about the presence of AN or its actions, as illustrated in the therapist scripts and dialogue that follow.

Externalizing interventions expand over the course of treatment to help individuals narrate personal values outside of AN (e.g., "I know what AN wants, what do you want?") or to elicit a more adaptive behavioral repertoire in response to AN thoughts/feelings through the use of metaphor ("AN is like . . ."). For example, AN may be likened to a friend that gives nonstop advice (cueing skepticism), to a child (e.g., cueing kindness or compassion), or to a dictator (cueing defiance). These interventions must be appropriately matched to the client's experience and the clinical situation.

IN PRACTICE

Therapist Script A

"AN is really strong today."

Therapist Script B

"How did AN convince you not to eat?"

Therapist Script C

"AN has been with you for a long time . . . like a traveling companion. Do you remember what it was like before AN was around . . . ?"

Therapist Script D

"There is AN, and then there is you, but sometimes it is hard to know the difference. Right now, I can see you. . . . I can hear what you care about outside of AN [*with gratitude*]. It is nice to see you."

Dialogue

CLIENT: My eating [and thin body] is all I have. Why do people want to take this away from me? I worked so hard. And there are other people who are much thinner and no one says a word to them! That girl that comes to the clinic . . . everyone just lets her get away with it. Besides, I am eating. A lot more than I was before. And no one has been straight with me about when I am done. I don't think Dr. S will stop pushing me to gain weight until I am 300 pounds!

THERAPIST: It sounds like it is really hard to think about losing AN. It has meant a lot to you. You know, sometimes all I can hear is AN's voice—and its fight to survive. AN takes over everything and leaves little space for Katie . . . and I can sense you [Katie] in there. And I wonder, if we weren't so focused on what AN wants, could we begin to think about what Katie wants?

CLIENT: What do you mean? This is me.

THERAPIST: I hear you, it's like this (*interlocks fingers*) and it's hard to know what it would even be like if there was a little separation (*pulls fingers apart, creating a little space between the hands*) . . . like who you might be (*offers one hand*). . . . I wonder, too, if it is frightening to think about that . . . about there being some space between you and AN . . .

CLINICAL GOAL 7: *Increase Contact with the Undesirable Consequences of AN*

The emotional benefits of AN are powerful and currently dictate the client's choices. The therapist works to create a context that allows the client to *also contact* the less desirable consequences of AN (or of rigid, punitive self-regulation). This work is not the same as cognitive challenging. It is densely experiential. The goal is not to change the client's beliefs; rather, it is to slow her down enough that she is able to contact her direct experience, fully and without defense. In many cases, eating disorder thoughts (e.g., thoughts about the need to restrain eating) will persist at the same time that there is increasing experiential dissonance and drive for change.

Although it might be tempting to ask clients to examine the pros and cons of AN (a common strategy in second-wave CBT), we find that this falls short for a couple of reasons. First, pro and con lists for AN often pit the deep emotional motivations for AN behavior (e.g., certainty, mastery, control) against the less compelling negative consequences of low weight or some possible future outcome (e.g., hyperthermia or risk of osteoporosis later in life). Second, this approach encourages clients to make choices of actions based on logic and reasons, rather than deeply held personal values.

Below we outline several possible consequences of living with AN and illustrate how the therapist might create a context for the client to come into contact with these aspects of her experience. Use of the word *sense* and frequent ellipses is purposeful and meant to convey a slow, curious exploration of the client's *experience*. Importantly, this is an early stage of loosening attachment to AN, and the ultimate aim is to help clients contact the *costs* of AN for *deeply held, personal values*. This may include, for example, the way in which AN is interfering with her relationships (or making it difficult for her to be the person she wants to be in her relationships). See Clinical Goal 8 in this chapter. We describe strategies to help clients clarify personal values in Chapter 8.

Contacting a Loss of Choice

The therapist helps the client contact the experience of restriction as a *must* or a *have to* rather than a choice. The client is encouraged to notice what happens when she tries to go against the demands of AN (e.g., AN gets louder and more insistent). Clients may still have the thought "I am in control," at the same time that they experience the limits of their ability to choose. Both experiences are held in awareness. Scripts and dialogues below provide illustrations. Dialogue B includes a behavioral experiment with a homework variation.

IN PRACTICE

Therapist Script A

"Does it feel as though you can choose . . . or that you *can't*, you *mustn't* [eat, rest, speak, take *your* needs into account]?"

Therapist Script B

"I am wondering if you also sense (as a matter of experience) that the rules have taken over . . . and there is no way you can deviate . . . ?"

Therapist Script C

"If you *don't* ignore your needs, if you *respond to them*, "give in" as you say, will you be berated for it? Told you are weak or out of control?"

Therapist Script D (with the "Slot Machine" metaphor)

"Have you ever played slot machines? Casino owners want players to stay and play, and while it is ultimately our decision, they also create conditions that keep people locked in. . . . There are no clocks, they pump in oxygen. . . . You think about leaving and someone comes by and gives you a free drink, and you think: 'I'll just stay a few more minutes.' Then maybe you win a little more money, so, of course, you stay even longer. It's a trap. You can't walk away. The casino convinces you with the occasional wins, that if you walk away now, you'll lose the big jackpot. And so they have you, locked in . . . waiting to hit it, for the golden gates to open.

"I wonder if it is possible right now to allow yourself to sense whether you have the choice to walk away—or whether you are sort of stuck in this, taking smaller wins, hoping for the jackpot—that one day you will reach a place [a weight] where you can live inside your own skin . . . ?"

Dialogue A

THERAPIST: It seems we don't know what would happen if you didn't comply with AN because you never break the rules . . .

CLIENT: I don't really want to. Sometimes I am forced to by my father.

THERAPIST: Can you take me into those moments and what it is like for you?

CLIENT: (*Gives description of a recent time.*)

THERAPIST: I wonder if we can slow down into that moment and check in with your experience. . . . There is the anger at Dad, but what's going on with AN in that moment?

CLIENT: I'm not sure if this is what you mean, but I was thinking "I can't believe that I am having to eat this" and "I am just going to get fat, and maybe I deserve it anyway [to get fat] . . . and I should be stronger . . ."

THERAPIST: That is a very different experience than when you do as AN says.

CLIENT: Yes.

THERAPIST: AN might say, "Good for you. . . . You are doing something other people can't!"
    If you comply/conform/obey, then you get gold stars, and if you don't, you get a lashing . . . ? Is that your experience?

CLIENT: (*Nods in agreement.*)

THERAPIST: It is a great way to keep you locked in . . . doing what it says.

CLIENT: Yeah, I suppose so.
    (*long silence*)

THERAPIST: And both of these things can be there. You can have the thought "This is what I want to do; this is my choice," at the same time that you experience what happens when you break the rules [you get a lashing].
    I wonder what it is like to touch the edge of that experience. To allow yourself to notice that . . . ?

Dialogue B (with a Behavioral Experiment)

The therapist and the client "experiment" with what AN does when the client even considers the possibility of going against the rules.

THERAPIST: Would you be willing to try a little experiment with me? OK, for this experiment I would like you to choose a snack we could eat together today, right now.

CLIENT: (*Nods her head but makes a disgusted face.*)

THERAPIST: I can see from your face that your mind is already getting busy. Can we just explore what your mind is doing? What does AN have to say about this?

CLIENT: Well, I mean that's unfair—and it's not time for me to eat anyway. I just had a snack. I also didn't bring anything, and I can't eat what you have there. I can just eat something later, when I get home. It kind of feels like a trick to do it now—we didn't talk about doing this last time.

THERAPIST: So AN is getting really busy trying to figure out a way to get out of this—and it even says maybe it's a trick or something?

CLIENT: Yeah, well if I do it, I prove something, but if I don't do it, then you'll think that means AN is in charge or something. I mean, I see what you're getting at, but I just don't know if I want to do that really.

THERAPIST: I remember you saying that you loved cheese crackers (before AN). What does your mind have to say about sharing some with me right now?

CLIENT: No—I mean, my mind is just really loud, shouting about the calories and telling me I'm disgusting for thinking about it.

THERAPIST: So, right now, what is your lived experience about choice?

CLIENT: Well, I don't want it . . . so . . . (long pause)

THERAPIST: And it's not allowed? (long pause)

CLIENT: (Affirms.)

THERAPIST: It isn't that there is any special virtue in eating cheese crackers (or any other food per se). What we are talking about here is freedom to choose; freedom to choose to have them or not. . . . Do you sense a loss of freedom (whether you want them or not) in how hard it is for you to choose something that goes against the rules? What that feels like, right now . . . ?

Behavioral Experiment: Homework Variation

This can also be a homework assignment when a client insists that she can eat at any time. The client identifies an action that would be inconsistent with AN (e.g., eating 50 or 100 additional calories at a meal, eating a forbidden food). She observes what happens when she attempts to complete this task. If she is successful, then this is a therapeutic win in facing fears and increasing flexibility—you have evoked a new response, and now reinforce and repeat. If she is unsuccessful, the therapist highlights the experienced lack of freedom to choose.

Dialogue C (with the "Popular Girls" Metaphor)

CLIENT: I felt better not eating dinner. I could focus on my work. Then my mom said I had to have a nighttime snack. I ate it, but it was horrible. All I could think is "You fat pig" . . . I felt awful about myself.

THERAPIST: AN got pretty brutal. It kind of reminds me of the popular girls that you were telling me about. If you are on their good side, it is great; they treat you well, but they can turn on you on a dime. That is how they keep you in line; following their lead . . . that's how they keep the upper hand.

Dialogue D (with the "Dictatorship" Metaphor)

CLIENT: I don't know . . . it is what I have done for so long. I don't even remember where some of these rules came from.

THERAPIST: You've just sort of followed along with AN? Got in step and stayed in step?

CLIENT: Yes.

THERAPIST: Less like a democracy, and more like a dictatorship?

CLIENT: Huh?

THERAPIST: In dictatorships, people are often so used to following the rules that they don't question things. They just go along because that's how it is, and how it has always been. Even when things become more brutal or extreme.

CLIENT: Yes, then.

THERAPIST: In dictatorships, there are also structures in place (like harsh punishment) to keep people compliant. It seems you know this space, too?

CLIENT: (*Describes it.*)

THERAPIST: In some ways it is really nice to have someone else making the decisions . . .
(*Pauses to allow the client to have this element of experience.*)
And I wonder if there is a cost in there, too . . . a cost in just doing what you have been told to do?
[An alternative version of this metaphor likens AN to a kidnapper. The therapist describes famous cases in which the captive adopted the kidnapper's worldview (e.g., Patty Hearst), potentially as a survival strategy (i.e., Stockholm syndrome).]

Metaphors that liken AN to an oppressive or demanding force can be useful in cueing a behavioral repertoire of defiance or disobedience. However, they should be used cautiously and timed effectively. Interventions that are too critical of AN, or are not paired with an appreciation for its positive elements, encourage clients to defend it.

As described by a client late in treatment:

"I've lived with a dictator for most of my life. I was told what to do, when to do, and how to do. There is no freedom living with a dictator. Your every action and behavior is controlled by them. You start out maybe questioning the rules, then you begin to follow without question, and then the rules wash out any semblance of you, so that you cannot differentiate between the two. You become the dictator. In the midst of treatment, you learn everyone wants to change the dictator. It feels like they are trying to change you, since you lost you when you succumbed to the dictator. It could be your therapists, your doctors, your parents, friends, family, and so forth. At times you get lost in the war, and forget why you're in it. Were you fighting to uphold the dictator who became 'you'? Or are you fighting because it seems everyone is coming at you like a dictator, and it's an impossible fight to win? I fought to uphold my dictator for decades. I ensured its safety. I protected it. It wasn't until I defied my dictator that I was able to start finding me again."

Contacting AN's Lack of Satiation

The client is put in contact with the experienced insatiable appetite of AN (e.g., there is no weight that is low enough or anything else that she could "achieve" that would allow her to rest). The client may be gently directed to notice whether she feels constricted or constrained by the mounting demands of AN for less food and more exercise or whether as AN has taken more space, there is less space for other aspects of her life. We provide several illustrative therapist scripts, along with dialogues that include metaphors of AN as unrelenting.

IN PRACTICE

Therapist Script A

"It sounds like AN will let you work as hard as you will until you die (*pause*). I'm wondering if you can sense that—like there is no end—not in a logical way (like your mind knowing it), but in an experienced way. Your experience tells you that . . ."

Therapist Script B

"As you talk about this now, it feels as though AN keeps piling up restrictions . . . and you keep inching back into a smaller and smaller space. Do you feel that?"

Therapist Script C

"Do you ever feel done; able to rest? (*pauses for response*) Could it be that your experience is telling you that the situation is rigged—that there isn't a weight that will be low enough to satisfy [AN] or make you feel like you are truly worthy?"

Therapist Script D

"Is this a familiar feeling . . . that nothing is ever [good] enough?"

Dialogue A (with the "Hungry Lion" Metaphor)

CLIENT: I don't know why, but I am set on 98 [pounds]. . . . I can't imagine being more than that. It feels like too much.

THERAPIST: That is different than the number you had before.

CLIENT: Yeah, before I just wanted to get down to 100. But then I got there . . . and . . .

THERAPIST: Is this familiar to you; that nothing is ever enough?

CLIENT: I suppose so . . .

THERAPIST: What is that like for you?

CLIENT: (*Describes.*)

THERAPIST: It just keeps going . . . one goal gives way to the next. . . . It's like a hungry lion. It is never satisfied, and the more you feed it, the more it grows. Demanding a bigger piece of meat. (*long pause*)

I'm not asking you to *believe* that AN will not be satisfied. I actually don't think your mind is helpful here at all (*smiles gently*). I am asking if you experience it to be so . . . ?

Dialogue B (with the "Demanding Boss" Metaphor)[*]

THERAPIST: Seems AN's demands never stop. It's more, more, more. Imagine if you started a new job, and your boss assigned you a project. It's important to you to do well, so you work extra hard: cancel plans with friends, stay up late, and get the project in early. Rather than a pat on the back or some time to recuperate, your boss demands the next assignment and expects it in a shorter time frame. And it keeps going like that. You start working overtime, nights and weekends, stop going out with friends, give up sleep. He ups the ante, and every time he does, you rise to the challenge, give more and more of your life to meet his demands.

CLIENT: Shouldn't we all strive to be better?

THERAPIST: I am not asking you to believe that it is good or not good to strive to be better or "perfect" (whatever that means; *smiles warmly*). I am asking you to notice your experience of doing that—the unrelenting pursuit of better . . . what it's like for you to live under constant and higher demands . . . and whether there is any cost in there . . . ? I don't know if there is . . . but it seems worth checking out.

Contacting the Brevity of Relief

The therapist helps the client notice that the relief provided by AN behaviors is temporary and does not solve the deeper problem (of emotional pain). Clients might also notice the persistent threat of losing control over eating or weight. Therapist scripts and dialogues are provided below as illustrations. The example in Dialogue B can be used with subjective or objective binge eating, although it is important to be sensitive to this distinction, which has treatment implications. If *objective* binge eating is present, behavior change goals will include reducing these discrete periods of uncontrolled eating. Objective binge eating might be a risk at certain stages of recovery, but is relatively uncommon among individuals with AN.

IN PRACTICE

Therapist Script A

"There was some sense of relief . . . when you ate only half [of the meal]. . . . How long did that feeling last (before you began to worry again about eating or weight)?"

Therapist Script B

"Is every day like that . . . just a restart . . . ?"

---

[*] This can be adapted to "teacher" or "coach" for younger clients.

Therapist Script C

"It sounds like your experience is that you can never put your guard down . . . that you have to keep constant watch [over your body or food] . . ."

Therapist Script D (with the "Groundhog Day" Metaphor)

"Have you seen the movie *Groundhog Day*? It is about someone who keeps waking up to the same day, over and over. Every morning starts exactly the same way, and the day progresses just like the previous one (until he decides to change what he does and change his fate). It seems that there is some comfort in the familiar; at first he is quite happy to get up and start the same day again. But then there is also a tedium and exhaustion. . . . I wonder if it ever feels like that, like the day is on repeat (you are going through the motions, following your schedule . . .). And maybe (likely) there is some comfort in that familiarity, but also some tediousness about it . . . ?"

Dialogue A

THERAPIST: What happens to your concerns about your body after you restrict?

CLIENT: I feel a little better.

THERAPIST: Does that last?

CLIENT: Sure, I mean, until I am triggered again.

THERAPIST: What do you mean by "triggered"? When I think of trigger, I think of a gun going off. If it is triggered, the bullet will come out—it's inevitable.

CLIENT: Yeah, I think that's what I mean. When I see someone else who is thinner than I am or I see my body in the mirror . . . it's disgusting. . . . I'm triggered, so I throw up.

THERAPIST: (*Gently introducing a functional formulation and choice.*) So, in these situations, you experience thoughts and feelings (like "I am disgusting") that feel intolerable and AN offers you a solution, a way to feel better again for a moment . . . ?

CLIENT: Yes, and I usually do . . . feel better after I throw up, I mean.

THERAPIST: Immediately, it's relief. What is it later?

CLIENT: I might be good for a little while . . . and then I feel bad again . . .

THERAPIST: Like medication for pain relief. . . . As soon as it wears off . . . the pain comes back?

Dialogue B

THERAPIST: Did AN leave you alone after you restricted lunch?

CLIENT: Um. For a little while, but I worried about what would happen at night . . . if I would overeat or binge . . .

THERAPIST: I imagine you watching the door (like a guard) to make sure that no urges come in. It seems like it would be hard to be vigilant or on guard all the time. Not really the kind of relief you would hope for.

CLIENT: Well, it didn't help. Because I binged and then I felt awful.

THERAPIST: So you were either consumed by the possibility of bingeing or consumed with guilt and shame. Is that your experience?

CLIENT: Yes, and it's awful. I don't know how to stop it. If I could just control myself better, this wouldn't happen.

THERAPIST: So it's this sense that you are not working [hard enough] and that if you just worked harder at controlling yourself and your body, it would all work out.

I get that there is a wish that it could work, yet I am wondering if your experience says that this is unworkable—that it promises relief but does it deliver?

Whether you binge that night or not, you are either bingeing [or feeling like you are] or worrying about bingeing.

You might get a little relief if you get through a night without breaking your rules, but then it starts again . . . ? (*long pause*) I wonder if there is another way, you know?

Dialogue C

CLIENT: I kind of want to see how far my body can go.

THERAPIST: And then what?

CLIENT: Yeah, that's the thing. I don't know.

THERAPIST: What if it's just empty. Like you got to see that wow, I can really push it . . . beyond human limits and then you have a moment of mastery. And then what?

Contacting the Costs of Preoccupation

Food, eating, and weight occupies considerable mental space of individuals with AN. This may make it difficult to focus on other things or be present with other people and in situations. The context is set such that the client may make contact with the costs of preoccupation for full living, as illustrated in the therapist scripts that follow.

IN PRACTICE

Therapist Script A

"So much time and energy (emotional and mental space) is given to AN . . . I am wondering what's left over. . . . Is there any space for anything else?"

Therapist Script B

"It seems like it felt nice to only think about food and calories; everything was so overwhelming at the time, and this was just simple." (*long pause*)

"And now this is all that life is [calorie counting, meal planning]."

"I wonder what that is like for you? Whether you wish for something more?"

Contacting the Loss of Autonomy or Personal Control

Some clients will not allow themselves to contact the undesirable consequences of AN. They may maintain that life is exactly as they want it to be, and that they can live fully with an exceedingly low weight, possibly with one exception: unwanted oversight. In this case, the therapist helps the client contact the loss of autonomy and personal control that comes with low weight, as illustrated in the therapist scripts and dialogues below.

Therapist Script A

"It sounds like your eating has brought a lot of unwanted attention, and that you feel less free to make your own decisions in your life. . . . What would it mean to you to get that back?"

Therapist Script B

"I hear what soccer and your scholarship has meant to you, and you don't want to lose those things (which are threatened with your low weight) . . .

"I guess I am wondering if these things can be worth it, worth facing fears of eating?"

IN PRACTICE

Dialogue

THERAPIST: I wonder what it has been like for you to have all of these people intruding in this way?

CLIENT: I wish that they would just leave me alone. I was fine until they stuck their noses in things. I can't do anything without getting 50 questions.

THERAPIST: That is one thing that you can sense very strongly . . . that AN has taken away some of your personal freedom, which is important to you. What would it be like for us to work to get that back?

Contacting the Consequence of Binge Eating

Some clients may be extremely attached to restriction (and unable to accept that it has undesirable consequences), but be horrified by their episodes of binge eating. In this case, stopping binge eating might be used to leverage other changes (until other reinforcers become available). The therapist helps the client contact binge eating as a consequence of restriction, illustrated in the script below.

IN PRACTICE

Therapist Script

"I hear you. It feels like there is nothing more important than your ability to restrict. I also hear that your binge eating is causing you incredible pain . . . and I think it is quite likely that these things are related . . . that restriction is creating the conditions for binge eating. This is what the research suggests, but I wonder about your experience . . . ?"

CLINICAL GOAL 8: *Contact Consequences for Personal Values*

Clients have varying degrees of awareness of their personal values (or what else they care about besides AN), particularly in the earlier stages of treatment. The therapist builds upon any available insight, elaborating clients' values and contacting how AN might interfere. As the client becomes better nourished and more aware of herself and what she cares about most deeply, this clinical goal is reengaged.

This clinical conversation is focused on the present moment and how AN is interfering with the *process* of living a valued, vital life *now*, rather than on how AN might interfere with *future goals* (e.g., getting a particular job, marrying or having children). The therapist helps the client make experiential contact with these lost moments of personal meaning. Therapist scripts are followed by sample dialogue that includes in-session exercises. Dialogue A includes the "AN Moment" exercise. Dialogue B includes the "Before–After AN" exercise.

IN PRACTICE

Therapist Script A

"AN has taken away guilt and shame (if only temporarily). I am wondering if it has taken away anything else . . . other things that you care about? What is your experience of your time with friends or family? Your work?"

Therapist Script B

"You have described how important it is to you that you are present, truly present, with your children. I am wondering whether that is possible with all the calculations and planning of AN . . ."

Dialogue A (with the "AN Moment" Exercise)

The therapist asks the client to slow down into a moment in which she was entangled with AN and explore the potential impact.

THERAPIST: Yesterday, when you were in that space, counting calories and worrying about dinner . . . what else was going on?

CLIENT: What do you mean?

THERAPIST: Well, that was what was happening in your head. . . . You were having a conversation with AN, but what was going on around you? Were you by yourself?

CLIENT: No, I was with my sister. She actually said that I wasn't listening, but I was trying to.

THERAPIST: Tell me more about what was happening that day. Where were you and she sitting? What did you notice about your sister's demeanor, and so forth?

CLIENT: (*Elaborates.*)

THERAPIST: What did you notice about your own experience of sitting with your sister, but being somewhere else in your head?

CLIENT: I don't remember anything other than feeling my thighs spreading on the chair . . . and thoughts about dinner . . .

THERAPIST: In that moment, AN took you away from your sister and the conversation with your sister. . . . Was that your experience?

CLIENT: Yes . . .

THERAPIST: Some moments of lost connection . . . How is this for you? Is this OK with you?

Dialogue B (with the "Before–After AN" Exercise)

The therapist helps the individual contrast life before AN and now.

THERAPIST: I wonder if we can go back in time, before AN . . . back before you started trying to change your eating and weight . . . well before that, if you can.

CLIENT: OK.

THERAPIST: Tell me about the time period that comes to your mind. How old are you?

CLIENT: 9 or 10.

THERAPIST: Young.

CLIENT: Well, I started getting worried about my weight in the sixth grade, so when I was 12 or so . . . 9 or 10, I don't remember this being something that I was thinking about then.

THERAPIST: OK. I would like to invite you to look around. What is going on around you? Who is there or not there? What are you doing? What does it feel like in your skin? . . . See if you can sense yourself . . . who you are and what you want. What is it like to be you?

CLIENT: (*Gives description.*)

THERAPIST: And now, what do you notice about your experience of yourself and your life now? How is it the same or different? Is there anything that you miss? Like maybe it is a younger expression of it, but something that you miss about yourself or your life.

Is Something Missing?

Individuals with AN are often unaware of their values or what they care about beyond conventional measures of success (e.g., thinness, high marks). For some clients, this is because rigid rule following (and risk aversion) emerged early and interfered with experimentation and the formation of likes, dislikes, opinions, and preferences. Other clients may have simply lost touch with what they cared about before life became centered on eating and weight (or other achievements). A lack of clarity regarding personal values is a major clinical issue in AN; strategies to comprehensively address this issue are discussed in Chapter 8. When the client's personal values are unclear, the therapist may simply invite curiosity about whether something is "missing," as illustrated in the therapist scripts below. Therapist Script E includes the "Gripping" metaphor, which may be useful to evoke throughout treatment.

IN PRACTICE

Therapist Script A

"I'm wondering though, is feeling relieved enough? Or do you have the sense that you want something more . . . ?"

Therapist Script B

"I know weight and shape—and doing your best—is important to you. I am also wondering, do you have the sense that something is missing? That there are other things that you might want in your life?"

Therapist Script C

"I hear you saying, 'I just want to be what I weighed in 2012. I was happy then.' I wonder though, were there other things that you had *then* that you don't have *now*, things that were different, other than body weight?"

Therapist Script D

"It seems you have lost yourself in AN, and in that, have lost what else you used to care about . . . other things that mattered. . . . Can you sense that?"

Therapist Script E (with the "Gripping" Metaphor)

"You've been holding onto AN . . . hoping it will deliver [a better life]. And when it doesn't, you tighten your grip, do more [restrict more, exercise more], like, "maybe that will do it." Can you sense that of holding, gripping, hoping? (*waits for client's response*)

"I also wonder, if you can sense that, with your hands gripping AN . . . they aren't free to do other things that could bring meaning (*therapist gestures gripped fists and then opens hands to pick up something nearby*). You can't pick anything else up. Can you sense that?

(*The therapist invites the client to grip a clipboard that represents AN, and then ask her to try to pick up something else [e.g., the tissue box].*) "Imagine this clipboard is AN and that this tissue box represents other things that are important in your life . . ."

Waiting to Live

Clients might be clear about their values, but be fused with the idea that thinness (or confidence) is a prerequisite for valued living. For example, clients may report that once they are thin enough, they will be able to do the things that are important to them (e.g., engage more socially or apply for a particular job). Thus, they keep working (on the goal of weight loss) and waiting for life to feel meaningful. In this case, the therapist helps the client explore how life has been put on hold and the costs of waiting. With younger clients, stories and poems may be useful, such as the passage in Dr. Suess's book *Oh, the Places You'll Go*, which describes "The Waiting Place." Therapist scripts and dialogue that help the client explore the workability of waiting are provided next. Unlike second-wave CBT strategies, the goal is not to change whether the client has the thought that she must lose weight to do things, but rather to explore the workability of choosing to make weight (or confidence) a prerequisite for engaging in her life.

IN PRACTICE

Therapist Script A

"I guess one thing that I am wondering is: How long are you willing to wait? It has been since 2002 . . . 18 years? Longer?"

Therapist Script B

"And what does your experience tell you? You have felt like it is just around the corner before. . . . Has any weight felt low enough? Your mind can say whatever it wants. I am interested in you (your heart, your experience). What does it say?"

Therapist Script C

"You are waiting for thinness to make you more confident, so then you can talk to people. I wonder, what if you can't control how you feel, only what you do? . . . What is your experience?

Dialogue

CLIENT: I really miss my friends. But I just can't stand myself right now. Once my body is better, I will start hanging out again.

THERAPIST: How long are you willing to wait?

CLIENT: I just want to lose a few more pounds . . .

THERAPIST: Is this familiar to you . . . this idea of "just a few more"? . . .

CLIENT: Yeah.

THERAPIST: I'd like to invite you to slow down here (*pause, gentle tone*) . . . and imagine what it would be like if things continue like this for the next several years of your life. Imagine next year, 5 years, or maybe 10 years from now, you are still trying to lose weight [still trying to feel different in your body, first, before you live your life]. . . . You are still waiting . . . to go out on a date . . . or to try to meet new people. . . . You are still avoiding any social interactions with friends . . . still missing birthday parties, brunches, afternoon movies, hikes . . .

Is this OK with you?

Foreshadowing Losses

Some clients have not experienced any costs of living with AN. This is often the case with recent onset of adolescent AN. It might also be observed among high-functioning adults who, despite a persistent energy deficit and low weight, continue to meet all their obligations and maintain social relationships at a reasonable level. In this case, the therapist may simply be foreshadowing that, at some point, AN will become unworkable for personal values (or a life well lived), as illustrated below. This type of intervention is facilitated by a strong relationship between the client and therapist—in which the client is completely clear about the therapist's interest in her well-being. The therapist is essentially lending her vantage point and inviting the client to experience the situation through her eyes.

IN PRACTICE

Dialogue (with the "Mountain Climbing" Metaphor)

CLIENT: I think it is fine. Everyone is overreacting. I haven't even had bad labs. I'm not losing my hair . . .

THERAPIST: Yeah, I hear you, it doesn't seem as if there is a problem. . . . You remember when we talked about mountain climbing? When we are climbing a mountain, our nose is right up against the rock wall—all that can be seen are the rocks right in front of our face. [*Illustrates with hand to face.*] . . . Our climbing partner has the advantage of a more distant vantage point though. He or she can see things that we can't see because we are up against it—up against the rock wall. He or she can see things like sharp protrusions or a ledge somewhere nearby . . .

> You know how it looks and feels up close. I am back here. I can see things that aren't available to you simply because of the difference in our vantage point, and perhaps you can see things about my side of the mountain that I can't see . . . (*smiles gently*). Can you imagine what your situation looks like to me? Can you see from my eyes in this moment?

CLIENT: (*Looks as though she senses this experience.*)

THERAPIST: From here, it is like a train is slowly and steadily barreling toward the wall, and eventually it's going to hit . . . and I can feel myself wanting to stop it before it happens, before you crash into it. . . . Because I care about you. I care about what happens to you.

> [In an alternative version of this metaphor, the client and therapist cross the room together and look back at where the client was sitting to get a more distant vantage point on the client's situation.]

Refining the Treatment Contract

As the client makes greater contact with the unworkability of current behavior patterns, it may be possible to refine the treatment contract (see below). Refining the treatment contract may include a greater commitment to working on improving eating and weight, or the inclusion of other treatment goals that are consistent with the client's values.

IN PRACTICE

Therapist Script

"We have been working to get your doctors and coaches to back off—so that you can regain your sense of autonomy and independence. I wonder if it might now be time to shift to a different sort of work—to diminishing the impact of this whole thing on your friendships. It has become clear how important that is to you, and how AN (and just generally working so hard to achieve goals at the expense of your well-being) has been getting in the way of being in relationships the way that you want to be . . ."

CLINICAL GOAL 9: *Expand to Other Behaviors that Serve a Similar Purpose as AN and Offer an Alternative*

As described previously, the core features of AN are often part of a repertoire of behaviors that function for avoidance and control. For example, dietary rules might reduce uncertainty, but so might a number of other behaviors, such as making lists or planning conversations in advance. The therapist is compassionately curious about these other behaviors and *when* and *how* these behaviors may serve the same purpose of AN. The ultimate goal is to examine the workability of avoidance and control *more broadly* and shift the entire system, offering acceptance as an alternative. The therapist conveys that the client's behavior is wholly sensible in the context in which it emerges and, at the same time, there may be costs, and perhaps there is an alternative (i.e., allowing emotional discomfort in order to behave effectively and be consistent with personal values). An illustrative script and several sample dialogues are provided next. Dialogue C includes the "Toolbox" metaphor, which might be evoked throughout treatment as clients reengage old "tools" (of avoidance and control).

An "Avoidance Card" exercise is also provided. This exercise may be particularly helpful when an individual has an extensive avoidant repertoire. In this exercise, avoidant behaviors are written on note cards to form a "deck." This makes it easier for clients to identify behaviors of diverse topography as a functional class and explore the broader workability of avoidance and control. The therapist might also write clients' avoided content (e.g., unwanted thoughts, feelings, body sensations) on note cards, potentially in a different color. This encourages clients to take an observer stance to unwanted internal experiences and may be used as a prop for acceptance and defusion work.

IN PRACTICE

Therapist Script

"We all have 'ways of being' . . . things we do to keep ourselves safe [from painful feelings]. It seems yours are "be small" (take up less space), be smart, be prepared, be quiet. . . . These are all the same in a sense—they all serve the same purpose. Perhaps all of these 'ways of being' are helpful (*long pause*) and maybe they cost something too . . .

"What if you didn't *have* to be those things—you could choose to—but you didn't *have* to?"

"You could choose to be quiet, or to speak up, for example, depending on what served you best in the situation. It seems that would require facing fear and discomfort . . ."

Dialogue A

The client is describing how AN makes her feel better about herself. The therapist probes for other behaviors that serve a similar purpose.

THERAPIST: What else do you do . . . to feel worthwhile or good about yourself?

CLIENT: I make good grades . . . do well at track meets. . . . That makes me feel good, for a little while, anyway. Until the next [exam, meet] . . . then I am sure that I will fail . . .

THERAPIST: So you have restriction and weight loss, but also "doing well" in these other domains that you turn to [to feel worthwhile or good about yourself]. . . . And it helps for a little bit, but not for long. Am I getting that right?

CLIENT: Yes.

THERAPIST: Are there other things that you do? I guess I am wondering whether "doing things" (e.g., favors) for other people is another thing that you do [to feel worthwhile or good about yourself]?

CLIENT: I haven't thought about it, but now that you say it . . . I suppose it is. I also just like doing things for my friends.

THERAPIST: What if you *didn't* do these things? Like, does it feel like a choice [to do them]?

CLIENT: Nah, I pretty much have to. . . . I worry that if I didn't, they wouldn't like me or something and maybe they wouldn't want me around . . .

THERAPIST: That must be hard, to feel like you are not likeable or valuable to your friends unless you are doing things for them . . . and because you always do things for them, you never find out.

OK, let me see if I am getting this . . . so focusing on your weight and doing really well in school and track are things that help you feel good about yourself, and that is really compelling . . . it is really nice to feel that way . . . even if it's just for a moment (*pauses, gentle tone*). . . . And the way you are with other people is about this too . . . kind of earning your worth. *And* none of it lasts . . . with people, you are not really sure if it is real . . . like if they really like you. You doubt your friendships and whether your friends would want to be around you if you weren't doing things for them. . . . Is that right?

CLIENT: Yes.

THERAPIST: And so these are all the same in some ways. . . . And they work for what they work for: You feel better for a little while . . .

CLIENT: Yeah, but then I am right back where I started . . .

THERAPIST: I wonder if there is another way [of living], a way that doesn't include earning your worth . . . ?

Dialogue B

CLIENT: I just can't walk into a situation and know what to say. . . . I feel so stupid . . . so I plan in advance. I am constantly planning conversations in my mind.

THERAPIST: That is about protection too then [just like AN]—protecting yourself from judgment.

CLIENT: Yeah.

THERAPIST: What do you do when faced with spontaneous interactions, like someone talking to you in the hall?

CLIENT: Oh, I keep my head down. I try not to make eye contact.

THERAPIST: So you either plan or avoid it . . . (*long pause*) What is that like for you? I guess I am wondering if it feels limiting? Like there are only certain times and certain ways that you can engage with other people. Do you ever feel like you are missing out on opportunities to connect . . . ?

CLIENT: (*Shrugs, looks sad.*)

THERAPIST: That feeling of being judged is powerful. So much so that you have been willing to give up something that is important to you (being with other people). . . . All humans do that. . . . We all do things that ultimately do not serve us to avoid painful thoughts and feelings . . . I wonder though, what if there is another way?

Dialogue C (with the "Toolbox" Metaphor)

THERAPIST: You've been trying so hard to feel better about yourself (like you are "not a wreck"). You have a toolbox full of strategies, and AN is right on top . . .

CLIENT: (*Gives knowing look.*)

THERAPIST: I wonder if we can unpack this a bit. Imagine that we have an actual toolbox here (*gestures the structure of a box*) . . . maybe it's labeled "Tools to not feel like a wreck." . . . What's in here (*gestures pulling "a tool" out of the imaginary toolbox*)?

CLIENT: (*Describes various strategies to feel better. Each strategy is examined with curiosity until the "toolbox" is empty.*)

THERAPIST: OK, nothing else in here (*pretends to look in an empty box*).

CLIENT: I don't understand why nothing is working. I feel better for a little while, but it never lasts . . . and in some ways, things have gotten worse . . .

THERAPIST: I wonder if it is like trying to get out of a hole with a shovel . . .

CLIENT: When you are in a hole, don't dig (*smiles*).

THERAPIST: Yeah, digging makes bigger holes. The funny thing is, we've all been given shovels and have been told shovels are the way to go! What if the solution is something completely different (*pause*). Finding a way to live inside your skin? Finding a way to live with yourself and your thoughts and feelings . . . ? Could it be?

CLIENT: (*Sits thoughtfully.*)

THERAPIST: You have seen those Chinese finger traps. What happens when you pull?

CLIENT: It tightens . . .

THERAPIST: How do you get out?

CLIENT: Push in?

THERAPIST: Yeah, it is so counterintuitive. Everything in you says, "Pull [away]!" But it tightens . . . chokes you.

Dialogue D

THERAPIST: I am wondering if medical school is kind of like AN in a way, it is about avoiding judgment . . . avoiding the shame you would feel for choosing something different.

CLIENT: Yes, I suppose it is. I know that it is not right for me. It's really awful, actually.

THERAPIST: I guess I am wondering if avoiding judgment is workable . . . sort of more generally . . . or whether the costs are too great?

CLIENT: (*Describes costs as she experiences them.*)

THERAPIST: I wonder what it would be like to try another way . . . something counterintuitive . . . like, instead of working to avoid judgment in all these different ways, opening up to it (or the possibility of it) . . . or really to the thoughts/feelings you would have if others don't agree with your choices.

"Avoidance Card" Exercise

The therapist works with the client to make a deck of cards. Each card lists a strategy that the client uses to change internal experience (i.e., behaviors that minimize contact with painful thoughts/feelings, make things more predictable or controlled, etc.). The act of creating the deck is an intervention in itself and helps to separate the behaviors from the client, making it easier to evaluate the workability of avoidance/avoidant repertoire. It also increases the extent to which the client experiences her behaviors as a collection of responses defined by their function. Grouping the cards together on a table or on the floor allows the therapist and client to refer to the behavioral repertoire in shorthand or to compassionately point to avoidance or control behaviors showing up in session (see Figure 6.1).

Cards may also be made for difficult internal experiences (i.e., thoughts/feelings/body sensations that are intolerable to the client). On cards, it may be easier to see how difficult internal experiences may be "held."

Avoidance/control cards typically include:

- AN behaviors (including fat talk, body-related worry, calorie counting, etc., in addition to restricting food, overexercising, or other behaviors).
- Behaviors associated with comorbid clinical problems such as OCD or social phobia (e.g., counting in 3's, cleaning, avoiding social situations).
- Behaviors of poor self-care (e.g., not taking breaks).
- Interpersonal behaviors (e.g., looking away, not expressing feelings or opinions, attending exclusively to others' needs).
- Clinically relevant behaviors observed in session, such as asking "Why?" (e.g., "Why am I like this?"; "Why do I have to gain weight?"), or reporting, "I don't know."

Dialogue (with the "Avoidant Card" Exercise)

CLIENT: Wow! I had no idea that I had so many things that I do . . .

THERAPIST: Does it feel overwhelming?

CLIENT: It's a lot.

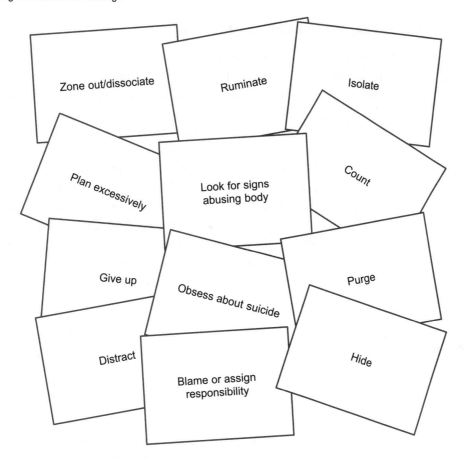

FIGURE 6.1. Avoidant repertoire on notecards.

THERAPIST: Well, I would say that it speaks to how hard it is to have feelings of uncertainty or being out of control, and how hard you have been working to keep it away. What else shows up for you?

CLIENT: I just wonder why I can't be normal. These things don't bother other people.

THERAPIST: If it is OK with you, I say we add that thought to our deck of experiences that are hard to have.

CLIENT: (*Agrees and makes a card.*)

THERAPIST: I also wonder, what if this is part of being human? We move away from things that are painful. I don't expect your mind to accept that—it has been telling you that there is something wrong with you for a long time, and we don't have to convince it otherwise.

I wonder if instead we could look at whether this is what you want—what you want to be doing. I can feel the cards kind of boxing you in. That with all the musts and have-to's, there is little room for anything else . . .

CLIENT: (*Describes her experience of this.*)

THERAPIST: The funny thing is that the way out may actually be in—into experience of uncertainty, for example. Making friends with it, in a sense.

An Unworkable System, Not an Unworkable Person

When clients contact the costs of avoidance and control (or realize the ways in which they are stuck), this may generate guilt and shame. It is important to emphasize that all behavior can be understood in the context in which it is situated—and this is an issue of an unworkable system, not an unworkable person. Indeed, AN is *wholly sensible* in a social–verbal community that highly values self-discipline (defined as "the act of disciplining or power to discipline one's own feelings, desires, etc., often for the purpose of improving oneself") and external markers of success. Indeed, individuals with AN are doing *exactly* what society has told them makes a good person or a good life. This is why onlookers are often so confused by AN. It appears as if life is going well for these individuals, yet their suffering is often profound, as evidenced by the extraordinary high suicide rate. As such, it can be extremely validating for the therapist to verbalize the client's felt sense that despite her effort, life lacks vitality. She is doing all of the things that society tells her will lead to a "good life," yet this has not enhanced her life meaning. We illustrate this point with the dialogues and case example below.

IN PRACTICE

Dialogue A

CLIENT: I don't understand. I have no reason to feel this way. . . . Nothing bad has happened to me . . . I got into law school . . .

THERAPIST: It isn't OK to just *feel how you feel*—it needs to be justified or something . . . ? (*pause*) Our minds want to evaluate everything (including our feelings), and maybe it's just not helpful. . . . Our minds are overextending themselves (*long pause*).

It seems we have all been told a story, a story about what makes for a good life or makes us good people. I wonder, though, in your experience, has (conforming to these ideas, disregarding yourself and your feelings along the way) led to a valued, vital life?

Maybe you feel "better" because you feel as though you are doing and being "good," but this is relative to the bad you feel otherwise. It is not more meaningful, as far as we have been able to tell . . . ?

CLIENT: Sometimes I feel like maybe it will click into place . . . and maybe that it is me if it doesn't . . . that I am doing something wrong.

THERAPIST: Yeah, there is this sense that it should work—after all, that is what we have all been told! Like you imagine this book "How to Succeed in Life and Be a Good Person," blah, blah.

CLIENT: (*Smiles.*)

THERAPIST: It is completely sensible that you have been doing this. . . . This is the world that we live in. I wonder if what you have to do is put down this book and look around—to decide for yourself what makes a "good life"—what kind of life *you* want to live, or who *you want to be* in the moments of your life?

Dialogue B

The client in the dialogue that follows has a history of suicidal ideation and self-harm.

THERAPIST: You have been doing exactly what society says will lead to a good life . . . "Work hard (really hard). Be the best. Be perfect. Your needs don't matter. . . . In fact, if you need to rest, that just means you are lazy, weak, . . . pathetic . . ."

And I hear you saying that in many ways, this has been working. . . . You make the grades. You lose weight, you feel like you look the part . . . it makes sense that you keep doing it . . . (*pause*) an incredibly human thing to do . . .

CLIENT: Everyone complimented me when I first started losing weight . . .

THERAPIST: . . . and yet.

CLIENT: (*Knowing sigh.*)

THERAPIST: . . . Sometimes you wish that you could die . . .

CLIENT: It's tedious, you know. . . . Everything must be counted. Accounted for. And nothing is ever good enough really. I used to be able to stop at 8 miles . . . now I have to do 16 or a feel terrible about myself . . .

THERAPIST: The demands are unrelenting . . . (*long pause*). And never in kindness. Never very nice to yourself. I wonder if you can have compassion for yourself in this moment, that you are trying to do "good" . . . the problem isn't you. The problem is it's a sham . . . a promise that your experience tells you doesn't deliver.

Case Example 6.1

Brittney is a 34-year-old woman who at the time of presentation was only consuming baby food from jars, reporting that she could not swallow anything other than pureed foods. She was vomiting regularly and abusing laxatives and diuretics. At her worst point, she refused all food and was spoon-fed by her sister. She had an esophageal tear due to repeated vomiting and extreme iron deficiency that required transfusions. She described not feeling "good enough" in any domain of her life, including the "eating disorder"; she either felt like a failure because her weight was not low enough or because of her poor compliance with treatment.

Brittney was a volleyball star in high school, but she struggled somewhat academically, in part due to a processing issue that also made it difficult for her to understand oral communication. She often misunderstood others and their motivations. She was known to be shy and earned the nickname "Smiley" when she was a kid because she would smile when any attention was directed to her. Often, her sister would answer for her. She described trying to mimic her peers in order to be accepted (including in small ways, like how to hold a pencil). She had considerable conflict with her mom and always felt as though she was being judged. Her history is notable for unwanted sexual encounters, including an assault by a boyfriend in high school. Brittney described being frozen in fear during the encounter, while also having confusing body sensations (that felt like arousal). She felt as though she should have been stronger or that she had made a mistake in trusting this individual. She evidenced hypervigilance to interpersonal threat and would often assume malintent. She described feeling as though she should punish herself and would carve words into her flesh (e.g., *fat*) and purposefully ignore basic needs or health maintenance (not taking prescribed vitamins in order to damage her body).

Brittney presented as highly ruminative and spent inordinate amounts of time thinking about what had happened in the past and what she should have done differently, in major situations (e.g., the assault) and minor interactions with other people. She described not trusting herself to make good decisions and not trusting her body. She was often interpersonally sensitive (perceiving criticism) and reported fear of wearing the wrong clothes, or saying or doing the wrong thing. In session, she often asked "Why?" (why was she the way she was). She often felt depressed. Brittney also was highly ritualized in other areas of her life—planning activities and conversations excessively, and presenting with obsessional behaviors, mostly surrounding the cleanliness of her body. Her primary social outlet was health care providers.

The initial functional assessment focused primarily on feelings that Brittney should be able to control her body, and the feeling of being dirty and wrong for her history, and for

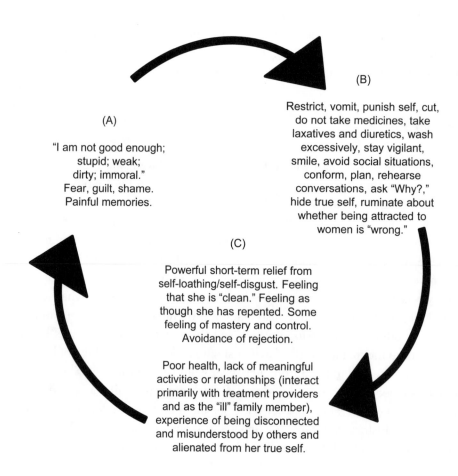

(B)

Restrict, vomit, punish self, cut, do not take medicines, take laxatives and diuretics, wash excessively, stay vigilant, smile, avoid social situations, conform, plan, rehearse conversations, ask "Why?," hide true self, ruminate about whether being attracted to women is "wrong."

(A)

"I am not good enough; stupid; weak; dirty; immoral."
Fear, guilt, shame.
Painful memories.

(C)

Powerful short-term relief from self-loathing/self-disgust. Feeling that she is "clean." Feeling as though she has repented. Some feeling of mastery and control. Avoidance of rejection.

Poor health, lack of meaningful activities or relationships (interact primarily with treatment providers and as the "ill" family member), experience of being disconnected and misunderstood by others and alienated from her true self.

FIGURE 6.2. System that has trapped Brittney (Case Example 6.1).

not being able to predict every situation. Later information revealed that she was avoiding disclosure of information about her sexuality (i.e., that she was gay). She feared rejection (as well as abuse) for her sexuality and was spending a lot of time ruminating about whether she was "wrong" (a morally bad or corrupt individual). Her consensual sexual encounters with men were made more painful by the incongruence with her identity. Over 5 years of prior treatment, Brittney had been diagnosed with AN–binge/purge subtype, OCD, social phobia, posttraumatic stress disorder, and personality disorder "deferred."

This case example clearly highlights how a complicated clinical presentation is simplified in its formulation and treatment targets by orienting to functional classes of behavior (see Figure 6.2). It also highlights how extensive systems of avoidance and control can become, and how this might perpetuate the narrative of ineffectiveness. The therapist does not try to talk the individual out of this narrative, but does frame the behavior as a human response to pain, as illustrated in the dialogue below.

IN PRACTICE

Dialogue

THERAPIST: It seems that you have been really scared—scared to be yourself and what that would mean, and so you have been hiding out and stacking strategies on top of each other hoping for some relief.

CLIENT: I know, I am such an idiot.

THERAPIST: That is something that your mind gives you frequently, so it's no surprise that it's coming up now. (*pause*) And I wonder if this is just what it is like to be a human being: to have a deep desire for belonging and in pain when we think something threatens that. . . . And to move away from that pain, in whatever ways we do it, maybe that is human, too.

Looking Ahead

We describe interventions to build the client's capacity to allow internal experiences to be what they are, without unnecessary attempts to change their form, frequency, or situational sensitivity in Chapter 7. This includes emotional pain (e.g., feelings of sadness, guilt, or shame), as well as other signals arising from the body that the client might judge and reject (e.g., feeling physically satisfied or full). The ability to allow experience to *be what is* permits individuals to engage in behaviors that are effective in meeting their needs and consistent with their deeply held personal values.

CHAPTER 7

Acceptance

ALLOWING UNWANTED INTERNAL EXPERIENCES

Listen with your heart. Learn from your experiences,
and always be open to new ones.
—CHEROKEE PROVERB

The overarching aim of intervention is to help individuals with AN open up to experience. This includes motivational states (e.g., hunger, emotions) and, more generally, the experience of living in a way that is less predictable and well controlled. With increased openness to experience, an individual with AN is better able to meet her physical and emotional needs and take risks that enhance life vitality.

Acceptance of internal experience is discriminated from wanting or liking (i.e., we do not have to like how our gut turns to allow the experience to be what it is). Acceptance is also discriminated from more passive responses, such as giving up or giving in. Instead, acceptance is an active choice to end the struggle with internal experience and invite what is already there (as the product of being a conscious human being with a history).

It is important to note that acceptance does not mean allowing unhealthy situations. In fact, accepting how we feel often allows us to make much-needed changes to our external circumstances (e.g., leaving an abusive relationship). Because *acceptance* has various connotations for clients, the therapist might use another word that conveys the same meaning. Alternatives to *accept* include:

Allow
Permit
Be willing
Make space for
Open up to

Acceptance is facilitated by the client's personal values, and a clear articulation of how being open to internal experience allows the individual to engage in life in a meaningful way. Acceptance is also facilitated by defusion and self-as-context. When thoughts are not what they *literally* represent (but instead products of thinking or mental activity), it is easier to accept their presence. Similarly, when the client is able to take the *perspective of the observer* (and observe her thoughts/feelings as separate and distinct from herself), she is able to hold all experiences lightly. She is not threatened by the presence or absence of any particular thought or feeling, and all internal experiences may be allowed. Values are described in Chapter 8. Defusion and the observer self are described in Chapters 9 and 10. Acceptance interventions are engaged throughout treatment, and whenever experiential avoidance interferes with the individual behaving in ways that are flexible and effective or enhance life vitality. If acceptance work is difficult or stalled, this indicates the need to more fully engage these other ACT processes (e.g., values to facilitate greater willingness, defusion to reduce the power of thoughts) or to return to creative hopelessness (Chapter 6).

Clinical Goals

We describe seven clinical goals for building acceptance among individuals with AN. Acceptance begins with clients simply *noticing* unwanted feelings (Clinical Goal 1). This is particularly important for individuals with AN who exert such oppressive control that they may not even be aware of the presence of emotions underlying their preoccupations.

CLINICAL GOAL 1: *Help the Client Notice Unwanted Feelings*

Individuals with AN may suppress their emotions so effectively that they are barely detectable by themselves or by the therapist. Table 7.1 lists common indicators of emotion in individuals with AN, and thus opportunities to build acceptance, initially by simply eliciting curiosity about whether a feeling is present and what that feeling might be. Emotion in individuals with AN is signaled by momentary exacerbations in eating, food, or body preoccupation. This might be intuitive; however, there are also less intuitive indicators. For example, individuals with AN may become very cerebral or logical when experiencing emotion, or as emotion intensifies. The dialogue that follows illustrates one way in which the

---

TABLE 7.1. Indicators of the Presence of Affect among Individuals with AN

- Obsessing about food, eating, or the body.
- Rationalizing behaviors (providing "reasons" for eating less, studying long hours, or leaving a social situation).
- Debating about the need to eat or gain weight.
- Becoming very cerebral and detail focused (e.g., providing inordinate amount of detail about mundane activities).
- Orienting to rules, or trying to identify a rule.
- Focusing on the feelings or needs of other people.
- Abruptly changing topics.
- Physically constricting (e.g., avoiding eye contact, crossing arms, taking up "less space") or "shutting down" (e.g., getting quiet, reporting "I don't know").

therapist might draw the client's attention to the possible presence of emotion, beyond what is directly expressed in body weight and shape concerns. After the sample dialogue, we provide direction for homework that is assigned between sessions to achieve this clinical goal.

Noticing feelings can be intense acceptance work for individuals with AN. Clients may not only find it difficult to allow *themselves* to be aware of their emotions, but also to allow the therapist to know that they have feelings. Initial exposure to feelings may be brief and only consist of labeling the emotion. As clients gain a greater capacity for acceptance, they may be exposed to uncomfortable emotions for longer periods of time.

IN PRACTICE

Dialogue

The therapist is observing a change in the content and process of the client's communication and is inquiring about the presence of emotion.

THERAPIST: What happened there?

CLIENT: Huh?

THERAPIST: Well, we were talking about your work, and then you brought up weight. I am wondering if something showed up for you in that conversation . . .

CLIENT: I was just noticing how my thighs felt. So gross . . .

THERAPIST: I'm wondering what else might have been happening, moments before you noticed your thighs—was there an emotion rising up?

CLIENT: I don't know. (*Fidgets. Long pause.*)

THERAPIST: Perhaps you could identify where your mind went . . . right before it turned to your thighs? . . . You were talking about work . . .

CLIENT: (*Long pause.*) I feel like I am doing a bad job . . . I'm not good at anything . . . I'm not even good at having an eating disorder.

THERAPIST: So, you were noticing a feeling of "not being good [at things]" . . . a feeling of failure . . . or maybe shame? . . .

CLIENT: (*Sits quietly.*)

THERAPIST: I appreciate your willingness to slow down here . . . (*pause*) It is courageous, you know . . . to allow yourself to pause in these moments and notice what you are feeling. (*Therapist conveys gratitude and respect in tone and body language.*) It is the process of opening up (to your emotions) . . . and perhaps it makes other things (in life) accessible to you too . . .

Between-Session Practice (Homework)

Clients can practice noticing feelings between sessions by recording eating disorder episodes. The client makes an entry when she engages in a target behavior (e.g., restricts a planned meal, overexercises, purges). She identifies the day/time and immediate situational factors (e.g., trying on clothes). She also practices expanding awareness to the broader emotional context in which the AN behaviors emerged. This includes identifying events unrelated to food and body that happened earlier in the day and may have impacted her mood. Expanding awareness to this broader context is an act of willingness and puts the client in contact with difficult feelings. The ability to observe the broader emotional context is also a skill that will evolve over time. Initially, clients' diary entries may be impoverished, reporting only external factors or relying on vague descriptions of internal experience.

Figure 7.1 provides an example of a diary card entry. The client completed the card after skipping lunch. In this example, "feeling stupid," anxiety, and shame were the unwanted internal experiences that prompted restriction. Restricting lunch likely functioned to redirect the client's attention from this feeling to a more solvable or preferred problem (of weight control) and/or provided the client with a mastery experience (an experience of being effective or making a "good decision"). By describing the broader emotional context of restriction, the client is allowing momentary emotional discomfort, and thus building acceptance. A blank diary card (Handout 7.1) is available at the end of this chapter; a copy you can download and use in your work with clients is provided on the publisher's website (see the box at the end of the table of contents).

The "Eating Disorder Volume" Metaphor

In many cases, there will be little variation in AN behaviors across the day(s) or throughout the week, making it difficult to identify proximal emotional antecedents. Thus, clients might also use "Eating Disorder Volume" as an alternative prompt to complete a diary card entry. The client practices discriminating relative increases in the intensity of food and body preoccupation and uses this as a signal to "check in" (i.e., observe the situation and what else they might be feeling). This approach is illustrated in Therapist Scripts A and B. A reproducible diary card using Eating Disorder Volume (Handout 7.2) is available at the end of this chapter; a copy you can download and use in your work with clients is provided on the publisher's website (see the box at the end of the table of contents).

Day/Time Situational Factors (Where were you and who were you with?)	Eating Disorder Behavior	Eating Disorder Thoughts/Feelings	What else happened earlier in the day that may have influenced your mood? Observations (any other thoughts and feelings that you notice)
Monday, 12:00 p.m. At work, alone at my desk.	Skipped lunch.	I feel fat.	I was not able to solve a problem. I think it irritated my boss. I feel stupid for not knowing the answer. I am afraid that I am going to be fired. I am a bad employee that makes bad decisions.

FIGURE 7.1. Example of an entry on a diary card tracking eating disorder episodes.

Discriminating Eating Disorder Volume can reveal more subtle increases in AN behavior that are driven by the presence of unwanted emotions. The "Eating Disorder Volume" metaphor is also useful in helping clients differentiate themselves from their internal experience (e.g., thoughts/feelings). Thus, it also functions as defusion and strengthens the observer self.

IN PRACTICE

Therapist Script A

"Sometimes when things are really frequent, they can feel constant; like the steady hum of an air conditioner. And we stop noticing the fluctuations . . . small deviations that rise and fall a bit, especially when it is a welcome, kind of comfortable buzz. AN has been a near constant presence, yet if we listen closely, we can hear a little rise and fall. It's like a radio that is always on, but the volume turns up or down based on what is going on in our lives. One of the things that we are going to do is learn to tune in to these more subtle changes. Now, your job will not be to turn the volume down. The volume will do whatever it does as a result of life. Your work will be about noticing . . . noticing these fluctuations and what is going on in and around you at these times . . ."

Therapist Script B

"Do you ever notice that sometimes the eating disorder feels really loud, like a bullhorn or megaphone in your ear, and other times, it is a little quieter?" [If this is familiar to the client, elicit examples to practice this discrimination. If the client does not observe fluctuations, you might follow up.]

"Sometimes we get so used to hearing something that we don't notice these kinds of changes anymore. It's like one of those games where there are two pictures and the task is to 'find the differences'—at first glance, the two pictures look the same. But if we study them a bit, we start to notice the subtle differences. One of the things we are going to do together is learn how to hear differences in the volume of your eating disorder thoughts and feelings. It might take some practice. Maybe we can practice together now. Right now, how loud are your eating disorder thoughts and feelings? [Draws a scale from 0 to 10; waits for a response.] Now, imagine that I suggest we eat a snack together. . . . What happens to the volume?

"Now, our job will not be to turn the volume down. The volume will do whatever it does as a result of life. Our work will be about noticing . . . noticing the Eating Disorder Volume and also what might turn it up or down: what might be stressful and what other feelings you might be experiencing. Sometimes the volume was changing earlier than we think; after something that happened much earlier in the day."

Lack of Emotional Language/Differentiation

Earlier in treatment, clients' emotional language may be vague and less differentiated (e.g., clients may report feeling "upset" or "stressed" rather than discriminating feelings of fear, sadness, or guilt). Clients' emotional language may also be limited to somatic descriptors of affect (e.g., feeling fat, heavy, or sluggish). As clients practice labeling feelings, diary entries may evolve to include richer descriptions of emotions and a broader range of experience. Therapists can help clients identify how they are feeling using emoticons, emotion wheels, or other psychoeducation materials (e.g., emotion regulation handouts that describe the different emotions, including common physiological responses and action urges; e.g., Linehan, 2014). Additional strategies to help clients label feelings are described in Chapter 10. Learning to label feelings is essential in treatment and allows clients to meet their physical and emotional needs. Similar to other interventions, teaching clients with AN to label internal states is iterative as nutrition improves and body mass has less of an impact on hunger, satiety, and the somatic constitutes of emotion.

CLINICAL GOAL 2: *Provide a Frame for Acceptance Work*

The therapist provides a frame for how allowing feelings (or other unwanted internal experiences) might permit the client to behave in ways that enhance her life. The therapist also sets a tone of permission and personal ownership in acceptance work. The goal is for the client to appreciate that, at times, therapy will be uncomfortable or bring up uncomfortable feelings, and that this occurs only with her consent (as illustrated in the dialogues below). Permission and personal ownership are particularly important with acceptance interventions, which have a strong exposure element. The client should never feel that acceptance is being done "to her"; rather, she is choosing to approach difficult thoughts/feelings in the service of her values. The therapist should keep in mind that individuals with AN may be compliant and mask their discomfort with in-session activities. This may necessitate more frequent checking in. The dialogues that follow use metaphor, which is intentional, and might be relied on even more in practice, along with physicalizing strategies (e.g., the Clipboard Exercise) to enhance experiential learning.

IN PRACTICE

Dialogue A (with the "Dentist" Metaphor)

THERAPIST: At times, this work will be hard because we will be staying with feelings that you have avoided for a long time . . . that maybe you have not ever allowed yourself to have . . .

CLIENT: Isn't this supposed to make me feel better? I could feel terrible on my own . . .

THERAPIST: Imagine that you went to the dentist and he poked around at your teeth but he didn't touch the sore one, so it was pretty painless. You might think: "WOW! That was a great visit!" It was painless, but not really helpful. To do this work, we will have to go where things are tender (or feel hard) because that is what will be the most helpful to you. By having the feelings in here, it might make it possible to have them out there . . .

Know, though, that this is always with your permission . . . and for what you want in your life—the life you would choose if you could live fully inside your own skin. . . . Not because it is somehow virtuous to feel hard things.

CLIENT: (*Looks thoughtful.*)

THERAPIST: As we do this work [of approaching feelings], it will be important to have your permission. I want you to know that you can say "no," or you can say "yes" and then change your mind. You can also tell me when you have reached your limit or when we need to slow down . . . I know that sometimes you might feel as though you should go along with things, so I will be looking out for this, and I will ask you directly sometimes, if that's OK. The question will be are you *willing* (in this moment) . . . rather than, do you *want* to . . .

Dialogue B (with the "Chinese Handcuffs" Metaphor)

The client is describing discomfort with uncertainty.

CLIENT: I just don't know what I am supposed to do.
    I hate this feeling . . . of not knowing what is right.

THERAPIST: You have been struggling with this feeling for a long time . . . this feeling that things are messy, unpredictable. And how intolerable that feels . . .

CLIENT: Yes. It's awful.

THERAPIST: I can feel you pulling away from it now. Do you sense that?

CLIENT: Yes, I suppose so.

THERAPIST: And that feeling of constriction.

CLIENT: (*Affirms.*)

THERAPIST: What if it is like one of those Chinese finger traps, when you pull . . .

CLIENT: It gets tighter . . .

THERAPIST: Yeah, the more you pull, the tighter it gets . . . (*Demonstrates.*) Do you know how you get out of one of those?

CLIENT: You push your fingers in, like this.

THERAPIST: Yeah, and it loosens, right? Weird but true.
    Fighting with uncertainty . . . maybe that's what gets you stuck? Trying to take all the guesswork out of your life? (*long pause*) (*Client nods.*)
    There are things you can't do because uncertainty might be there . . . like being with other people. It's hard to be with people because it is so uncertain and relationships are messy.
    I wonder if our work could be about finding a way to *live* with uncertainty. To allow it as a feeling . . . ?

CLIENT: How do I do that?

THERAPIST: Well, we start by looking for places that uncertainty can show up and practice turning toward it. Spending some time with it—anything other than avoidance really . . .

CLIENT: That sounds awful!

THERAPIST: I hear you; it will be hard. And I appreciate that your mind will not like what I am suggesting at all. . . . Any work that we do would be with your permission and as slowly as you want. You set the pace . . . and you can say "yes" and change your mind. I will be checking in with you all along the way . . .

Dialogue C (with the "Tug-of-War with a Monster" Metaphor)

The client is describing her ambivalence about letting go of AN.

CLIENT: If I start eating more . . . I won't have anything that sets me apart, makes me special. . . . So even though I know it is hurting my family, I kind of go back and forth with this in my mind, trying to figure it out.

THERAPIST: It's like on one side is "you" and on the other side is the fear and the thought "I am not special or interesting in any way." You have been in this tug-of-war for a long time, hoping to win and know that you are OK . . . that you are special [cared about? worthwhile?]. And AN has been part of that, one way in which you pull.

CLIENT: (*Agrees.*)

THERAPIST: What if the answer is not to pull harder but actually to drop the rope? To open up to the fact that sometimes you have these thoughts and feelings . . . and allow them (as thoughts and feelings) . . . I imagine if you let go, you will feel afraid . . . and maybe it will also free you. Like, what might you do if you were not stuck in this tug-of-war?

Dialogue D (with the "Dam" Metaphor)

The client is describing her preoccupation with food and eating.

CLIENT: I am just tired of it. All I can think about is food. I want to be able to think about other things that are important to me.

THERAPIST: It sounds like filling your head with meals and planning allowed you some reprieve, but now there is not even the "good" stuff. By "good" stuff, I mean stuff that feels vital, meaningful, and life giving. . . . Is that your experience?

CLIENT: Yeah. And I want there to be. I'm really sick of it.

THERAPIST: Part of this is probably the effects of undernourishment: As long as you are in this state of deprivation, your mind and body will be oriented to food.

But the other thing is: What if you can't have one without the other? What if in order for the good stuff to be able to come in, the hard stuff has to be welcome, too? That is the place that we can work . . . in opening the gates, not in deciding exactly what comes through . . .

(*pause*)

It's like you have built a dam. Dams are built to control floods. And I am sure that sometimes it feels like you are drowning and the water needs to be dammed. While dams provide protection (and other benefits, such as powering a turbine), they destroy the natural flow of the water. You lose diversity, native species, and the natural beauty of the waterway. Rather than currents and swirls, there are just these still areas of water. Stillness is calm, but it is also lifeless. In places where the water has been completely cut off, the land becomes dry and barren. De-damming restores the natural flow—the water can move freely again. We lose some control in doing this, but we gain things too—the waterway can come back to life. I wonder what it would be like to de-dam . . . whether this will bring things back to life again. Maybe we start with just a small crack . . . see what it is like [to do that] . . . to open up a bit.

Dialogue E

The client is talking about her friendships.

THERAPIST: You've told me how important your friends are to you. And it occurs to me that you know them, but they don't really know you. You sort of hide yourself from them. Don't fully let them see you. You do a lot for them, but you don't share yourself.

CLIENT: I want to let them in. I'm just scared . . . scared that, I don't know. It sounds stupid when I say it out loud, but I guess I'm scared that they won't really like me . . .

THERAPIST: So you're scared that if you show more of yourself, are more open and vulner-able, then you'll experience rejection . . .

CLIENT: Yeah. I am. I know this keeps me at a distance from them, though, and I don't like that.

THERAPIST: So there is fear and there's something meaningful in there—in opening up to them?

CLIENT: Yes.

THERAPIST: And so, by allowing the feeling of fear—creating a space for the physical sensa-tions in your gut or your chest, allowing the thought "They won't like me" to be present *as a thought*—you open up the possibility of being closer to people you care about . . . ?

CLINICAL GOAL 3: *Teach the Client to Discriminate Initial Reactions from Secondary Responses*

The therapist teaches the client to discriminate emotional pain (i.e., reactions that we have to events just as a product of being a conscious human being with a history) from the suf-fering that occurs as we evaluate, judge, or reject our experience. This occurs in session, as illustrated in the dialogues below, and may be practiced between sessions using Handout 7.3, which appears at the end of this chapter; a copy you can download and use in your work with clients is provided on the publisher's website (see the box at the end of the table of contents).

IN PRACTICE

Dialogue

THERAPIST: I am wondering how you are feeling?

CLIENT: I don't know . . . I feel really upset about it . . . It's so stupid [to be upset].

THERAPIST: You almost let yourself have that emotion: Allowed yourself to be upset . . . and then your mind stepped in. You started judging yourself for feeling that way. Did you notice that?

CLIENT: I do feel that way . . . stupid, I mean . . . for being upset.

THERAPIST: I hear you . . . and I also notice there are two things in there. There is the experience that you have just as a product of being a conscious human being, with a pulse. Life hits you with something hard and you feel upset.

And then something else happens. You hit yourself again with "stupid." You respond to your reaction with judgment. It's a very human thing to do . . .

So there are two things in there. The initial experience (which is painful) and then the additional struggle that comes as you evaluate or judge your emotional response.

I guess I am wondering, does that actually make it harder to carry, rather than carrying upset, you are carrying "upset" + "stupid"? Imagine that each one is a boulder on top of you (*therapist gestures placing an imaginary boulder representing "upset" and then adding a second imaginary boulder representing "stupid" on the client*).

CLIENT: (*Agrees and elaborates on her experience.*)

THERAPIST: I wonder if you would be willing to just start tracking this: Practice noticing when you have an emotion, and also noticing when you are judging or rejecting that experience as bad or wrong?

CLINICAL GOAL 4: *Continue to Shape Acceptance of Unwanted Internal Experience*

As clients gain a greater capacity to notice and allow feelings for brief durations, the therapist elaborates this practice, shaping willingness to allow a broader range of experience for longer periods of time and at varying degrees of intensity (when doing so serves the client's personal values). This might include allowing a simple somatic sensation (e.g., pit in the stomach) or a coordinated system of responses (body sensations, thoughts, memories, urges) labeled as an *emotion*. For example, in working on shaping acceptance of anxiety, the individual is working to allow the presence of feelings of tightness in the chest, turning in the gut, the thought "I am going to mess this up," memories of the last time she "messed up," urges to run, and so forth.

We provide some examples of acceptance-building strategies in Table 7.2. Clients are encouraged not only to allow feelings but also to interact with them in new ways (ways other than avoidance and control). The goal is broad and flexible repertoires in the presence of any and all thoughts and feelings. With a greater capacity to allow internal experiences, individuals with AN may come to know themselves more deeply and meet their needs.

For many individuals with AN, opening up to their feelings (even something as basic as the breath moving through the body) can feel overwhelming. It is the therapist's responsibility to titrate this experience accordingly. The therapist is aiming for the place where the client is challenged but not unable to cope without avoidance or escape. For some clients

TABLE 7.2. Sample Acceptance Strategies

Strategy	Sample dialogue
Label the feeling.	"I am noticing the feeling of [fear/anxiety, sadness]."
Describe the qualities of the feeling.	"Can you describe it to me like you might describe the texture of this fabric? Is it a knot, a pit, or butterflies? Is it sharp or dull?"
Describe the location of the feeling in the body.	"Where do you notice it most? Is it in your chest, your throat, or somewhere else in your body?"
Breathe air around the feeling.	"I wonder if you could practice breathing air around it, giving it some space."
Release around the feeling.	"We often tighten when we have a feeling we don't like. Could we practice releasing or softening your body . . . neither holding in the feeling, nor bracing against it or holding it out. Let's start with your toes. . . . Can you release your toes . . . ?"
Have the outside match the inside.	"I notice that you often smile when you feel something hard. I wonder if you could let your facial expression match how you are feeling; see if you can melt the smile and allow the feeling to come through . . ."

Make an invitation.	"What would it be like to . . .
	    "Welcome this feeling?
	    "Allow what is already here to be here?
	    "Permit this experience as it is?
	    "Invite this feeling in . . . maybe offer it a seat, like you would a guest in your home?"

Assume a receiving posture.	"Would you be willing to open your hands, like you would if you were going to receive a gift? This feeling is here anyway. Can you receive it?" The therapist might gesture a gentle handing of something to the client.
Physically turn toward or allow physical closeness to an experience (e.g., using objects in the room as representation of the internal experience).	"Imagine that this [object] represents this feeling that you have, and everything in you wants to turn away. . . . What would it be like to turn toward it, could you allow it?" "Can we practice letting it sit here next to us? Can you allow it to be closer, maybe hold it in your hand or place it on your lap? We can hold it together, if you like . . ."
Cue a behavioral repertoire of gentle holding.	"Imagine holding this feeling like you might a pup or a precious gem." "Maybe you could bring it to your chest (with your hands) and hold it close to your heart."
Cue a behavioral repertoire of appreciation.	"What would it be like to observe this feeling . . . like you might a sunset (rather than treating it like a problem to be solved)?" "If this [emotion] was an abstract painting . . . what colors and patterns might you notice?"

(continued)

TABLE 7.2. *(continued)*

Strategy	Sample dialogue
Cue a behavioral repertoire of observation or curiosity.	"Let's assume that you are a reporter or a scientist. What would you describe?
	"Imagine this experience like a checklist. Tightness in chest. Check. Turning of stomach. Check. Warmth or heat in face. Check. The thought that I am going to screw this up. Check. The urge to run. Check."
	"Imagine that I have never experienced this before, and it is your job to describe it in rich detail—from how it feels at the bottom to the top of the emotion wave. . . . If this feeling could speak, what would it say? What is its communication about what you need (if anything)?"
Take it with you.	"We have written your experiences on cards (your thoughts, feelings, body sensations, urges, memories, etc.). I invite you to take them with you . . . in your backpack or pocket. They are coming with you anyway, but it is a different sort of thing to *choose* to take them. . . ."

(or at some stages of therapy), it might be appropriate to observe internal experience for 30 seconds; for others it might be 15 minutes. The therapist starts "where the client is" and reinforces successive approximations to experiential willingness. Helping clients label experiences can also make the experiences more manageable. As previously mentioned, acceptance work is always in the service of values (or what the individuals wants for her life) and values should be palpable during this work. Below are several sample dialogues illustrating how the therapist might help the client open up to unwanted experiences. Dialogue C uses the metaphor of a wave, which mirrors the natural rhythm of emotion (i.e., the rise and fall that would naturally occur if there were not unnecessary attempts to change the experience).

IN PRACTICE

Dialogue A

THERAPIST: It looked like you tensed up just then. Did you notice?

CLIENT: Not until you mentioned it, but yeah.

THERAPIST: Is it hard to talk about friendships and how alone you have felt?

CLIENT: Yes, and I do feel tense.

THERAPIST: Where do you notice the tension?

CLIENT: (*Gestures.*)

THERAPIST: So here and here (*gesturing*). I am wondering what else you notice? . . . Another sensation in your body (like your heartbeat), or maybe something you would label an emotion?

CLIENT: I feel a lot of things. It's all kind of jumbled up . . .

THERAPIST: I wonder if we could just take an inventory, unpack it a bit—see what's in there?

Like imagine you have a box of little treasures . . . items of interest, and imagine we could take them out one by one—and be curious about each of them? (*Gestures as if they are unpacking a box—with a gentle, kind motion.*)

CLIENT: (*Describes each experience with the therapist guidance*) . . . This is really hard.

THERAPIST: And you have mostly stayed away from it—but not today (*with gratitude*). I wonder if, in this moment, you can connect with (or sense) how this might be meaningful to you . . . how allowing these feelings might make it possible for you to take risks and be with people in the way that you wish for . . .

Dialogue B

CLIENT: I haven't heard from my sister in a while. I wonder if she is mad at me or . . . (*Goes on at length with detailed content that lacks emotion language.*)

THERAPIST: You sound worried, but is there also a hint of sadness in there?

CLIENT: I don't know, I shouldn't feel sad about it. She is allowed to have her life! Her husband is . . . (*Goes on at length giving details of her sister's life.*)

THERAPIST: I notice that when sadness shows up, you move away from it quickly. You also invalidate your experience—saying that you shouldn't feel that way or it doesn't matter if that is how you feel. I am wondering if we could do something different this time. . . . If instead we can take time to acknowledge the feeling, allow it, and see if there is something in there for you? Like maybe it communicates something about what you value—what is important to you?

CLIENT: Yes, I suppose we can.

THERAPIST: You can say no. . . . It is always up to you . . .

CLIENT: It's all right. I want to . . . well, I don't really want to, but if you think it is important . . . I can see how it might be.

THERAPIST: Does the feeling exist somewhere in your body?

CLIENT: (*Nods.*)

THERAPIST: Where can you feel it most?

CLIENT: In my chest and stomach . . .

THERAPIST: Can you tell me about its qualities . . . what it is like?

CLIENT: It feels like a pit.

THERAPIST: Like a gaping hole kind of pit, or a pit like the center of a fruit?

CLIENT: Like a solid pit. And like I can't breathe.

THERAPIST: It looks like it might be coming into your throat too . . . like it is hard to swallow.

CLIENT: Yeah, feels like choking, kinda. (*Drops shoulders as if a weight is on her back.*)

THERAPIST: Sometimes sadness has a heaviness to it. We say we "have the weight of the world on our shoulders" because of this quality of sadness.

CLIENT: (*Nods.*) (*A little teary.*)

THERAPIST: What would it be like to allow that feeling . . . allow yourself to feel sad and heavy in the body, maybe you could actually breathe air into or around that feeling?

CLIENT: I don't want to feel this way.

THERAPIST: I know. The only way to do that is to not care about your sister, though . . . to not care about relationships. And, even then . . .

This is how it feels when we care about someone and miss closeness with them.

CLIENT: (*Holds her breath.*)

THERAPIST: Can you breathe air into your chest? Can you create some space for that feeling in your throat? . . . Allow sadness (it is here anyway). (*Motions to the client an invitation to raise her chin up and make eye contact.*) I wonder, even in the presence of this emotion, can you stay with me . . . ?

Dialogue C (with the "Wave" Metaphor)

CLIENT: I feel so anxious. It's awful. I just want it to go away.

THERAPIST: Have you ever stood on the beach and allowed a wave to just wash over you? (*Gestures.*) Allowing the wave to wash over you is different than diving into it (jumping in and body surfing; letting the wave knock you about). It is also different than fighting against it (trying to hold the wave back). It is standing there on the shore, allowing the rhythm of the wave to move through you while your toes are buried in the sand. The wave rises up and falls, and rises again.

It is similar to the rhythm of the breath moving through your body.

You might feel a little pull of the undercurrent (or sometimes a big pull) . . . and you can stand there, toes in the mud. What if we could do that . . . right now with this emotion? Practice this kind of arms-open stance, practice moving with the rhythm of the waves, using the breath as an anchor.

Would you be willing? This would be doing something different with that feeling than what you may have done in the past—it would be having it, instead of it having you. Allowing it to move through you.

If you can do it in here, you are more likely to be able to do it out there, when it matters most . . .

Dialogue D

THERAPIST: (*Noticing a change in the client's body language.*) What is coming up for you right now?

CLIENT: I guess I just feel anxious.

THERAPIST: Can you also notice what you are doing with that feeling? Are you fighting with it, trying to push it away (*gestures pushing something away*)?

CLIENT: I don't know. I do want it to go away. . . . I have felt like this for so long.

THERAPIST: I notice that it looks as though you are physically braced against it, like you are tensing your muscles in your body and face to either keep it out or keep it in. Can you feel that?

CLIENT: Yeah . . .

THERAPIST: What do you notice—in particular?

CLIENT: (*Describes sensations with some assistance.*)

THERAPIST: So it seems this is what it feels like to fight, at least at this moment, with this feeling.

> I wonder if we can also sample the alternative (what it feels like to open up to this feeling)?

> Could you release your muscles and allow the feeling to flow more freely through you . . . ?

Dialogue E (with an "Avoided Events" Card Exercise)

THERAPIST: It occurs to me that there are all these thoughts and feelings that are hard to have, and I am wondering if we can create a deck of cards together, representing these different experiences.

CLIENT: Uh, OK.

THERAPIST: We can then use the deck of cards to practice opening up to these experiences. What should we put on the first one?

CLIENT: Feeling fat?

THERAPIST: Absolutely. What else?

CLIENT: (*Gives other examples.*)

THERAPIST: I am also thinking about other experiences that you have described . . . like feeling "off" or awkward.

CLIENT: I hate it. I never know the right thing to do or say. I feel like such an idiot. . . . I think people think I am a "try hard" . . . I don't know what I am doing with my life either. . . . I feel like such a wreck . . . my eating is the only thing that I can get in line.

THERAPIST: So there are all these thoughts and feelings about whether you are doing good or right, if people like you and if you are going anywhere in your life. Feelings of uncertainty—fear and some shame? This thought about being a wreck seems particularly powerful. (*Writes single words on a card summarizing the client's experience.*)

> What do you want to do with these?

CLIENT: Burn them?!

THERAPIST: Ha ha! And you've kind of been trying that! I wonder if we can try something different, like what if we first just give each a nod . . . and place it in your lap? "There is thought *X* or feeling *Y*." (*Coaches at a slow deliberate pace. The client has a reaction to "wreck," which feels overwhelming.*) Maybe we can hold this one together? As a thought or feeling that feels powerful. (*Holds one end and offers the other end to the client.*) What is it like to hold this experience?

Acceptance Work Is Not Always "Serious," but It Is Always Compassionate

Acceptance may include relating to experiences in a playful manner. For example, difficult thoughts and feelings can be personified, can be given character, a voice, mannerisms, or a name. The client may welcome or open up to this character in some way (e.g., offering a place to sit or offering tea). These interventions, which also function as defusion and strengthening the observer self, can help clients stay with uncomfortable experiences longer and relate to them in a new way. Playful interventions should always be engaged in a compassionate manner that respects the power that these thoughts and feelings have in other contexts.

Cueing an Unwanted Internal Experience for Acceptance Practice

The most compelling acceptance practice is often in the moment, as unwanted internal experiences naturally arise in session. However, the therapist can also cue unwanted internal events for practice. This can be accomplished through structured exercises that block avoidance behavior and increase contact with unwanted thoughts and feelings. For example, clients might be asked to imagine relinquishing AN (or punitive self-control; e.g., breaking a rule) and notice the thoughts/feelings that arise, or to release the physical constriction of the body, which often functions to constrain affect (illustrated in Dialogues A and B).

The therapist can also cue unwanted internal experiences for acceptance practice via retrospective recall of difficult events that occurred over the last week. Clients may be invited to enter into a moment of difficulty during the past week and "look through" their eyes, describing the scene in detail with five senses (what they hear, smell, etc.). If the client coped with the experience by restricting, purging, or exercise, the therapist might ask the client to imagine that she was not able to engage in these behaviors. Difficult internal experiences might also be cued by repeating a key phrase that captures the experience, or asking the client to repeat the phrase or tell the story at a slower pace (frame by frame, as if it was a movie in slow motion). Dialogue C illustrates this approach with a client with limited emotional awareness. Dialogue D illustrates this approach with an aware client and is able to progress to a deeper expression of acceptance (i.e., the practice of allowing difficult feelings for a longer period of time).

IN PRACTICE

Dialogue A (with the "Giving Over" Exercise)
The client is talking about herself in a derogatory manner.

CLIENT: I don't know why I don't just get up and do something. I am so pathetic.

THERAPIST: I wonder if you notice how you talk to yourself. . . . From this chair, it sounds really painful. Like can you imagine saying that to a child—maybe a younger version of yourself?

CLIENT: (*Makes a disgusted face.*) I see what you mean, for a kid, but I deserve it . . .

THERAPIST: So there is compassion for a younger you, but not you now . . .

It's a funny sort of thing (that happens to humans) . . .

The "you" who was *there and then* is the same "you" who is *here-and-now* . . . not in a logical way, but as a matter of experience . . . it is the same you . . .

I wonder if we can do something. . . . Imagine that all that stuff you say to yourself, like:

"You're fat."

"You're lazy."

"You just want to get out of doing things."

"What's wrong with you? You are so gross, disgusting. Get up!"

Imagine that I could take it from you. That you could hand it over to me, and I could just put it over here, with all these things that are not being used. (*Gestures to stacks of papers and books in the office.*)

CLIENT: (*Looks worried.*)

THERAPIST: I will give it back to you. . . . You won't leave session without it, but imagine for a moment that you could give them over (*Holds hands out to receive something.*) What shows up?

CLIENT: Terror.

THERAPIST: Terror. Tell me more. What specifically do you notice [thoughts, feelings, body sensations, memories, etc.]?

Dialogue B (with the "Releasing the Body" Exercise)

The client is asked to release her muscles to open up to experience in the moment.

THERAPIST: Would it be OK if we tried something? I wonder what it would be like to uncross and drop your arms (*pauses with invitation*) and drop your shoulders. . . . Would you be willing to try this with me? You don't have to; it is completely your choice. I bring it up because when our physical bodies are held that way, it is often to hold something (like an emotion) in or hold something (like the world) out.

I am wondering, what would it be like to allow your physical body to soften right now? So that it isn't clamped down or braced against anything . . . ?

CLIENT: (*Starts to drop arms, crosses them back.*) I feel better like this . . .

THERAPIST: Can you describe what feels better? What do you notice?

CLIENT: Letting my arms down feels so exposed . . .

THERAPIST: Something shows up there—"exposed," "vulnerable," even in just the idea of doing it. . . . I wonder if we can just pause here.

Dialogue C (with Retrospective Recall; Client with Low Awareness)

The therapist is reviewing the client's homework. The client completed a diary card of AN behaviors.

THERAPIST: Tell me about these days when it was hard to eat dinner. What were you feeling?

CLIENT: I don't know, really.

THERAPIST: Can we do something together? I want to see if we can drop into one of these moments . . . enter in through memory.

CLIENT: OK.

THERAPIST: I want to see if we can notice what thoughts and feelings you might have been experiencing. Maybe we could enter at the mealtime, but then go back in time a bit. Would that be OK?

CLIENT: Yes.

THERAPIST: Let's first slow down to arrive here in this moment, with your breath . . . (*Leads a brief centering exercise.*) And then let's see if we can go back to this moment. The moment when you were faced with this choice . . . "Do I or do I not eat?"

See if you can paint a picture clearly in your mind and drop into this memory, looking from your own eyes. Can you describe the scene for me? What do you see? Hear? Smell?

CLIENT: (*Describes.*)

THERAPIST: OK, and now I want you to check in with your experience. What do you notice happening in your mind? Tell me a thought you notice?

CLIENT: (*Describes.*)

THERAPIST: OK, great. What do you feel in your body?

CLIENT: (*Describes.*)

THERAPIST: If you were going to give it an emotion label, what might it be?

CLIENT: (*Describes.*)

THERAPIST: Now, let's take a step backward. What was happening earlier in the day . . . ?

CLIENT: (*Describes events.*)

THERAPIST: What were you thinking and feeling?

Dialogue D (with Retrospective Recall; Client with Awareness)

THERAPIST: Take me into that moment at dinner, when you decided, "I've had enough."

CLIENT: I was feeling so guilty. Like I didn't deserve to eat.

THERAPIST: This is something that you feel quite a lot . . . that you don't deserve things . . .
Can you drop into this space and really pull up that feeling [of not deserving things, guilt]?

CLIENT: It's hard to do. I can't really. I think I just shut it down.

THERAPIST: Tell me in detail about that moment. . . . Paint the scene, as richly as you can . . .

CLIENT: I was sitting at the kitchen table. My husband was staring at me. I know what he was thinking. The look on his face . . . but all I could think about was how I am screwing everything up.

THERAPIST: Can you imagine his face; trace it in your mind.

CLIENT: Yes.

THERAPIST: Can you see the table . . . your plate?

CLIENT: Yes, the table is kind of this wood grain. I hate it, actually.

THERAPIST: And the smells, maybe you could feel yourself in the chair . . .

CLIENT: Yeah, I am starting to feel my stomach upset.

THERAPIST: Can you notice that feeling of guilt . . .

CLIENT: Yeah. (*Looks down.*)

THERAPIST: I wonder if we can notice that feeling without having to push it away or channel it into the eating disorder. You have the feeling, not the feeling having you. (*pause*) I wonder if you can look up at me, if we can hold this together. . . . Guilt . . . this set of thoughts and feelings, maybe urges, memories . . . experiences that can be held tightly.

It might be that by having (and holding) this feeling in here together, we make it possible for you to have it "out there" too . . . without having to do something to make it go away.

Ending Acceptance-Focused Sessions

It is useful to end sessions that focus heavily on acceptance (or willingness) with a clear directive of how to generalize the work to the client's daily life. The therapist encourages the client to practice acceptance in difficult moments outside of the session and identifies committed actions for the week, as illustrated in the following therapist script and dialogue.

IN PRACTICE

Therapist Script

"This feeling is going to show up over the next week as you are living your life.

"I suspect that it will show up when you return your friend's call, for example . . . and rather than push it away, I wonder if you can practice what we did in session today? Maybe you can use the mantra 'Welcome anxiety, I thought I might see you here' and breathe air around the tightness in your chest.

"The goal is not to make the feeling go away, but to give it some space, to allow it to be, so that you can do the things that matter to you."

Dialogue

THERAPIST: What would it be like to carry this experience forward—so the next time you are faced with this feeling, you don't have to be pushed around by it? You don't *have to* run away. *You* get to decide (what you do or don't do).

CLIENT: I would like that.

THERAPIST: Let's think together about when the next opportunity will be. What does the rest of your day look like [activities/schedule]?

CLINICAL GOAL 5: *Leverage Acceptance to Meet Needs*

Allowing internal experience (e.g., feelings of fear, guilt, or shame) increases the client's ability to meet her needs. This includes not only her physical needs (e.g., the need for food or rest) but also her emotional needs (e.g., the need for comfort or social support, or joy). As the client practices allowing feelings, she not only comes to know herself and her signals, but she is also better able to take effective action (breaking "rules" when doing so would be effective, e.g., resting when tired despite feelings of guilt). The following dialogues illustrate how acceptance may be leveraged to meet needs.

Dialogue A (Leveraging Acceptance to Facilitate Eating)

THERAPIST: We can bet that overwhelmed will show up the next time you are faced with a meal . . . and I wonder, could you open yourself up to it, like we have here? Allow overwhelmed?

CLIENT: How?

THERAPIST: Let's see if we can actually walk through this together. It is 4 o'clock now. When will you be eating dinner? Who will be there?

CLIENT: Probably 6:30 . . . Mom and Dad, maybe my brother.

THERAPIST: See if you can put yourself there now. Imagine that overwhelmed comes to dinner, too. You think it is likely?

CLIENT: Yes.

THERAPIST: See if you can imagine offering overwhelmed a seat (since it was coming anyway).

> Imagine allowing overwhelmed to be there . . . as a feeling . . . (*pause*) . . . maybe a tangle of feelings . . . it might be useful to see what all is in there. Thoughts, feelings, urges. . . . See if we can allow them to be present while you choose to eat dinner with your family.

Dialogue B

THERAPIST: It sounds like you knew you were tired, but you just couldn't let yourself sit down.

CLIENT: Yes, I just felt so lazy. I wasn't sure that I had done enough to warrant sitting.

THERAPIST: So there was the thought "I am lazy" and guilt . . . and this sense that you needed to earn rest before you could allow it. What would it be like to rest, earned or not? To choose to be kind to yourself and responsive to your needs . . .

CLIENT: Uhh.

THERAPIST: Can you just allow that feeling right now, that feeling of "Uhh"? Breathe air around it . . .

> (*Later in session*) I would like to invite you to try this the next time you notice you are tired; see if you can allow the thoughts and feelings (as thoughts and feelings) and do what would be effective (rest). . . .

Advanced Acceptance

Clinical Goals 6 and 7 involve more advanced acceptance work. This work is engaged as the therapeutic focus continues to broaden beyond AN and clients have some additional clarity about their personal values. Clinical Goal 6 focuses on helping clients discriminate when they are moving *away from* unwanted internal experiences versus *moving toward* something that is meaningful or in the direction of their values. Clinical Goal 7 expands clients' capacity for acceptance using behavioral challenges. Behavioral challenges create conditions for clients to experience emotional discomfort and practice willingness. Behavioral challenges increase the client's capacity to behave effectively in evocative situations and, when explicitly linked to a value, are considered committed actions (see Chapter 8).

CLINICAL GOAL 6: *Help Clients Discriminate the Motivations of Their Actions*

It may be difficult at times to determine whether behavior is motivated by experiential avoidance or personal values. This might be particularly true for individuals with AN, whose avoidant repertoires include prosocial interpersonal behaviors. For example, sometimes orienting to another person's preferences is driven by *avoidance* of conflict; other times, it might be in service of the *value* of giving to others. Behavior that is motivated by avoidance will feel rigid and compelled, rather than flexible and free (or freely chosen). This can be an important discrimination to teach and practice in session, and it will clarify targets and opportunities for acceptance work. Figure 7.2 might be a useful discrimination tool to aid in this practice and may be revisited during values clarification (Chapter 8).

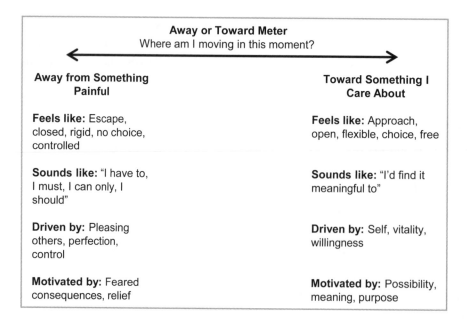

FIGURE 7.2. Away and Toward Meter that discriminates whether actions are motivated by moving *away from* emotional discomfort (e.g., anxiety, guilt, or shame) or *toward* something meaningful (i.e., values). Figure contributed by Ashley A. Moskovich, PhD.

CLINICAL GOAL 7: *Expand the Client's Capacity for Acceptance with Behavioral Challenges*

Behavioral challenges create conditions for clients to experience emotional discomfort and practice willingness. This expands the client's capacity to allow unwanted thoughts and feelings when doing so would be effective or life enhancing. Some behavioral challenges center on food or eating (e.g., Dialogue A), while others do not (Dialogue B). Often, they include breaking rules. Table 7.3 provides a list of behavioral challenges relevant to clients

TABLE 7.3. Behavioral Challenges That Build the Client's Capacity to Allow Unwanted Thoughts and Feelings

Behavioral challenge	Description
Stopping before a deadline	The client practices stopping preparation in advance of a due date or sets a time limit for studying in the evening.
Making a mistake	The client practices not correcting a mistake (e.g., not rewriting something or apologizing for a minor transgression) or making a new one (e.g., writing with her nondominant hand).
Engaging in play	The client practices engaging in activities that are not achievement oriented (e.g., playing a game in session, going to a park).
Expressing freely	The client practices not filtering expression (e.g., free word association, journaling, impressionistic art).
Having an opinion	The client practices expressing opinions (to the therapist or to other people in her natural environment).
Making eye contact	The client practices making eye contact in and outside of session (e.g., when passing in a hallway or during a conversation).
Setting a boundary	The client practices setting a boundary (e.g., saying "no," limiting her availability for something).
Taking up space	The client practices releasing rather than constricting muscles, or purposefully assuming a "bigger" body posture (spreading out).
Inconveniencing someone	The client practices inconveniencing someone (e.g., reschedules, asks someone to wait).
Communicating a need	The client practices expressing needs to other people (e.g., asking to change the temperature of the room, indicating the need to stop for lunch when out with friends).
Doing something spontaneous	The client practices engaging in activities that are unplanned (e.g., stops at another store, takes an invitation to join someone for coffee).
Inhibiting overapologizing	The client practices not apologizing for things that were not under her control.
Taking compliments	The client practices saying "thank you" without downplaying or caveats.
Allowing disarray	The client practices allowing her physical space to be out of order, or allowing something in session to be "unfinished" or "unclear."

with AN. Many of these challenges can be practiced in session, as well as being assigned for homework. If a client sets an intention to complete a behavioral challenge as homework and is unable to complete it over the week, this provides fodder for acceptance work and the opportunity to practice in session (as illustrated in Dialogue C).

Behavioral challenges are are not entered into lightly. Willingness comes from a deep sense that this is *for something* (i.e., the life the individual wants). As such, this practice may only be possible after the client has further clarified her personal values (see Chapter 8). It may also be necessary to shape successive approximations to the target behavioral challenge (i.e., identifying smaller steps).

IN PRACTICE

Dialogue A

The client's weight has improved and she has added variety to her diet. The therapist is inviting the client to introduce flexibility in her eating schedule.

CLIENT: I am scared to do that. I have already made so many changes.

THERAPIST: You have, that is absolutely true. And it has been possible because you have been willing to face fear . . . to allow fear to be present and to walk in the direction of your values. This is another practice in that—a little different in that it is focused on increasing flexibility in your eating schedule (rather than increasing the amount or types of food you are eating), but at the process level, it is the same. It is you saying "yes" to fear or discomfort in order to expand your life space . . . so that you don't have to live constrained by *when* you must or mustn't eat . . .

CLIENT: I want to be able to do that . . . but what you are suggesting is too much.

THERAPIST: What would feel like the right practice for you? We are looking for something that is challenging but does not exceed your willingness.

CLIENT: Well . . . I could have dinner a little later . . . maybe 30 minutes or so, 5:30 instead of at 5:00 . . .

THERAPIST: OK, that sounds great! Let's plan for that. What thoughts/feelings do you imagine will show up as 5:00 approaches . . . and passes?

Dialogue B (Discussing a Behavioral Challenge Homework)

THERAPIST: You set an intention to speak up in class. How did it go?

CLIENT: I did it, but it was awful.

THERAPIST: Even better. It was hard *and* you did it. Good for you! Tell me more about "awful."

CLIENT: I just felt stupid . . . everyone was looking at me . . .

THERAPIST: "Stupid" is familiar to you . . . something that shows up a lot . . . especially when you are in these situations. Sometimes it keeps you from getting your needs met (you don't ask questions, for example). This time it didn't (*smiles*).

CLIENT: I suppose . . . (*Expands on "stupid."*)

THERAPIST: I hear you . . . these thoughts/feelings are still so powerful (*pause*) . . . I wonder if we can practice holding these experiences lightly now, with compassion . . .

Dialogue C

The therapist and client are discussing the behavioral challenge of dropping off a job application. The dialogue that follows highlights how a behavioral challenge that was not completed provides an opportunity for reinforcement of successive approximations and in-session practice. It also illustrates how acceptance work can be playful and references a variant of the "Passengers on the Bus" metaphor.

CLIENT: I didn't do it. I went to the store but just sat in the parking lot with my application.

THERAPIST: You went to the store! That is great!

CLIENT: Yeah, but I didn't turn in the application.

THERAPIST: Notice how your mind likes to take things from you. Can you allow yourself to pause and notice that you went to the store?

CLIENT: (*Smiles.*) Yes, I suppose . . . (*long pause*) My mom was there and she wasn't helpful. She kept saying, "Why can't you just do it" and "It isn't that hard." People who don't deal with social anxiety just don't understand. My mom tried to show me how to do it, but she said it in a way that I would never do. Kind of rude. Just "I am turning in this application," really abrupt or something.

THERAPIST: Did you ask your mom to show you?

CLIENT: Yeah.

THERAPIST: That felt safer [to have an example]. . . . This is the process of opening up to anxiety or fear, it doesn't happen all at once.

CLIENT: Yeah.

THERAPIST: Being able to turn in this application is important to you?

CLIENT: (*Nods.*) I have to be able to do these things.

THERAPIST: Are you willing to practice with me now? I'll pretend to be the store clerk.

CLIENT: Um . . . (*long pause*)

THERAPIST: You don't have to. . . . It is always your choice. I would encourage you to consider whether you are willing, not whether you want to, though. (*Smiles.*) It might be useful.

CLIENT: OK.

THERAPIST: Here, you can use this. (*Hands the client a piece of paper.*) Pretend it's your application.

CLIENT: (*Pauses, looks unsure.*)

THERAPIST: There is no right way; in fact, do it wrong!

CLIENT: Can you show me first?

THERAPIST: I'm wondering what feelings are coming up for you.

CLIENT: (*Describes.*)

THERAPIST: Asking me to show you now . . . is it the same thing as asking your mom then . . . driven by fear?

CLIENT: (*Agrees.*) (*Long pause, unable to do it herself without an example.*)

THERAPIST: (*Moves to shaping an approximation.*) How about if I do it silly—do it how you would never do it?! (*Engages in a series of role plays. Pretends to hand in the application using a loud, rude tone. A quiet, mousy tone. Waves it around. Makes funny gestures during the exercise, etc.*)

CLIENT: (*Smiles.*) Ha ha, that is helpful.

THERAPIST: Now, you give it a try.

CLIENT: Can I do it serious?

THERAPIST: Absolutely! However you want.

CLIENT: "Hi, I am here to turn in my application. I also completed the materials online. If you are not hiring right now, can you keep my application on file, please?"

THERAPIST: You did it!

CLIENT: (*Smiles.*)

THERAPIST: Let's go back to the moment in the car . . . and take a look at what got in the way. What thoughts/feelings did you notice (when you were sitting in the car with your mom)?

CLIENT: "They are going to laugh at me. . . . They are going to laugh at my outfit. They are not taking me seriously . . ."

THERAPIST: (*Writes content in thought bubbles and puts paper above head playfully.*) Like this?

CLIENT: (*Smiles.*)

THERAPIST: How about you read these thoughts, really get with them (let them hook you and let the emotion show up), and then do it again?

CLIENT: I would rather leave on a high note!

THERAPIST: How so?

CLIENT: You said I did a good job!

THERAPIST: Oh! I see! You don't want to practice again because it might not work out as well. Notice this is your mind evaluating your performance (as good/bad).

This is not really about the outcome, but the process of doing it. If you are willing, I suggest doing it again with these thoughts and feelings really present. I realize it is a massive act of willingness. And it is always your choice.

CLIENT: OK.

THERAPIST: Great! (*Helps the client contact these thoughts/feelings.*)

CLIENT: I can feel tightness in my chest and my heart beating . . .

THERAPIST: Perfect!

CLIENT: (*Repeats the exercise.*)

THERAPIST: You did it! *With* anxiety! I love it!

Maybe we could think about other times anxiety has been getting in the way this week . . . stopping you from doing something you want to do.

CLIENT: Well, I went to the coffee shop near my house, but I wasn't able to order coffee. I was going to go in, but there were a lot of people my age in there . . . so I decided not to . . . I just walked by.

THERAPIST: At that moment, when you walked by the coffee shop, anxiety was deciding . . . what you get to do and what you don't get to do. It was driving the bus.

CLIENT: Yes, and I was just sitting in the back! (*Laughs together.*)

THERAPIST: Anxiety at the wheel! Anxiety can come along for the ride, but it doesn't get to drive. . . . You get to drive the bus!

CLIENT: Yeah, it's my life! (*Smiles.*)

THERAPIST: Yes, it is! . . . So how about coffee sometime this week? . . .

Other Considerations in Acceptance Work

Acceptance as Exposure and Response Prevention

In acceptance work, clients make nondefended contact with unwanted internal experiences, and in this sense, acceptance is exposure. However, rather than aim for habituation (as in traditional exposure paradigms), the goal of acceptance is to facilitate broad and flexible behavioral repertoires in the presence of a feared stimulus. Instead of SUD ratings, clients may be asked to report on willingness to allow an experience, such as an emotion. The therapist may also track evidence of greater breadth or flexibility in the client's repertoire in the presence of an unwanted thought or feeling (e.g., the client talking about the experience in new ways, sitting in a more open posture, etc.).

In working with individuals with AN, treatment also commonly includes planned, in-session exposure to feared foods, mirrors, or breaking dietary rules (Dialogue A). It might also include exposure to traumatic memories (Dialogue B). Dialogue C illustrates how the therapist might use the "Avoidance Card" exercise during an exposure to block the entire class of avoidant responses (rather than a single avoidant behavior common in more traditional exposure and response prevention).

Dialogue A

THERAPIST: You brought your oatmeal for the food exposure, excellent! Is this the type of oatmeal that you used to have as a kid?

CLIENT: Yes, this is it. I haven't had it in years. It was my favorite. I didn't put butter in it though.

THERAPIST: Well, I think this is great—and I hope you can appreciate your hard work in approaching this. . . . I also want to say that there is not any virtue in *eating* or *not eating* any particular food (or eating it in any particular way). . . . What we are working on is freedom to choose. (*pause*) What's coming up for you now?

CLIENT: I guess I am just worried that this will make me gain weight . . .

THERAPIST: You are noticing anxiety or fear.

CLIENT: It feels even harder than I imagined. I don't know if I can do it.

THERAPIST: And the thought "I don't know if I can do it." . . . that is coming up too. Maybe we can take a moment to notice what else might be here . . . like what does eating oatmeal represent? . . . What does it feel as though it means?

CLIENT: (*Describes feelings of failure.*)

THERAPIST: And so those thoughts and feelings, too. The thought X. The feeling Y.

CLIENT: I want to do it. I'm just scared. I don't know. Maybe we can do it next time . . .

THERAPIST: We often have the urge to run away when we are afraid. . . . I wonder if we can just take a moment to acknowledge that the urge is here—and also sit with this question of what might be here for you—what might be important about being able to do things that scare you (not just in this moment, but in other moments of your life). . . . (*long pause*) What might that mean for you and your life? And then we can choose to do it today, or not.

Dialogue B

The client has a past experience of unwanted touch. She identifies this experience as central to the development of AN, but has also developed a fairly extensive avoidant repertoire that includes behaviors such as "looking for reasons" (why the event happened), collapsing into self-criticism and self-blame, dissociation, and ritualistic counting.

THERAPIST: I wonder if we can talk about this painful history?

CLIENT: Yikes . . . OK . . .

THERAPIST: I notice that we have both had the urge to avoid it a bit . . . and yet it seems important to do. This memory comes up for you . . . and brings with it other painful thoughts and feelings . . .

We have also noticed that this often coincides with restriction and other behaviors that diminish the quality of your life . . .

CLIENT: Yes. That's true.

THERAPIST: One thing that I want to mention (before we get started) is that as we do this work, you may feel more compelled to engage in these strategies (or other ones) to manage painful thoughts and feelings. In session, we can expect, for example, that you might feel the urge to collapse into guilt or to ask "why," or to do other things that take you out of the moment, like dissociate or count in your head.

With your permission, I would like to see if we can gently set these urges aside, and come back—back to these difficult thoughts/feelings. . . .

Of course, you get to set the limit and the pace. . . . I will be checking in with you throughout and making sure that you are still willing and with me (present in this moment, rather than in some past moment).

Between sessions, it will be important that you continue with your meal plan and that you let me know if you start to struggle.

Unlike other exposure, our goal will not be to make discomfort go away (you have plenty of ways to do that). Our goal will be to help you have the life you would choose *with* your history and your reactions . . .

Dialogue C (with the "Avoidance Card" exercise)

THERAPIST: Right now we have five cards [that represent the strategies that you use to escape or avoid painful thoughts/feelings]: restrict, plan, do for others, stay quiet, and criticize yourself. What is missing? What are the other ways that have gotten you away from the feeling that something is wrong with you?

CLIENT: Well . . . sometimes I distract myself with work. . . . Is that what you mean?

THERAPIST: Absolutely! Let's add that one.

CLIENT: Throwing up . . . although I haven't done that in a long time.

THERAPIST: Yep, I'll write that one. We have also noticed that sometimes you overapologize for things. Does that seem like one?

CLIENT: (*Smiles.*) Yeah, we should probably add it.

THERAPIST: Next time that we are going to a place that is hard (like talking about the divorce), we can expect that some of these things might show up.

If it is OK with you, I'm going to have these cards out so that we can recognize them ("Oh, there is the 'apologize' card") and maybe we can practice setting those behaviors aside and coming back to feeling. . . . Sound OK?

Guilt

Individuals with AN report frequent guilt. Guilt is often a signal that we have violated our personal values. However, among individuals with AN, guilt also often signals fear. For example, clients with AN may feel guilty for not being available to a friend one evening or not completing a work task before leaving for the day. While guilt is related to their personal values, guilty feelings are often driven by fear that these minor transgressions will have severe consequences (e.g., loss of a relationship or a job). Acceptance work includes allowing guilt (which may reflect values), but also opening up to fear. An illustrative dialogue is provided below. Defusion will also be important: helping individuals with AN "unhook" from guilt if there is nothing to learn (about values) and come to the present moment (rather than living in the future of feared consequences).

IN PRACTICE

Dialogue

The client is describing a recent day at work during which she was not particularly talkative.

CLIENT: I don't know, I just feel guilty about it. I should have been more friendly or something.

THERAPIST: It seems like this guilt is a common experience for you, and that it comes up a lot in interpersonal situations.

CLIENT: Yes, especially at work, I often feel bad that I am not talking to people more.

THERAPIST: I am wondering whether this is connected to a value for you . . . like it is important to you to be engaged with other people?

CLIENT: Yes. It is so important to me.

THERAPIST: I wonder what it would be like to hold this guilt gently, like, "Oh, this feeling is reminding me that I care about X."

CLIENT: (*Discusses.*)

THERAPIST: I also wonder about your needs. Maybe at times you need less interaction. . . . And then, maybe, guilt is driven more by fear (fear that you won't be liked or something) . . . (*pauses for response*) I wonder whether there would be something useful about allowing fear, while you do what is best for you . . . ?

Positive Affect

Clients with AN often avoid or suppress positive, as well as negative, affect. Most typically, this is out of fear that if they allow themselves to feel good, this will make them selfish, greedy, or egotistical. Difficulty allowing positive affect might manifest as immediately negating positives (e.g., "I could've done better"), anticipating good things will end, or avoiding things that are pleasurable (e.g., only allowing bland foods). Thus, acceptance with individuals with AN *also includes* opening up to positive internal experiences or allowing pleasure.

Dialogue

THERAPIST: It seems it is hard to allow yourself to feel good (feel proud, take a compliment), enjoy things . . .

CLIENT: Why should I do that? That just seems hedonistic or selfish or something.

THERAPIST: I don't mean to suggest that it is important to feel *any particular* way, but it seems that not allowing yourself to feel good is the same as not allowing yourself to feel bad. It is a continued battle with your emotional life—to control how you feel, rather than allowing it to be as it is.

I get that your mind has things to say about the implications of allowing yourself to feel good . . .

And I also wonder how it might change your life, if you were able to pause in a moment of uplift? Or allow a compliment? Or receive love?

Lack of a Valued Context

There is no special virtue in experiencing painful or uncomfortable thoughts/feelings. However, willingness to do so often makes it possible to engage in things that are meaningful in our lives. If the therapist is feeling stuck in acceptance work, acceptance may not be sufficiently situated in a valued context (i.e., the client is unable to appreciate how being willing might enhance her life). Sometimes acceptance is not situated in a valued context because the client's values are not well articulated or accessible. For example, the client might be unsure about what she cares about other than thinness. In this case, the therapist is pointing to the possibility that allowing feelings may allow for "something more" and building from this foundation as values clarity improves. As mentioned earlier, it might also be necessary to revisit interventions in Chapter 6, which help the client make experiential contact with the unworkability of avoidance and control and prepare for change.

Looking Ahead

In Chapter 8, we describe interventions that help clients author personal values. Values provide an adaptive alternative to using rigid, punitive rules to guide behavioral choices. Rather than action dictated by what one "should" or "must" do, actions are guided by what is personally and deeply meaningful. Values engagement also creates patterns of activity that are incompatible with AN (e.g., it is difficult to maintain rigid exercise routines when richly engaged with family, friends, and meaningful work) and enhances overall quality of life.

Diary Card for Tracking Eating Disorder Episodes

Instructions: Record eating disorder episodes (i.e., times when you engaged in an eating disorder behavior, such as restricting a meal, bingeing, purging, or excessive exercise). Describe the situation: Whom were you with? What were you doing? Describe thoughts and feelings that coincided with the episode, or occurred immediately prior. Were there events earlier in the day that might have influenced your mood (i.e., how you were feeling about yourself or your situation)? Record any observations. There are no wrong answers.

Day/Time Situational Factors (Where were you and whom were you with?)	Eating Disorder Behavior	Eating Disorder Thoughts/Feelings	What else happened earlier in the day that may have influenced your mood? Observations (any other thoughts and feelings that you notice)
Example Monday, 12:00 p.m. At work, alone at my desk.	Skipped lunch.	I feel fat.	I was not able to solve a problem. I think it irritated my boss. I feel stupid for not knowing the answer. I am afraid that I am going to be fired. I am a bad employee that makes bad decisions.

(continued)

Diary Card for Tracking Eating Disorder Episodes *(page 2 of 2)*

Day/Time Situational Factors (Where were you and whom were you with?)	Eating Disorder Behavior	Eating Disorder Thoughts/Feelings	What else happened earlier in the day that may have influenced your mood? Observations (any other thoughts and feelings that you notice)

Eating Disorder "Volume" Diary Card

Instructions: Complete an entry when you notice a change in your eating disorder "volume." Describe the situation and make observations about your internal experiences and events earlier in the day that might have influenced your mood (i.e., how you were feeling about yourself or your situation). If the eating disorder "volume" is high for the majority of a day, consider how this day might be different from other days and record your observations. There are no wrong answers.

Eating Disorder "Volume": Rate 0–10 0–barely there 10–megaphone	What was the situation? (Where were you? What were you doing?)	Observations (any other thoughts, feelings that you notice)
Example 10	I was dress shopping with my mom.	I look so fat. It is no wonder that no one has asked me to go to the dance. I'm disgusting. I think everyone at school hates me.

(continued)

Eating Disorder "Volume": Rate 0–10 0–barely there 10–megaphone	What was the situation? (Where were you? What were you doing?)	Observations (any other thoughts, feelings that you notice)

Initial Reaction and Secondary Response Diary Card

Instructions: We have reactions to the things that happen in our lives. For example, if we lose something important to us, we may feel sad. We also have reactions to our reactions. For example, we might not only feel sad but also feel guilty or upset that we are having an emotion, or that we feel a particular way.

Record your initial reactions to events, as well as your secondary response. Secondary responses might include eating disorder thoughts, feelings, or behaviors that may signal struggle with your emotional experience.

Situation	Initial Reaction to the Situation (thoughts, feelings)	Secondary Response (thoughts/feelings about your reaction). Include any eating disorder thoughts, feelings, or behaviors.
Example Friend cancels plans.	I was really looking forward to seeing her. Maybe she doesn't like me. Sad.	I have no right to be sad. There are so many people who have it worse than I do. I need to stop feeling sorry for myself. I wouldn't blame her for not liking me. I don't deserve dinner.

(continued)

Initial Reaction and Secondary Response Diary Card *(page 2 of 2)*

Situation	**Initial Reaction to the Situation** (thoughts, feelings)	**Secondary Response** (thoughts/feelings about your reaction). Include any eating disorder thoughts, feelings, or behaviors.

CHAPTER 8

Helping Clients Author and Engage Personal Values

He who has a why to live can bear almost any how.
—FRIEDRICH NIETZSCHE

Many individuals with AN have not defined personal meaning, but rather have organized behavior based on rules of what is good or right or will achieve conventional measures of success. While this approach is safer, it also limits life vitality. The overarching goal of values interventions is to help individuals with AN clarify what is most central or meaningful to them personally (unencumbered by their fears) and choose actions consistent with their values in daily life. Although individuals with AN may seem as though they have defined values (e.g., selflessness, perfection), these are often morals or convictions that they have adopted to avoid negative experiences and maintain emotional and behavioral control.

The relationship between values and acceptance is symbiotic (see Figure 8.1). First, as described in Chapter 7, values increase willingness to have unwanted internal experiences. For example, if we value being emotionally close to people, we may be *more willing* to experience the vulnerable feelings that come with creating and maintaining that closeness. Second, acceptance of internal experience facilitates values authorship and engagement. By opening ourselves up to experience (including positive feelings), we accumulate self-knowledge: We learn our likes/dislikes, preferences and opinions, and, ultimately, what we find deeply meaningful. We might also be better able to use personal values to guide decision making and take risks that enhance our lives.

Clinical Goals

We describe seven clinical goals aimed at helping clients with AN author personal values and establish patterns of behavior aligned with those values. Values are leveraged to not only facilitate behavior change in the domain of eating and weight, but also to generally

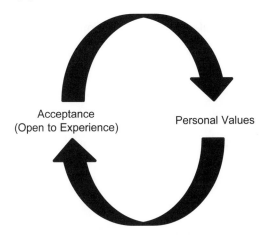

FIGURE 8.1. The mutually facilitative relationship between acceptance and values. Values increase acceptance, or willingness to experience the emotional discomfort inherent in living, and acceptance of internal experience makes it more possible to clarify and pursue one's values.

improve the ability of clients to meet their needs. Values are also used to enhance life meaning and build patterns of behavior that are incompatible with AN.

CLINICAL GOAL 1: *Introduce the Concept of Values and Set the Context for Values Authorship*

Values are defined as freely chosen qualities of purposeful action or *how one wants to be in the moments of his or her life*. Values are discriminated from rigid morals or convictions (e.g., rules or "shoulds"), and from attachment to thinness, perfection, or control driven by the removal of anxiety, guilt, or shame.

Values are also discriminated from the more familiar construct of goals. While goals are discrete, values are ongoing and may guide an individual's choices or actions in a variety of situations and across time and place. For example, an individual might have the *goal* of reading to her child at night. Engaging in this behavior may align with her value of being present for her children, but it is not the same thing. The value of *being present* is also never "completed"; it is something that one can strive to be in each moment of her life. Dialogues A–C illustrate making these distinctions with common AN content.

In introducing the concept of values, the therapist also offers personal values as a guide for life choices. This function of values is particularly useful for clients with AN who may be overwhelmed by making daily decisions. Metaphors that liken values to a guiding light or compass are often useful in helping clients orient to values as a general direction in which to move (see Dialogue D).

Values authorship is facilitated by a slow, deliberate pace and *therapist presence*, which includes a clear interest in the client and what she wants in her life, and being "real" or genuine and in the moment. The next therapist scripts provide values prompts, which can be used to begin a conversation about values or personal meaning. The therapist is looking for expressions of genuine caring or true "mattering."

IN PRACTICE

Therapist Script A

"I know a lot about what is painful to you and what you *don't* want. I know less about what you *do* want [other than thinness]. What you value. What's important to you and might be missing in your life. . . .

Therapist Script B

"If I could lift the pain (all the hard thoughts and feelings), then what would you be doing (or caring about)?"

Therapist Script C

"If I could look deep in your heart, past what you think you should or ought to be, and past fear and concerns about eating or your body, what would I find there? . . .
    "Who or what is important to you?"

Therapist Script D

"Who do you want to be in [relationships, work, etc.]? Not what do you want to accomplish or achieve, but *who* do you want to be?"

Therapist Script E

"If you were to look back at your life today, are you living exactly as you would like to be (or is there something else you wish for)?"

Therapist Script F

"If you could live inside your own skin, what would you do then? How would you want to invest yourself, your energy, or your time?"

Therapist Script G

"If you or the moments of your life could 'stand for something,' what would that be? What would you want your moments to have been about—Managing anxiety? Thinness? Or something else?"

Therapist Script H

"What could dignify the discomfort inherent in living? What would dignify facing fears regarding [eating, rejection, etc.]?"

Therapist Script I

"I know what AN wants. What do *you* want? What is important to you?"

Dialogue A

THERAPIST: I guess I am wondering what you care about most deeply . . . what is important to you, deep in your heart . . .

CLIENT: I don't know. I care about being thin.

THERAPIST: I hear you. . . . I know that this is important to you. That's a little different from what I meant to ask you though. . . . Thinness or a particular weight is more like a goal.

CLIENT: What's the difference?

THERAPIST: Goals are much more familiar to people, and something that has played a key role in your life. . . . Goals are a little different from values, though. Goals are something that you want to achieve. Values are more like a quality—a quality of your actions. I know this probably sounds a little strange. (*pause*) One way to determine whether it is a value or a goal is to consider whether it could be "checked off a list" [of accomplishments] in a sense. If so, it is a goal. A specific weight . . . that is a goal. Being someone who [fill in the blank with a potential value of the client] is different. You don't check that off a list. We never get done being a person who [insert value]. (*pause for reflection*)

   The other thing that is important here is that thinness or being a particular weight is strongly about changing how you feel . . . maybe not exclusively, but much of it is that. It takes away pain and comforts you. . . . And there is this rigidity to it, you know, like it *must be.*

   I want to know what you would choose to "be about" if you could live inside your own skin . . . who and what would be important to you . . .

Dialogue B

CLIENT: I value being [perfect, selfless; not greedy or wasteful, not taking or using too much, not taking up too much space in this world].

THERAPIST: I wonder if we could check in with what "caring about that" is about? . . . like, I wonder if there is fear in there driving that? . . . I ask because it feels like it is a "must," a "have to" . . .

CLIENT: (*Sits thoughtfully.*)

THERAPIST: Let me ask you in this way: Imagine you could wrap "be perfect" as a gift in a package with a bow, and imagine giving it to someone you love: Here is "be perfect." Is this a gift that you would give someone?

Dialogue C

CLIENT: I value being in control.

THERAPIST: I can see that this is important to you . . .

CLIENT: Yes . . .

THERAPIST: I wonder, does it feel flexible and free? . . . like you are moving toward something that is life giving? (*Client appears confused.*)

One way to know is to ask yourself, "Does it feel like it *enhances* my life, or is it like *a must*?" Like, "I must be in control; I can't *not be* in control. That would be intolerable." Kind of clamped down . . .

CLIENT: I hate the feeling of things being a mess. I can't stand it.

THERAPIST: And being in control . . . keeps things from being a mess?

CLIENT: Yes, I'd say, yes . . .

THERAPIST: So you value control because it saves you from this feeling. That's important, but a little different from the kind of valuing that I am talking about. . . . I am looking for something that you care about, *not because* it gives you relief, but because it means something deeply to you, like deep in your heart. We don't have to know what that is now, only that it might not be "control" . . .

Dialogue D (with the "Lighthouse" Metaphor)

The client is considering making choices for herself.

CLIENT: I don't know what to do. . . . I have always just done the next thing required of me. . . . If I am not supposed to do that, what am I supposed to do?

THERAPIST: You sound terrified.

CLIENT: I am!

THERAPIST: I know this is so hard—and at times you might feel lost, not sure which way to go [without AN or rigid rules]. Do you know how sailors find their way home when they are lost at sea?

CLIENT: Lighthouses?

THERAPIST: Yeah . . . they look for the light. Values are like that. They light the way: Provide a direction for us to move in.

What is your guiding light (or what would you like it to be)? . . . (*pause*) This is a big question and one that we can explore together . . .

CLINICAL GOAL 2: *Help the Client Author Personal Values*

Ideally, values emerge organically, as individuals reflect on their struggle and identify the ways in which they want their lives to be different. However, this is more likely to happen with other presenting issues than AN. For example, a client with irritable depression might report, "I want to stop yelling at my kids and withdrawing from family life." This individual is clear about the changes he or she would like to make, and it is not difficult to identify the value that motivates the individual's desire for change (i.e., personal values related to the type of parent or family member the client wants to be). An individual with AN, however, is often not distressed by her behavior and unlikely to perceive it as a violation of her personal values. This also might be the first time she has considered anything other than punitive self-discipline or self-control, or that she might determine the direction for her life (rather than simply doing what she believes is expected of her).

Below we provide several strategies to facilitate values authorship among individuals with AN. These strategies may be used along with other existing resources including values inventories such as the Valued Living Questionnaire (VLQ; Wilson, Sandoz, Kitchens, & Roberts, 2010), values card sorts, values compass or bullseye exercises, or other prompts. The epitaph exercise might be particularly useful, albeit evocative, with individuals with AN given the dangerousness of continued low weight. Strategies to facilitate values authorship should be matched to the client's age and developmental stage.

Values authorship is ongoing and evolves over time. The aim is not for the client simply to name a valued domain (e.g., "family"), or even a value within that domain (e.g., "I value being a parent who is present"). Rather, it is to engage the client in a conversation that helps her make experiential contact with what living in accordance with a particular value would mean to her (most deeply).

We describe 10 in-session strategies to help individuals with AN clarify personal values. This is followed by a homework activity (the "Mission Statement" exercise) and additional prompts for younger clients. We also describe varying clients' daily routine, which might increase opportunities to contact meaning and aid in values authorship. Finally, we describe how clients' values are leveraged to facilitate behavior change.

Drilling Down

Individuals with AN might report that they value being perfect or "in control," or that being thin is the most important thing to them. The therapist can "drill down" from this top layer, which is most accessible, to identify a value. This will require working through layers of avoidance. For example, attachment to thinness might be driven by fear of rejection. However, it also suggests a desire to be liked or accepted by others, and while this itself is not a value, it does reveal that the individual cares about relationships (possibly connection) or being part of something larger than oneself. This is illustrated in the dialogues that follow.

IN PRACTICE

Dialogue A

CLIENT: I want to be thin. That is the most important thing to me. Everything would be better if I was thinner.

THERAPIST: Tell me about everything being better. What would be different?

CLIENT: I'd be more confident for one thing.

THERAPIST: What would you be able to do if you were more confident?

CLIENT: I don't know. I wouldn't be so quiet and I'd probably have more friends . . .

THERAPIST: Friends are important to you?

CLIENT: I just feel like I am not noticed by people. They forget I am there . . .

THERAPIST: You want to be with people, be part of things . . . feel like you mean something to someone or to a group?

CLIENT: (*Affirms.*)

THERAPIST: Can you tell me what would it mean to you in the deepest sense? To be part of something—to matter to people?

CLIENT: (*Describes.*)

THERAPIST: Wow, yes, I get that. . . . It's such a basic need, isn't it? I can sense how important that is to you; that one thing you are caring about in all of this is connection to other people . . . and I get that your mind has made weight and confidence a prerequisite for that . . .

[Later, the therapist might say: I wonder what that would look like for you to value that *now* . . . to be someone who values connection with other people (*with* or *without* confidence). How would it affect what you do (or your actions in your daily life)?]

Dialogue B

Therapist is trying to elicit a conversation about values and has asked the client who or what is important to her.

CLIENT: I want to be able to wear my old clothes. . . . I keep trying them on, hoping they will fit again.

THERAPIST: First, if these are the clothes that you wore when you were severely undernourished, then we need to think about getting rid of them . . . it would be like a cancer patient wanting to wear clothes from when they were going through chemotherapy and their body was weak, depleted, and fighting to survive. . . .

Second, my question would be, where do you want to go in those clothes?

Dialogue C

The client is talking about the importance of good grades. The therapist repeatedly probes to get beneath layers of avoidance and closer to a value.

THERAPIST: Grades are one of the most important things to you.

CLIENT: They are . . .

THERAPIST: What is important about getting good grades?

CLIENT: I want to go to medical school. . . . Both my mom and dad are doctors. . . . People respect doctors, you know.

THERAPIST: So caring about your grades is important for your future goals [of medical school], and that is about people thinking highly of you, looking up to you. What's important about that?

CLIENT: What do you mean?

THERAPIST: Well, why is it important to you that people think highly of you, look up to you . . . ?

CLIENT: You have nothing if you don't have a good reputation. It is important what people think . . .

THERAPIST: Why is that important?

CLIENT: That's just how the world is . . . you need people to refer patients to your practice or you'll never make it. . . . Sometimes I worry that I might end up a bum or something . . . on the street.

THERAPIST: It's either a doctor or a bum. Everything you do is high stakes then. . . . (*pauses*) So, for you, good grades is about being secure . . . secure in your future? I wonder if we could dig in a bit more . . . and explore which part of that is driven by fear (of being insignificant or destitute) and which, if any, is driven by your values and who you want to be in the deepest sense . . .

Exploring Time Investment

The therapist helps the client explore the activities in which she is investing time, and the factors influencing this investment. The goal is to identify whether there is a value guiding this participation and, if so, to name it. Activities might have been meaningful initially, but no longer bring joy or a sense of vitality because of fear of failure, obligation, overcommitment, and so forth. This discrimination may help inform client values, as illustrated in the sample dialogue below.

IN PRACTICE

Dialogue

THERAPIST: You invest a lot of time in tennis, between practice and games . . .

CLIENT: Yeah, I am there almost every night. I used to love tennis. Now I hate going. . . . I've been thinking about quitting, but I think it will upset my dad . . .

THERAPIST: Why do you hate it now?

CLIENT: I haven't been playing well . . . it's embarrassing.

THERAPIST: So tennis has lost its appeal because it feels painful to not play well (or as well as you would like to). . . . I am wondering, if we put that aside, is there something in there that is meaningful to you (about playing)?

CLIENT: (*Long silence.*)

THERAPIST: I don't know if there is. . . . You certainly have been going since you were very young . . . so it might be just what you have always done . . . or that it is for someone else (like your dad, for example) . . . ?

CLIENT: I don't know. . . .

THERAPIST: That's one of the questions for us to dig into. You've devoted a ton of time to tennis. And one question is what has that been about? For example, is there a value in there that is truly yours and dow we need to sort through feelings of failure, obligations, and so forth, for you to reconnect to that? Or is this you "going along with things" that aren't really meaningful to you . . . and there is another value that might be expressed by stepping out of tennis . . . and investing time in other things.

Mental Experimentation: Imagining That the Desired Outcome Is Achieved

Clients are invited to imagine what life would be like if they achieved their weight or shape goal. The therapist explores this imagined future and generates hypotheses about what the client might value. Sometimes mental experimentation requires drilling down as well. For example, if a client describes how achieving a particular body size/shape would increase her "popularity" or "confidence," then additional probing is necessary to determine what is important about these outcomes. A therapist script is provided below.

IN PRACTICE

Therapist Script

"I want you to imagine that you reach the goal you have in mind. See if you can really imagine that you are exactly where you want to be. Look around and see what you notice. In what way is life different? In what way are you different? Are there things that you imagine doing that you are not doing now? Are there people in this vision? How are you in relation to them?

"What about other domains—like work or school—what is happening in these other domains?"

Mental Experimentation: Imagining That Life Continues as It Is Now

Clients may also be asked to imagine what life will be like if things continue just as they are for the next year, or the next 5 or 10 years (i.e., what they lose as they continue to struggle with eating and their body, or center life on achieving a particular weight). This exercise was first described in Chapter 6. When used in this context, it functions as fodder to help the client identify what is important to her, or what she values. The key question is, if it continues like this, what is the cost; what is missing or lost?

Entering through Pain

Clients may be able to report what is painful, but not what is meaningful or what they value. The therapist can work backward from pain to identify what is important to the client. Pain and values are often related, and may even be "two sides of the same coin" (i.e., our worst fears may also reflect what is most important to us).

IN PRACTICE

Therapist Script

"We've been talking a lot about fear of rejection . . . and I wonder if, on the flip side, this tells us something about what is important to you (or what you value)? . . . Like the pain signals 'Hey, there is something important here. Something you care about.' . . . (*long pause*) I wonder if, for example, rejection is painful because you care about being with other people. . . . Could it be?"

Dialogue

The client is talking about an incident in which she spoke harshly to her husband.

CLIENT: I just feel so guilty [about what I said to my husband]. It wasn't called for. . . . He was just trying to help.

THERAPIST: I wonder if there might be something important in that feeling of guilt. That although painful, it communicates something really useful about your values . . . who you would like to be in relationships with people you love, even when (or especially when) it's hard . . . ?

Identifying Moments with Emotional Charge

Clients may be encouraged to scan the last days or weeks for moments (outside of eating and weight) that felt emotionally charged, as illustrated in the script that follows. These moments may provide information about the client's values, or what is important to her.

IN PRACTICE

Therapist Script (with the "Metal Detector" Metaphor)

"I wonder if we can just look over your past days and see if we can find the place that has a charge; Imagine that I have a metal detector wand, and I run it over your days. We want to find the place where it would beep and tell us 'something is here.' . . . It doesn't matter if it feels like a 'positive' or 'negative' charge, just that there is a signal of some kind . . ."

Exploring Memories before Preoccupation with Eating and Weight

Client values might also be clarified by accessing earlier memories, before the client became preoccupied with eating and weight. Clients are asked to recall a moment that felt vital or meaningful (although not necessarily good), a "sweet moment," or a moment when they felt free to "be themselves." Often this is when they were much younger, before they were so critical or hard on themselves or their body. A sample dialogue is provided below.

IN PRACTICE

Dialogue

THERAPIST: Let's see if we can go back in time together, back before AN. . . . Can you scan your memory for a moment that felt meaningful?

CLIENT: During soccer . . .

THERAPIST: That felt meaningful.

CLIENT: Yeah, until I started worrying about everything. It made it hard to play the game . . . and . . .

THERAPIST: What was it like before that, though?

CLIENT: I was just in the game. (*Describes this.*)

THERAPIST: Fully in the moment, it sounds like. . . . Being able to be present like that. . . . Is that important to you?

CLIENT: Yeah, I used to be like that. . . . Somewhere around the third grade that all started to change. I got so in my head about whether I was doing well in things, and what I could be doing better . . .

THERAPIST: You'd like to find your way back to the present moment—not so caught up in (or entangled with) performance fears . . . ? Here. Now. . . . We can work for that. I would love to work for that . . . for you to be able to be more fully in the moments of your life. . .

Exploring Memories Linking Weight and Happiness

Clients may describe a time in the past when they were happy and relate this happiness to their weight at the time: "I feel best at 105. When I was 105, everything was great." The therapist may help the client identify other things that were different at that time. Often, individuals were also more engaged in life (and the things that mattered to them). Identifying what the individual was doing differently can facilitate values authorship. This approach is illustrated in the dialogue below.

IN PRACTICE

Dialogue

CLIENT: If I could just get back to 105. . . . I felt great then.

THERAPIST: What else was going on at that time? Who were you surrounded by, what were you doing?

CLIENT: (*Describes full life engagement.*)

THERAPIST: Wow! That sounds lovely. It sounds like you were really doing things that matter to you. I know that it feels like your weight was responsible, and I wonder if you were simply doing and being the person you wanted to be, and so life felt vital and meaningful . . . ?

CLIENT: I think I was doing those things because I was thinner though. I felt better about myself . . .

THERAPIST: I hear you . . . a change in your body feels like a prerequisite to doing these things. And it sounds like these are the things that matter to you. I wonder, if just as an experiment, we can talk more about these things [your values, what is important to you] directly, rather than through weight.

Returning to Activities That Were Given Up

It is not uncommon for individuals to stop engaging in activities they used to enjoy as they become consumed by AN. For some individuals, this shift is accompanied by a narrative that exonerates AN from blame ("I just didn't feel like doing X anymore"). Clients are asked, in the spirit of exploration, to return to activities that they used to enjoy. The therapist guides the client in exploring whether there is something meaningful in the activity, as illustrated below.

IN PRACTICE

Dialogue

THERAPIST: Horseback riding used to be really important to you . . .

CLIENT: Yeah, I stopped that a while ago.

THERAPIST: When was that?

CLIENT: Umm . . . probably in 2006. I started working out more and I just wasn't interested in it anymore. I used to really like being around the horses.

THERAPIST: I wonder if you would be willing to approach this again . . . in the spirit of exploration. Our minds think they know what things will be like, but directly experiencing something, we learn a lot more.

You mentioned that your aunt has a farm . . . and horses, right? Do you think that over the next week you might be able to spend some time over there, just to see what it is like? See if there is something important in that for you?

Trying On a Value

Clients with AN may be asked to "try on a value" in order to gain a greater sense of themselves and what brings personal meaning. This is particularly useful for clients who identify values, but are unsure whether their values are genuine (i.e., are their own; reflect what is truly important to them). The client is encouraged to take a stand or "behave as if," then use their direct experience as data. The barometer is not whether it feels good to behave in a particular way, but whether it is experienced as vital or meaningful. This approach is introduced in the script below using metaphor.

IN PRACTICE

Therapist Script (with the "New Pair of Shoes" Metaphor)

"Trying on a value is kind of like buying a new pair of shoes. We have to put them on, walk around in them some . . . experience what it is like to have them on our feet, before we can decide whether they are right for us . . . whether to buy them.

"I wonder if you can do that with [X value]. Try it on . . . see what it is like to behave in ways that align with this value . . . see whether it suits you. You aren't committing to buying it, just to trying it out. Are you willing to give it a shot?"

Imagining That No One Knows

Individuals with AN often behave in ways that they perceive will meet the expectations of others. In some situations, the client might be clear that her behavior is inconsistent with her values, but suppress these ideas for fear of disappointing others or causing conflict. The client may be asked to imagine a situation in which *no one would know* or be affected by her choices, and explore how this would impact what she would find meaningful or important (illustrated in the dialogue below).

IN PRACTICE

Dialogue

CLIENT: I have always wanted to be a doctor or a lawyer. Or at least do something in math or science.

THERAPIST: Tell me more about that.

CLIENT: Well, everyone has an advanced degree in my family. . . . They are all doctors and lawyers. . . . It comes up all the time at family reunions . . . how everyone is really successful.

THERAPIST: So success is something that is important to your family . . . and it's defined by particular kinds of jobs.

CLIENT: Oh yeah. My parents always talk about me going to medical school or becoming a lawyer and how important it is to have an educational background and job that other people respect. They tell me that my life will be better if I go to medical school or become a lawyer, and they just want to make sure I can take care of myself.

THERAPIST: And what about you . . . do you want to be a doctor or a lawyer?

CLIENT: Yeah, uh huh.

THERAPIST: So let's just pretend for a moment that you lived on a remote island. And on this island nobody asks anybody about what they do for a living and nobody knows what anyone else does.

CLIENT: That would be awesome. There'd be no pressure!

THERAPIST: You feel pressure?

CLIENT: Well, I guess I am nervous about whether I will be able to make it, you know . . . about whether I will be able to be successful as an adult. . . . My parents try to help me . . . talk to me about what to do. And I appreciate it, but I also get overwhelmed. I've planned out the next several years of courses . . . and . . . I just have to get through it.

THERAPIST: So on that island . . . do you think you would be making the same choices?

CLIENT: Well, I am embarrassed to say it, but I think I'd be more interested in writing. . . . But I know this would worry my parents . . . and they're probably right anyway.

THERAPIST: I wonder if we can dig into what you care about in writing—what is important or appealing about that. . . . There might be a value in there . . . one that is all your own.

"Mission Statement" Exercise

A mission statement is a useful metaphor for values authorship. Mission statements are written by organizations and present a unifying vision of what is most important to each member of the organization. Like values, mission statements are personally authored (by the organization, in this case) and process-oriented (about what they strive to be). Mission statements may be more familiar to clients than "values," and examples may be easily found online. The "Mission Statement" Exercise (Handout 8.1 at the end of this chapter) is a homework assignment that can help individuals with AN clarify values. This exercise can be used anytime in treatment but might be particularly useful when clients are early in identity development or in a life transition (e.g., leaving for college, divorcing) or are transitioning from AN to more flexible living, serving as a manifesto for the next stage of their life. A copy of Handout 8.1 that you can download and use in your work with clients is provided on the publisher's website (see the box at the end of the table of contents).

Additional Prompts That May Be Particularly Useful for Younger Clients

We provide several additional prompts that might be particularly useful for younger clients below. These prompts are more sensitive to developmental stage or use ideas or mediums that might be more appealing to young people.

IN PRACTICE

Therapist Script A (People You Admire)

"Who do you look up to in your life? What are the qualities of these individuals and their behavior? You can include characters in stories or films."

Therapist Script B (Values of Your Parents or Other Influential Adult Figures)

"When you look around your life and consider the values of your parents or other influential adults in your life, what do you notice? What is important to them? Are there some values that you have passively adopted or staunchly rejected?"

Therapist Script C (Tweet)

"Imagine you get to tweet something, one time in your life. What would you want that tweet to be?"

"If no one sees anything else from you, what would you want them to see or know? What would you want to have 'stood for'?"

"What if no one could see it but you?"

Therapist Script D (Music/Lyrics)

"Sometimes it can be hard to verbalize what is important to us, but we can feel or hear it in music. I wonder if you would be willing to bring in a song (or a few songs) that feel meaningful to you?"

Varying Routine to Increase Opportunity to Contact Meaning

Individuals with AN tend to be behaviorally inhibited and to follow routines. As a result, they lack behavioral variability, and thus have fewer opportunities to contact things that might be meaningful and may not have any new ideas about their life or what they might want. The therapist can facilitate values authorship by helping the client introduce variability into her daily life. For example, the client might be encouraged to introduce small changes in daily routines, such as taking a different route to class or the office or reading in the break room rather than her car. It might also include allowing small amounts of unstructured (or "free") time. It is important to keep in mind that these types of changes will be extremely challenging for many clients with AN, and willingness to do things to help clarify values is facilitated by acceptance.

IN PRACTICE

Therapist Script

"It seems to me that doing the same things, in exactly the same way, every day might make it less likely that you will contact things that are meaningful. By varying things a bit, you might bump into something that enhances life (or would enhance your life if you had more of it, e.g., interactions with people). You might also start to have new ideas of what could be meaningful to you. You might be able to imagine things that you can't now (because everything is always the same, and so your mind follows the same pattern too). If you're willing, we can look over your day and find places where you might do something a little differently. Maybe one small change . . ."

CLINICAL GOAL 3: *Leverage Values to Restore Energy Balance/Meet Needs*

By this point in treatment, clients have likely made some changes to restore their energy balance and improve weight. However, these changes might have been primarily due to other supporting contingencies (e.g., weight restoration as a necessary condition for participation in some activity, parent facilitation of meals). With some additional clarity of personal values, it may now be possible to increase the client's ownership of weight restoration and the ongoing action of sustained nutrition. Eating adequately is put in a frame of coordination with values, or what the individual wants for her life.

IN PRACTICE

Therapist Script A

"It is clear how important it is for you to listen to your friends [family, spouse, children, patients] . . . to be there for them . . . and being consumed by thoughts about eating (what you are eating now or what you will be eating later) has taken you away from that. I wonder if facing fears, to normalize your eating and decrease preoccupation (with food, calories, etc.), can be about that: About being present with the people in your life who you care about and want to be there for . . ."

Therapist Script B

"It is so important to you to be someone who does 'the hard thing.' . . . It seems eating (or responding to your needs) *is* the hard thing. In a very real way, eating is about living this value . . ."

Therapist Script C

"It seems your work really means something to you . . . and I am wondering if taking care of you allows you to be in it, fully, the way you want to be?"

Therapist Script D

"I wonder if eating (and meeting your needs) can be about honoring your value of treating people with kindness and respect (without exception, that includes you) . . . ?"

Therapist Script E

"I can't think of any value that you have mentioned so far that would not be served by your basic needs being met. Not a single one. How about you?"

Therapist Script F

"Eating allows you to be in your life (physically and emotionally). You are alive and aware and engaged in a way that you can't be when you are starving yourself. . . . You can care about things. Can you sense that?"

Therapist Script G

"It is important to you to be someone who faces fears . . . it seems to me that eating may be living that value . . . about being someone who faces fears . . ."

Dialogue A

THERAPIST: Over the last several weeks, it has become increasingly clear to me how much you value being a parent—the kind of parent that you wished for when you were young.

CLIENT: Absolutely, that is so important to me.

THERAPIST: I can't imagine that this is not served by you caring for yourself and your needs. There is a reason the flight attendant tells you to put on your own oxygen mask first. We are able to be aware/alert and help (care for) others. In choosing to eat, to respond to your needs, you are also modeling for your daughter—you are showing her how to care for herself. What a beautiful thing.

Dialogue B

THERAPIST: Facing fears (regarding eating) will be hard . . . and we will need a "what for" . . . a meaning in that discomfort. Something that is about you, and what you want your life to be about in the deepest sense.

CLIENT: Well, I don't want to do it, but I know that if I don't, my mom will be mad at me.

THERAPIST: So one thing is that facing fears might decrease conflict with your mom . . .

CLIENT: I don't like fighting with my mom.

THERAPIST: It's painful. And that's not what you want your relationship with her to be like. What do you want [it to be like]? What do you want to be about in that relationship?

CLIENT: (*Describes past and current relationship and the desire for closeness.*)

THERAPIST: And what I hear you saying is that when you are locked in this fight with your body and eating, you are not able to "be about" that—to live that value. . . . So working on this stuff [facing fears] is also about living your relationship values . . . ?

CLINICAL GOAL 4: *Offer Valuing Oneself (Kindness, Compassion, and Attunement to One's Needs)*

AN is characterized by a failure to treat oneself as a person of innate worth, who is worthy of kindness or compassion or having one's needs met. Individuals with AN might feel as though they have to earn the right to eat, sleep, or rest, or that they must constantly forsake their needs for other people or conserve resources. Not only does this directly threaten the individual's life, but it also has a massive impact on her adaptability in daily life. Most individuals with AN do not spontaneously choose to value themselves or treat themselves with kindness and compassion. Not only is this so far outside their worldview, but it also induces guilt and shame or fear that they are selfish, greedy, needy, lazy, or out of control. Thus, the therapist needs to specifically encourage the client to experiment with this idea: to see if there is something important about treating themselves (and their needs) with respect, and whether they experience greater life vitality or well-being. In offering this value, the therapist is also introducing a behavior that is incompatible with rigid, punitive self-regulation. This is illustrated in the dialogues that follow.

Dialogue B includes the "Abusive Parent" metaphor. As described previously, self-parenting metaphors might also be presented as psychoeducation regarding the four parenting styles that emerge from the intersection of high or low parental expectations/demands and warmth (authoritative, authoritarian, permissive, and neglectful) (Baurmind, 1991). This terminology may be made more accessible by referring to an authoritarian parent as a "drill sergeant" and permissive parenting as "anything goes." The therapist helps the client identify what quadrant they are in (based on their behavior) and where they might move. Shifting from a drill sergeant to a warm, responsive (or authoritative) self-parent might be used as a broader metaphor for the overarching goal of the treatment of AN, an idea we return to in Chapter 11.

IN PRACTICE

Dialogue A

THERAPIST: I wonder if you would be willing to do something. We have been talking a lot about what you value—what is important to you—and it is clear that you are not on your list. And up to this point, your behavior has reflected that. I am wondering whether you would be willing to experiment with a different way of being; experiment with what it would be like to choose to value yourself—to choose to treat yourself as a person of worth?

CLIENT: I don't feel worthwhile.

THERAPIST: I know . . . and what I am asking is whether you would be willing to experiment with behaving that way—as a choice, not as a feeling—whether you would be willing to choose to treat yourself that way. You don't have to feel that way to choose it. I imagine that it will bring guilt and shame, and maybe fear, and I also imagine that there might be something else in there too . . . something important and life giving.

Dialogue B (with the "Abusive Parent" Metaphor)

THERAPIST: Do you notice the way that you talk to yourself? It is painful to hear.

CLIENT: I deserve it.

THERAPIST: You feel pretty attached to it. What comes up for you when you think about choosing to talk to yourself another way?

CLIENT: Why would I do that? I wouldn't get anything done. . . . I'm really lazy. I would just sit around and eat. I don't know why I love food so much. It's pathetic.

THERAPIST: So maybe there is fear (of what you would be like if you didn't talk to yourself this way) but a lot of this is driven by shame? You know, when we are young, our parents (or caregivers) have a big role in determining what we do (when we eat, sleep, etc.). They infer how we are feeling and then help create conditions to meet our needs (like giving us food when we are hungry). But when we get older, we assume responsibility for this. We become the parent (or caretaker), cueing in to determine how we are feeling and what our feelings communicate about what we need. There are lots of ways to do this. One way is as an authoritarian parent that is cold and has strict rules and emphasizes obedience and punishment . . . a drill sergeant. Another is a warm and responsive parent, who has guidelines for behavior but is flexible, responsive, attuned.

I wonder if we can do something: Can you imagine talking to a child the way that you talk to yourself? Like, "You aren't hungry! I don't care if you're tired! Get up! Run, you lazy bastard." Like really try to imagine you talking to the younger you, and saying these things. . . . Maybe it can't be you for this, maybe imagine you are talking to a younger child the way you are talking to you.

CLIENT: (*Engages in the exercise.*)

THERAPIST: I guess I am wondering . . . is this the kind of parent that you want to be? What if this is a choice? What if you can choose to be a different kind of parent (to yourself). . . . I wonder how life would be different if you didn't ignore your needs or berate yourself for having them. If you chose to be a kind, responsive parent/caretaker . . . not permissive (like, "anything goes"), which I know is what you fear, but kind, responsive, with gentle guidelines that flex in accordance with your needs . . . caring about the person . . .

CLINICAL GOAL 5: *Clarify Values Related to Others*

Individuals with AN tend to avoid conflict and try to please others. They often fear disappointing or being a burden to other people and may work hard to anticipate others' needs. While this likely serves to attenuate uncomfortable feelings, it also suggests a value in relating, belonging, or connecting with other people.

The therapist helps the individual with AN clarify what is important to her in relationships and how she wants to relate or to be in relation to others. The therapist also
helps the client explore whether her current interpersonal behavior paradoxically interferes
with these values (e.g., whether not sharing feelings limits emotional closeness). Clients
are encouraged to experiment with new behaviors (e.g., self-disclosure) that, while riskier,
might be more interpersonally effective and consistent with their values.

Some clients with AN feel as though they cannot simultaneously value others and
themselves (i.e., that to care for others, they must neglect their own needs). The therapist
might need to help the client reconcile these two seemingly competing values by addressing
fear of being selfish and identifying how she might behave in a manner that respects herself,
as well as the other person. This is illustrated in the dialogue below.

IN PRACTICE

Dialogue

THERAPIST: What about you in that situation? Did you consider what you needed or wanted?

CLIENT: I feel really selfish when I do that. I care so much about being kind and helping
others, and if I start thinking about myself all of the time, then I won't be doing that
anymore . . . and that feels wrong.

THERAPIST: So what comes up is that it is either you or them. It is really hard, or maybe
impossible to hold both . . . and you're afraid that you will lean too heavily into your
court and that will mean something about you . . .

CLIENT: Yes.

THERAPIST: You don't worry about leaning too much into theirs?

CLIENT: No! Not at all . . . although I do sometimes resent things. . . . Sometimes I feel like
I am giving 200% and I am not getting that in return.

THERAPIST: So there is also some pain in doing that [doing everything for others and neglecting you]. And it sounds like, in some ways, it creates distance, because you resent it.

I wonder what it would be like to allow fear . . . ? To know that your mind is going
to say that you are being selfish and choose actions that hold both you and the other
person in regard . . . like you both matter . . . ?

The Issue of Superiority or "Being the Best"

Occasionally, a client might describe a desire to be "better than other people" or to be "the
best." She might describe, for example, that she feels good when she sees other people eating particular foods or that she wants to be the thinnest one in the room. She might also
describe competing with other people on all other sorts of metrics (doing or being the best
at work, school, etc.). The desire to be superior to others, like other rigid attachments to outcomes, is likely driven by experiential avoidance. For example, outperforming others may
be the only way for her to know that she has worth, or being superior may make her feel
safe from criticism or interpersonal vulnerability. By bringing the function of this behavior

to light, the therapist can create an opening for the client to consider what else might be important to her. This is illustrated in the following dialogue.

IN PRACTICE

Dialogue (with the "Mountain Top" Metaphor)

CLIENT: Everyone was stuffing their faces with cake and ice cream. There was so much food around. It felt nice to not be eating like everyone else. . . . I felt like I was stronger or something.

THERAPIST: Do you feel that at other times?

CLIENT: Maybe in school. . . . I have the highest GPA. I like doing better than other people.

THERAPIST: It's like sitting on a mountain top. . . . It's safe up there in a sense. No one can get to you, you know? (*long pause*) I wonder if it feels nice because if you are on top, you are less vulnerable, less likely to be hurt?

CLIENT: (*Agrees.*)

THERAPIST: They also can't reach you, though . . .

CLIENT: No one really wants to be my friend anyway. I don't really care.

THERAPIST: (*Observes the change in client's demeanor.*) It looks like you might care some . . . and wouldn't that just be human—if you did care about having friends . . . about being with other people?

CLINICAL GOAL 6: *Help the Client Use Values to Guide Momentary Decisions*

The therapist helps the client practice using personal values to guide decisions of daily life. The client is encouraged to consider: *If I was living in accordance with my deepest values, how would I treat others, myself, or my body?* Clients can track whether their behavior was consistent with their values over the past week using a variety of tracking tools or diary cards. An example is provided in Figure 8.2. Handout 8.2 (at the end of this chapter) is a blank diary card for tracking value-guided action. A copy you can download and use in your work with clients is provided on the publisher's website (see the box at the end of the table of contents).

Clients will benefit from generating several examples of behaviors that align with their personal values. Specifically identifying value-guided actions across *different situations* can help with generalization. For example, a client might value connecting with other people; however, actions consistent with this value may vary based on whether the individual is with a spouse, with colleagues, or with a stranger in the elevator. With a spouse, this may look like intimate disclosure; with a stranger in the elevator, this may look like eye contact and exchanged small talk. This intervention is illustrated in Dialogue A. Identifying situation-specific examples of value-guided action might be particularly important for individuals with AN who tend to form rules for behavior that are insensitive to context, or who might respond with an extreme expression of a desired change, for example, shifting from "never" to "always" disclosing intimate information.

My Chosen Value	Examples of Actions Consistent with My Value
I value genuineness. I want to be a person who is true to myself and to other people. I want to choose to be honest and genuine, even when it is hard.	Telling my friends how I feel. Acknowledging when I am feeling sad (rather than hiding or denying it). Doing things that I enjoy, rather than going along with the crowd.

Weekly Tracking		
Day	Rating 0 = off track (my actions were completely inconsistent with my value) 10 = on track (my actions were very consistent with my value)	Notes
Sunday	8	I worked hard today. I was honest with my mom when I didn't want to go to my sister's play. I wore my boots, even though I wasn't sure if other people would like them.

FIGURE 8.2. Example of an entry on a diary card tracking value-guided actions.

In addition to using values to guide ongoing decision making, clients might also set specific intentions for the week, identifying a committed action that they intend to engage in that is linked to a personal value (as illustrated in Dialogue B). We provide some examples of values and corresponding committed actions in Table 8.1. Handout 8.3 (at the end of this chapter) can be used to help clients identify committed actions aligned with their values. A copy you can download and use in your work with clients is provided on the publisher's website (see the box at the end of the table of contents).

IN PRACTICE

Dialogue A

CLIENT: It is really important (to me) to be someone who is genuine . . . real. I feel like I have been faking it for so long—pretending to be something I am not.

THERAPIST: What would that look like, to live in accordance with that value of genuineness? If I was a fly on the wall, what would I see? What would you be doing [or doing differently]?

CLIENT: (*Describes what it would look like.*)

THERAPIST: I imagine that it might look differently when you are with your friends versus with your family, at work, or alone. . . . What would "being genuine" look like in these other situations?

TABLE 8.1. Examples of Values and of Behaviors Consistent with Those Values (Committed Actions)

Values "I want to be a person who . . ."	Behaviors consistent with the value (committed actions)
Is open and genuine with other people.	• "Tell my sister how I feel." • "Share things about myself that I wish others knew or understood (like my likes/dislikes, internal thoughts, opinions on topics)." • "Tell my friends or colleagues when I disagree with their ideas." • "When someone asks me what I want to do, I 'check in' and give an honest answer."
Participates.	• "Take invitations sometimes." • "Speak up in social situations." • "Be an active member of the group (rather than stand on the sidelines)."
Is present.	• "When I find myself lost in my head, come back." • "Work during work hours, not at other times." • "Pay attention to the conversation rather than planning what I'm going to say."
Cares more about learning than about getting it right.	• "Express ideas for feedback." • "Try something new."
Treats myself as an equal, and my body with respect.	• "Inhibit apologizing/prefacing." • "Set limits with others." • "Ask for something I need/want in a group, such as telling my partner I want to go to a specific movie, restaurant, or play." • "Respond to my hunger." • "Allow 'down time.'" • "Take a break from movement."
Is self-sufficient/independent.	• "Make choices that keep myself well (with food and rest)." • "Study for my driver's license." • "Explore my own interests and job opportunities."
Approaches hard things.	• "Try a new food." • "Talk to the neighbor."

Dialogue B (Processing Homework with a Specific Intention to Be Value-Guided)

THERAPIST: Tell me more about setting a boundary this week with your boss.

CLIENT: It was really hard, but I did it.

THERAPIST: Fantastic! Did the thoughts and feelings you expected show up?

CLIENT: My stomach hurt.

THERAPIST: And often, that shuts you down . . . this time it didn't, you made your boundary known—nice work!

CLIENT: Yes, I am glad I did it. . . . I do think that I could have said more.

THERAPIST: It sounds like, next time, you would like to practice taking it a step further. And this is a familiar feeling, that you could have (should have) done more. (*pause*) I wonder if, right now, you can just allow yourself to have this . . . ?

CLINICAL GOAL 7: *Help the Client Use Values to Enhance Life*

Value-guided behavioral activation (i.e., increasing participation in a valued domain) can increase clients' overall life vitality and create a sense of mastery, meaning, and purpose beyond AN. Value-guided behavioral activation might be particularly useful for clients with AN who may underparticipate in valued domains due to overcommitment to achievement or behavioral inhibition. The client is encouraged to choose a value domain that she ranks high in importance and to increase participation in that domain. For example, if an individual finds deep meaning in the care and welfare of animals or the earth, she might participate in a policy march or volunteer at a shelter. The goal is to build out the individual's life in a meaningful way. Value-guided behavioral activation is likely to be psychologically challenging; however, it also increases vitality and contact with alternative sources of reward (other than AN). Examples are provided in Table 8.2. Handout 8.4 (at the end of this chapter) is a worksheet to guide clients in considering how they might increase their participation in the domains of life they consider important. A copy you can download and use in your work with clients is provided on the publisher's website (see the box at the end of the table of contents).

Challenges to Values Clarification and Engagement

High Harm Avoidance and Perfectionism

Traits such as high harm avoidance and perfectionism are common among individuals with AN and can present significant barriers to values clarification. Clients may be afraid to care about something deeply (due to the potential for failure, loss, or other emotional pain) or to

TABLE 8.2. Examples of Life Domains and Possible Value-Guided Actions Associated with Those Domains

Domains	Actions
Friendship	• "Go to a meet-up group." • "Text a friend." • "Initiate plans with colleagues." • "Call someone." • "Accept an invitation."
Spirituality	• "Attend a place of worship." • "Read scripture." • "Meditate or pray." • "Spend time outdoors."
Parenting	• "Schedule special time with my daughter." • "Eat a family meal together." • "Attend my son's game."
Leisure	• "Take a slow walk." • "Go to yoga." • "Spend time each night pleasure reading." • "Go to a coffee shop."

experience positive feelings, such as vitality or joy. These barriers can be addressed with acceptance and defusion and by differentiating the process (of engaging values) from the outcome (illustrated in the dialogue that follows).

IN PRACTICE

Dialogue

CLIENT: Why care about relationships? No one will want to be with me. I will never get married and have kids.

THERAPIST: This idea that you are not good enough (for people to care about) and this imagined future of being alone . . . is painful. . . . These are thoughts and feelings that come up for you quite a lot, and have for a long time . . . and they keep you from pursuing relationships that are important to you. They keep you from caring (about others) or allowing yourself to be cared about . . .

I wonder, too, if valuing relationships is different from getting married or having children (which are more like goals). Like, what does that mean to value relationships *in each moment* . . . each moment choosing to be someone who cares about relationships, who opens up to the possibility of relationships (of caring and being cared for), with or without any particular outcome . . .

Getting Stuck on Outcome

Clients may behave consistently with their values and not have desirable outcomes; that is, they may be vulnerable and be rejected, they may stand up for themselves and not be listened to, and they may be more flexible in their study routines and make a "bad" grade. It is important to separate behaving consistently with values from outcomes. Things will not always turn out the way we like, and the aim of values is not to achieve any particular response from the world or others; it is being true to ourselves and the process. The reinforcement for valued action is in taking value-guided action. Often, when we stay true to the process, the outcome "takes care of itself," but this is not always the case.

If behaving consistently with values is repeatedly punished in the client's natural environment, this might suggest the need for an external change (e.g., change in a friend group or intimate partner; finding people who hold similar values or respect our values) or a skills deficit that needs to be addressed (e.g., difficulty setting boundaries in a manner that does not damage the relationship). Separating process and outcome is illustrated in the dialogue below.

IN PRACTICE

Dialogue

CLIENT: I really tried. It just didn't work.

THERAPIST: What do you mean by "It didn't work"?

CLIENT: Well, I told him how that made me feel, and he just kept doing it.

THERAPIST: Ah, I see what you mean. It didn't work in changing his behavior. Was it true to the process, though—true to you? By telling him, were you being the person *you* wanted to be?

CLIENT: Yes, I was.

THERAPIST: Well, that's it then! That's fabulous! You only get to decide on what you do. The world or other people will do what they do, you know?

Difficulty Discriminating Valuing from Avoidance and Control

Clients may have difficulty discriminating when they are behaving in a way that is value guided, versus when their behavior is motivated by avoidance and control. Behaviors that can serve both functions provide a unique opportunity to practice determining the motivations of one's behavior. For example, a client might consider whether in a particular situation, an action, such as "speaking up about her preference about where to go for lunch," was living her values or whether it was motivated by avoidance (eating at a safe place). When behaviors are motivated by avoidance and control, they feel narrow and rigid. Value-guided behaviors, on the other hand, feel flexible and free (although not necessarily "good" or easy). Revisiting Figure 7.2 can help clients make this discrimination.

Weak or Absent Ability to Speak from "I" or Determine Personal Preference

Some clients may struggle with identifying values due to limited experience speaking from "I" or determining personal preference. Often, this is related to a long history of basing decisions on the opinions or perceived expectations of others, or AN emerging at a key period of identity development. The ability to speak from "I" and/or identify personal preferences can be shaped in session and are described in Chapter 10.

Looking Ahead

In Chapter 9, we focus on defusion. Defusion strategies help individuals with AN decrease attachment to the content of mental activity and be more fully in the present moment. This allows behavior to be more flexible and dynamically matched to the individual's needs and the demands of the situation. These interventions build on earlier defusion work, including externalizing AN (Chapter 6) and observing the Eating Disorder Volume (Chapter 7).

"Mission Statement" Exercise: Authoring Personal Values

Introduction to the Activity

Personal values are like mission statements. They present a vision for our lives—guiding principles of what is most important to us and how we want to live the moments of our lives. This activity guides you in writing your own mission statement.

First, what is a mission statement? Mission statements are unifying visions for an organization. They serve to communicate the values of an organization to the public and to the organization's individual members, so that they can work toward a common aim or vision. Here are a few examples of mission statements of popular organizations:

Facebook

Founded in 2004, Facebook's mission is to give people the power to share and make the world more open and connected. People use Facebook to stay connected with friends and family, to discover what is going on in the world, and to share and express what matters to them.

Starbucks

To inspire and nurture the human spirit—one person, one cup and one neighborhood at a time. With our partners, our coffee and our customers at our core, we live these values:

Creating a culture of warmth and belonging, where everyone is welcome.

Acting with courage, challenging the status quo and finding new ways to grow our company and each other.

Being present, connecting with transparency, dignity and respect.

Delivering our very best in all we do, holding ourselves accountable for results.

We are performance driven, through the lens of humanity.

Life Is Good, T-Shirt Company

Spreading the Power of Optimism

Life is not perfect. Life is not easy. Life is good.

We see it when we believe it. Each one of us has a choice:

To focus our energy on obstacles or opportunities.

To fixate on our problems, or focus on solutions.

We can harp on what's wrong with the world (see most news media), or we can cultivate what's right with the world. What we focus on grows.

That's why the Life Is Good community shares one simple, unifying mission: to spread the power of optimism.

(continued)

Handout contributed by Lisa K. Honeycutt.

After reading these statements, it may be clear what each of the organizations cares about and the values that guide its interactions. Mission statements for an individual can serve the same purpose. They can:

- Provide direction in daily life choices.
- Encourage a focus on personal values.
- Identify life "goals" that are consistent with our vision of what is most important.
- Lead to change by pointing out when we are behaving in ways that are inconsistent with our valued oath.

Below we outline three steps to create your own mission statement.

Step 1: Brainstorm.

The brainstorming process is one that cannot be rushed, so take your time to consider what motivates and inspires you. Allow yourself to be creative and inclusive. Do not prematurely judge any idea. A few brainstorming activities are provided below.

Mission Statement Review. Identify organizations that you respect and find their mission statements. Identify themes that speak to you.

Thinking Cap Questions. Ask yourself a few BIG questions, and write down everything that comes to mind, questions like:

What roles are important to me in my life (daughter, friend, student, worker)?
What are some things that I am passionate about?
What is most difficult to me, and does this tell me anything about what I care about most deeply?

Quote Collection. Look over some famous quotes and write down ones that speak to you or inspire you. What is it about these quotes that really moves you? Are they inspirational, humorous, and so forth? Do you know anything about the person who uttered the quote? Sometimes knowing the author of a quote, and learning more about his or her life, can actually be quite inspiring!

Musical Marathon. Think about some of your favorite songs and lyrics with which you connect. Think about why these songs are some of the most moving to you. What is each song "about" to you? Does each song have a theme to which you relate? Are the songs all very different, or do they have many similarities? How do they make you feel when you listen to them?

Inspiring People. Make a list of at least five individuals you admire. It would be best if these are people you know pretty well. List each person, then list as many of their personal qualities (both positive and negative) as you can. Now look over the list and think about the qualities you have written. Of these qualities, how many are qualities you wish you could also possess? Why? Try to describe qualities that are not the individual's innate features but are chosen qualities.

(continued)

Step 2: Draft it.

Now it is time to start putting your mission statement into words. Reflect on the four objectives of a mission statement. Now start drafting a mission statement that sounds like you and reflects your vision for your life and what matters most to you.

Step 3: Make it your own.

Now that you have taken the time to draft the "words" of your mission statement, think about how you would like to display it. After all, the purpose of a mission statement is to have it visible to you—as a guide. You might decide to print it out with a few fancy fonts, make it a graphic image, create a painting that interprets your words—the sky is the limit!

Diary Card for Tracking Value-Guided Actions

Instructions: Identify a value that is important to you that you would like to focus on this week. Take a moment to reflect on this value and what it means to you. List some examples of actions that you would take if you were acting in accordance with this value in your daily life. Then, track for the week. Rate the consistency of your actions with your value each day and make some notes of the actions that you took that were value-consistent or, alternatively, the thoughts/ feelings that got you off track.

My Chosen Value	Examples of Actions Consistent with My Value

Weekly Tracking		
Day	**Rating** 0 = off track (my actions were completely inconsistent with my value) 10 = on track (my actions were very consistent with my value)	**Notes**
Sunday		
Monday		

(continued)

Diary Card for Tracking Value-Guided Actions *(page 2 of 2)*

Day	Rating 0 = off track (my actions were completely inconsistent with my value) 10 = on track (my actions were very consistent with my value)	Notes
Tuesday		
Wednesday		
Thursday		
Friday		
Saturday		

Values and Committed Actions

Instructions: Our personal values can help us choose actions in difficult moments. Below is an example value and committed actions that are consistent with that value. Consider your own personal values and identify actions that would be consistent with those values in different situations. Remember, values are not what others think you should or ought to do (or based on rules of good behavior). They are also not goals (things that you want to accomplish), but rather are *how you want to be* in the world, even when it is hard.

Values "I want to be a person who . . ."	Committed Actions
Example Is open and genuine with other people.	• *"Tell my sister how I feel."* • *"Share things about myself that I wish others knew or understood (like my likes/dislikes, internal thoughts, opinions on topics)."* • *"Tell my friends or colleagues when I disagree with their ideas."* • *"When someone asks me what I want to do, "check in" and give an honest answer."*

(continued)

Values and Committed Actions *(page 2 of 2)*

Values "I want to be a person who . . ."	Committed Actions

Value-Guided Behavioral Activation

Instructions: There are lots of different domains of life that might be important to us. However, due to a variety of reasons (e.g., academic or work demands), we might not be very active in these domains. Below is an example domain and the possible actions associated with that domain. Consider the domains of life that are important to you and how you might increase your participation in these domains. Consider any and all actions, even if you do not think that you can or will take these actions now (i.e., don't let your mind stop you).

Domains	Possible Actions
Example Friendship	• Go to a meet-up group. • Text a friend. • Initiate plans with colleagues. • Call someone. • Accept an invitation.
	• • • • •
	• • • • •
	• • • • •
	• • • • •

CHAPTER 9

Defusing Language and Contacting the Present Moment

May you live all the days of your life.
—JONATHAN SWIFT

Individuals with AN live life based on rules with concrete measures of success and engage in *near constant* evaluation of themselves and their performance. As a result, their behavior is often stilted and insensitive to the demands of dynamic situations, and they suffer profound feelings of inadequacy.

Defusion strategies increase clients' awareness of their ongoing mental activity and help clients discriminate when attachment to the content of cognition is helpful, and when it is not, based on workability for life values. Clients practice observing even the most evocative thoughts (e.g., "I am a waste of space") without attachment, diminishing their influence over behavior. As clients disentangle from the unhelpful mental activity, they gain greater access to the present moment and all that it offers.

Among individuals with AN, attachment to eating disorder content (i.e., dietary rules and body weight and shape concerns) functions as experiential avoidance. Focusing on this content attenuates negative affect by controlling the individual or the situation or directing attention to more concrete, solvable problems and solutions (e.g., counting calories, weight). Letting go of attachment to this content (or AN, more broadly) is an act of willingness and increases contact with more painful thoughts and feelings (e.g., fears, insecurities).

Clinical Goals

We outline eight clinical goals to decrease unhelpful attachment to the content of mental activity and to increase present-moment awareness among individuals with AN. Defusion strategies build on interventions presented in Chapters 6 and 7 that separate the client from AN (i.e., encourage the client to observe AN as a collection of thoughts and feelings that emerges in a context and are separate from the self). This includes externalization of AN and monitoring the Eating Disorder Volume (pp. 153–154) The final clinical goal of this chapter presents strategies to diversify the stimulus functions of food, eating, and the body.

CLINICAL GOAL 1: *Increase Client Awareness of Ongoing Mental Activity and Discriminate this Activity from Direct Experience*

The therapist helps the client observe her ongoing mental activity and discriminate this activity from direct experience. A key strategy is to use the "mind" as a metaphor for language, thinking, or thoughts. The therapist points to the presence of "mind" in session and helps the client "watch the mind at work" (e.g., comparing, evaluating, narrating, planning, analyzing, judging), as illustrated in Therapist Scripts A–C and the sample dialogue. Mental activity is discriminated from directly experiencing the world (through the five senses), as highlighted in Therapist Scripts D and E. Structured exercises may also be used to increase awareness of the presence of "mind" (e.g., "Taking the Mind for a Walk"; Hayes et al., 1999, p. 163). Exercises that are particularly relevant to the phenomenology of AN are provided in Therapist Scripts F and G. These include observing the mind (or mental commentary) during a body scan and during "play" (i.e., a non-goal-directed activity) and observing the mind's propensity to derive rules.

For younger clients, it might be helpful to observe "mind" as a character in a comic strip or in a dramatization (e.g., a brain that is always butting in with analysis, warnings, advice, or rules for behavior).

IN PRACTICE

Therapist Script A

"You have such a great mind . . . and you can hear it . . . working hard to solve problems, analyzing the situation. . . . And even analyzing you and your worth. . . . Am I OK, am I not OK (weight is just one of the criteria that it uses) . . ."

Therapist Script B

"Your mind is always giving you advice or warnings. . . . You notice that it does this about food, but it also does it about other things . . . like now, your mind is warning you that it isn't safe (to say what you are feeling) . . ."

Therapist Script C

"Your mind made sense of that experience, by telling you that it was because you aren't worthwhile or something. . . . The mind is always trying to figure out why things happen. . . . Its job is to tell stories, explain things. If we know why something happened, we might be able prevent it from happening again (at least that's the hope/promise).

"You might notice your mind explains 'good' things too . . . creates a narrative of why that 'good thing' happened and how you can make it happen again. Like: Study all night, that is how to make an A. It's like carrying around a playbook of how to achieve outcomes and prevent mistakes . . ." [Later, the therapist will explore the workability of blindly following scripts, particularly in novel or dynamic situations.]

Dialogue (with the "Watching the Mind in Session" Exercise)

THERAPIST: What is going through your mind right now . . . what thoughts do you notice?

CLIENT: I don't know. I'm wondering why you are asking me.

THERAPIST: Great! So you are having the thought "Why is she asking me this?" What other thoughts do you notice?

CLIENT: I don't know. . . . I guess I am thinking about what we are going to talk about today.

THERAPIST: Do you have other thoughts about that?

CLIENT: Well, I am hoping that we will talk about why I always say the wrong thing. . . . I want to stop doing that.

THERAPIST: So you are having the thought "What are we going to talk about?" and the thought "I need to work on 'saying the wrong thing.'" Maybe there are other thoughts, too—like "Saying the wrong thing is bad" and "I always do that," and ideas of what would be a better way to be.

I wonder if you would be willing to do something with me right now . . . a practice in observing the mind.

CLIENT: I don't know what you are going to ask me to do . . . and I might not want to do it.

THERAPIST: Great! So there is mind, giving you a word of caution . . . the thoughts "I don't know what this is" or "I might not like it." . . . Cautioning is familiar to you . . . something your mind does quite a lot . . .

Therapist Script D

"Your mind is busy today! Mine, too! I wonder if we can just take a moment to slow down . . . center. . . . And maybe notice the difference. . . . What it is like to be in words or images in our heads versus here-and-now, in this moment . . .

"We have access to this moment through our senses . . . what we can hear, see, feel, smell, and taste . . ."

Therapist Script E (with "Driving on Autopilot" Metaphor)

"The mind is running backward and forward in time . . . thinking about what you did wrong yesterday . . . deciding what to do tomorrow. Everywhere but here-and-now. Minds have a tendency to time travel. Mine, too. [*Smiles.*]

"Have you ever driven somewhere (to school, home, or work) and when you arrive, you have no idea how you got there? You don't remember anything about the drive? (*Waits for client to respond.*) Your mind was somewhere else, some other time or place: reminiscing/ruminating, worrying/planning, analyzing or problem solving . . . not in the moment, noticing the trees and what the steering wheel feels like to your hands. These are two very different ways of being in the world. One is in our head (in the world of words, thinking, and thoughts): mind-full. And the other is in the moment: mindful (present, aware of what is going on in and around us). . . .

"I wonder if we can just practice noticing mind-full versus mindful, just noticing what these two ways of being are like and how they are different . . ."

Therapist Script F (with the "Watching the Mind during a Body Scan" Exercise)

In this exercise, the therapist facilitates a body scan, drawing the client's attention to her mental commentary (which is typically continuous and unrelenting). The client is encouraged to observè "positive" (e.g., "My bones are visible here") and "negative" (e.g., "My thighs are spreading across the chair") commentary in a similar manner. She is also encouraged to notice the difference between the direct experience of her body and the mental overlay (i.e., the comparisons, evaluations, judgments, or predictions that she [or her mind] has about her body). Throughout the exercise, the therapist should be cognizant that a body scan also functions as exposure for individuals with AN.

"The mind is constantly running commentary, sometimes describing, but often labeling, judging, or evaluating (our experiences). . . . It is so pervasive that we often don't notice it, or notice it as mental activity. That is, we don't make a distinction between our direct experience (of things) and the descriptions, evaluations, or judgments (that come from our mind).

"If you are willing, I suggest that we notice the mind during a body scan. I will walk you through the exercise. . . . The aim is simply to let your awareness move over your body, observing the mind's ongoing commentary. . . ."

[The client expresses cautious willingness.]

"Let's start by letting your eyes fall closed, or if you prefer, keeping your eyes open, but finding a soft focal point (something to gently affix your gaze). Grounding your feet into the floor. . . . A gentle uplift with the crown of the head while the chin gently tucks. First finding your breath . . . just breathing normally and noticing the rise and fall of the breath. . . . And then directing your attention to your feet—pressing against the floor in your shoes, and noticing the sensations of your feet; the soles and the arches. . . . (*longer pause*) Notice also what the mind is doing. . . . (*longer pause*) It is attending, and it might also be labeling the sensation that it notices or judging it as good or bad. Maybe it has general commentary about the state of your feet . . . or when you wore these particular shoes last . . . and notice just for a moment that there is the direct sensation of your feet, and there are all of the things that your mind has to say about them—mental activity—thoughts about your feet or the sensation in your feet. And now I want to work our way up, allowing your attention to move to your calves . . . the sensation in your calves . . ."

[*Instructs throughout, to the crown of the head.*]

"Noticing the experience of your body (direct sensation) and your mind's commentary. Noticing where mind gets stuck and where it cannot linger. . . . Noticing what the mind has to say about the external body, but also the internal body and the sensations that arise from it. . . . The goal is not to change this commentary, or your experience in any way, just to notice that there is the direct experience of your body and then there is what the mind has to say about it . . . in the same way that there is the direct experience of the chair [that you are sitting in] and how you might describe or evaluate it, or even imagine this chair in your mind. Just noticing that these are two different experiences. One is the direct experience of the thing, and another is the experience of that thing through the mind—or with language . . ."

Therapist Script G (with the "Watching the Mind during Clay Manipulation" Exercise)

"There is the world inside our heads and the one that we can directly see, touch, taste, and smell. We often fail to make a distinction between the two . . .

"I wonder if we can do something a little different today. I have some clay (*offers some to the client*). I wonder if we can just take a few moments to notice its texture, smell, visual properties, and so forth—to observe it with the senses. I would encourage you to pick it up, manipulate it however you like. [*Therapist does this as well.*] Just allowing yourself to notice this as a direct experience . . . (*pause*)

"I wonder if we can also notice the mind's activities or commentary about the experience. This might include simple labeling ('The color of the clay is blue'), as well as evaluations or judgments ('This smells funny,' 'This is a weird exercise,' or 'Am I doing this right?') or thoughts about the past or the future ('When will this be over?').

"Just noticing these two different ways to be in the world. . . . Noticing your mind and noticing your direct experience of the clay in your hands. (*pauses to do this for several minutes*)

"We can manipulate the clay over and over—changing its shape. There is no specific thing to achieve. Just the experience in this moment. Noticing, perhaps, what the mind does when you engage in something without a specific end product or outcome/goal. Noticing what the mind has to say about that.

"Noticing what the mind has to say about play (*pause*). Noticing how this mental commentary changes your experience of the experience (if it does). . . . (*pause*)

"Maybe experimenting with what it is like to notice the mind's commentary and coming back to the five-sense experience of the clay . . ."

Therapist Script H (with the "Observing the Rules" Exercise)

In this exercise, the therapist invites the client to observe the rules that she has in different life domains.

"Our minds are always narrating what is happening. Even when coming here today, your mind probably was running commentary: 'I turn left here,' 'Oh, the elevator isn't working,' 'I wonder if I am going to be late,' and so forth. Some of this commentary is in the form of rules ('Don't go down that hall; it is a dead end'). . . . We have noticed before that your mind is particularly good at forming rules. . . . This is just part and parcel of being someone who is highly verbal . . . and rules are nice, too, because they are concrete and clear, and so you know what to do (and how well you have done).

"When we are afraid, our mind might more readily generate rules . . . about how to minimize risk and keep us safe.

"Take the example of eating. You have a lot of rules about this to avoid overeating, weight gain, or other outcomes that are feared (e.g., 'Don't eat more than 500 calories a day'). I'm going to invite you to notice the rules that you might have across domains of life—including eating, but also in areas such as work, play, rest, and relationships. For example, in your relationships, we have noticed this implicit rule of 'Don't be a burden to others,' and this is often what dictates how much you share your thoughts and feelings with other people.

"Rules work well for some things but not all things . . . Following rules, we might not adapt our behavior to changing conditions or try new ways of doing things. For example, we might take our umbrella because it said it was going to rain, even if the sky has cleared. Now, there is not really any hardship in this example. . . . Carrying an umbrella that we don't need is not that big of a problem. But in other situations, rules can cause us to be really out of sync with our needs—like in the case of not sharing your thoughts and feelings. When you hold back (don't share with others), you continue to feel isolated and alone . . .

"Let's see if we can identify the rules that your mind gives you in these different domains:

- Eating
- Movement/exercise
- Feelings (which are acceptable, when and whether to express them, what to do when feeling a particular way)
- Academics/work
- Relationships."

CLINICAL GOAL 2: *Identify AN as Content the Mind Produces in Times of Stress/Distress*

The therapist identifies dietary rules and body weight and shape concerns as content of the mind (produced in times of stress). AN thoughts/feelings are identified as arbitrary, in a sense, based on "programming" or learning history about what's important or how to get ahead in life (e.g., appearance, self-discipline/self-control). Therapist scripts and dialogues are provided below. Additional sample dialogue that is relevant to this clinical goal can be found in Chapter 6 (in the section "An Unworkable System, Not an Unworkable Person," pp. 146–147).

IN PRACTICE

Therapist Script A

"AN is one of the things that your mind gives you when you are upset: 'Control your eating. The problem is you are too fat.' This is familiar to you . . . familiar to a lot of people . . . people that grew up on this planet, anyway."

"We are inundated with messages that the body is a problem to solve . . . a way to feel better about ourselves or our lives."

Therapist Script B (with the "Mary Had a Little Lamb" Exercise)

"This is a well-worn path . . . When you are feeling upset or stressed, your mind suggests that you worry about your weight. This is its go-to. It feels meaningful . . . and I wonder if it is similar to the nursery rhymes that we grow up with. We've heard or said it so much (played it over in our minds), it is quickly cued up. Like 'Mary had a little . . .' (*pauses for client's response*). If you grew up here, your mind will produce 'lamb' . . . and if you grew up somewhere else, maybe not . . . or like 'Twinkle, twinkle, little . . .' (*pauses for client's response*). . . . Yeah, given this cue, 'star' pops into your mind . . .

"It is not that this content is important per se . . . it is just what you have heard all your life . . . the songs that you grew up with . . . "

Dialogue A (with the "Commercial" Metaphor)

CLIENT: I just don't know how to fit in, so why try? I can lose weight. . . . I'm not trying to brag, but I can lose 10 pounds easily by just not eating. I hate to say it, but it makes me feel special.

THERAPIST: Your mind often offers you AN as a solution to that feeling of not fitting in. Like, "Be different, just stand out then." Or maybe, "Be better" or "Be the best at this." In that way, your mind is trying to help you . . . save you from this painful feeling of not fitting in. It is giving you what it has been programmed to in a sense . . . like (*said in a commercial voice*): "Feeling bad about yourself? Lose weight, be thin and beautiful, and you will be lead a charmed life!" . . . (*shift to a gentle tone*) And yet . . .

Dialogue B (with the "Two Hands" Metaphor)

The therapist is using a physical metaphor to illustrate how AN content may provide a distraction from emotional distress (something else for the individual to focus on and fix or change).

The therapist holds both hands out, palms facing up.

THERAPIST: I want you to imagine that *in this hand* I have thoughts and feelings about your body (*offers hand*), and *in my other hand* I have your deeper insecurities . . . things that you might fear, like being a bad person . . . being unlikable, things like that . . . (*offers other hand*). I wonder, given those choices, which would you rather think about. . . . Which hand would you choose?

CLIENT: My body.

THERAPIST: Absolutely, it makes complete sense. Even though it is uncomfortable, it is somehow less painful to think about . . . a more acceptable problem . . .

CLIENT: I see what you mean, for sure. I really do hate my body, though.

THERAPIST: I hear you. . . . The discomfort with your body is real . . . and it's not hard to imagine why the mind focuses on the body as the problem. It's a much easier problem to solve (than deeper insecurities). . . . And it doesn't hurt that society sanctions it too . . . encourages us to focus on our appearance in order to feel better about ourselves (and solve deeper pain).

[This exercise can be expanded to build acceptance. In this variation, the therapist invites the client to *receive* the hand that represents his or her insecure thoughts and feelings and helps shape the capacity to do so.]

CLINICAL GOAL 3: *Introduce Workability as the Metric*

The therapist introduces *workability* as a metric for determining whether to listen to thoughts. The client is encouraged to consider whether acting in accordance with thoughts (or the advice that thoughts would give) takes her in the direction she wants to go, or otherwise enhances her life. The truth, rationality, or positivity of thoughts is irrelevant. Dialogues A and B provide illustrations.

Dialogues C–E illustrate how the therapist might also help the client apply the workability metric to rules in different domains, including eating. Observing rules with less attachment allows clients' behavior to be dynamically matched to the situation and their needs.

IN PRACTICE

Dialogue A

CLIENT: I'm not normal. No one else has to work so hard to figure out what to say. I watch other people and they just look so relaxed and everything. I am so uncomfortable and I just want to get out of there.

THERAPIST: That's pretty typical of your mind, and what your mind gives you in social situations it seems. . . . It looks around, evaluates the situation (compares you to other people), and warns you: "You are not normal . . . GET OUT!"

CLIENT: What if I'm not?!

THERAPIST: I hear you. . . . It's a scary thought. . . . Part of what makes it feel that way is that it feels like the literal event, like the actual event of not being normal (and the implications of that) . . .

CLIENT: (*Agrees.*)

THERAPIST: I know that it is hard to appreciate at this moment, but you actually have a great mind . . . one of those that allowed our ancestors to survive . . . one that is always on the lookout for danger, sizing up situations and erring on the side of caution. The question is whether listening to the warnings of your mind is helpful to you in this situation? . . . Does it take you in the direction that you want to go, or does it take you in a different direction?

Like the thought "You are not normal . . . get out, or even, don't go. You should stay home, and not interact with other people." . . . In your experience, does listening to that thought take you where you want to go—does it build your life out or narrow it down?

CLIENT: Narrows it down (I am alone). But what if it's true? What if my mind is right?

THERAPIST: Well, I suppose it could be. And there is always the possibility of being rejected, which is what I think you fear most. I guess the question is whether you want to live your life avoiding this possibility . . .

Dialogue B (with the "Don't Think about a White Bear" Exercise)

CLIENT: I went to the office party, but I spent the whole time comparing myself to the other people there. I know I'm not supposed to do that, but I couldn't help myself.

THERAPIST: Your mind launched into comparison mode. That is so like our minds . . . comparing/evaluating everything . . . including ourselves . . .

CLIENT: There was this woman there . . . and she was super skinny, but not eating any of the pizza, and I couldn't stop thinking about it. I just kept thinking, "I think she is skinnier than me . . ." and I just kept trying to figure it out.

THERAPIST: When you found yourself entangled with those thoughts (of how you compared to her, or other people), what was the effect of that?

CLIENT: Well . . . I don't think I talked to anyone . . .

THERAPIST: You withdrew into yourself and into your mind.

CLIENT: Yeah, I was trying to decide if it was true or not. . . . I tried to not think about it, but it didn't work.

THERAPIST: Maybe we can't control what we think, only what we do, or how we respond . . . (*Therapist invites the client to "Not think about a white bear" for one minute and processes this exercise.*) Like, maybe you can't stop that this thought pops in your mind (and trying to stop it might be part of the problem), but maybe you can decide if you follow it . . . chase it . . . ? It seems doing that took you out of the situation and away from other people. . . .

Dialogue C (Workability of Rules—Body Signals)

CLIENT: I don't know why I would be hungry. It wasn't even close to dinner yet, and I ate lunch. In the past, I skipped lunch, so how could I be hungry?! It's just not possible. And if I eat when I am not hungry . . . well, that's how people become obese.

THERAPIST: It feels scary. (*pauses*) Before we are verbal, this is a lot easier, you know? The more our mind gets involved in eating, the harder it becomes, to read our signals and know what we need. Our minds generate rules. Rules for what to eat when, that may or may not match our actual energy needs. . . . You have a particularly cautious mind that always errs on the side of needing less and doing more . . . and so you end up depleted.

CLIENT: It is overwhelming. How do I know what to eat [without rules]?

THERAPIST: I get your mind wants it to fit some sort of algorithm . . . that would feel so much safer. Uncertainty is so hard. . . . It holds the possibility of making a mistake.

The thing is, our needs are dynamic and changing in ways we cannot always predict (we use more energy when fighting illness, in subthreshold disease processes, and in menses and adjusting to changes in temperature, and so forth). . . . I wonder if this is a place for us to work on opening up . . . making space for uncertainty . . . ?

CLIENT: (*concerned, fearful*) If we don't have any rules, we might eat cake every day . . .

THERAPIST: I am not suggesting that we throw out guidelines (e.g., guidelines for balanced nutrition), but rather that the mind (and its largely arbitrary rules of what we can eat, when we can be hungry, etc.) doesn't override other sources of information; that we can also take into account our hunger, our preferences, the situation, or other factors . . ." (*Therapist goes on to work on acceptance of uncertainty.*)

A note on rules about eating. During active weight restoration, individuals with AN may have to continue to use rules to determine eating (e.g., following a meal plan). This is often necessary because, when undernourished, clients may not sense hunger or may experience premature fullness. This is an unavoidable complication of AN that will be upsetting for individuals who already mistrust their bodies and are confused by its signals. Reliance on rules or structured meal plans decreases over time as clients approach their target weight and eventually transition to more intuitive eating.

Dialogue D (Workability of Rules—Emotions, with the "Jury" Metaphor)

CLIENT: I have no reason to be sad. And then I think maybe I do . . . maybe anyone would feel this way, but I also . . . (*goes on at length*)

THERAPIST: It is like a jury deliberating whether your feelings are legitimate or not. Like, "Ladies and gentlemen of the jury, I would like to present to the court the events of the evening . . . and you will decide whether Julie had a right to feel [sad]."

CLIENT: (*Responds.*)

THERAPIST: Maybe mind isn't helpful here, deliberating about the rightness of the feelings . . . coming up with the conditions under which it is OK to feel [sad] and so forth . . .
    (*pauses for discussion*) It seems it would be painful to be so unresponsive to yourself and your needs . . . to reject and neglect your feelings. If we were to see a child sad, we would give him or her comfort . . . because that is what people need when they are sad.

CLIENT: (*Looks down.*)

THERAPIST: I wonder if we can start by just noticing that there are your feelings and then there are your judgments/evaluations of your feelings and the rules you have about when and why you can feel a particular way . . .

Dialogue E (Workability of Rules—Interpersonal)

THERAPIST: Our minds generate rules all the time . . . and they can feel important and meaningful . . . but maybe they are simply mental activity? . . . and sometimes mental activity is helpful and sometimes it is not. Like if I have the rule "I should dress warmly in winter" . . . it's not going to be helpful if I'm bundled up in snow gear when it's 80 degrees out just because it is December. If I instead notice the rule as a guideline and check in with how it *actually feels* outside, I'll probably dress most effectively for that situation. . . .
    It sounds like your mind has a rule: "Don't ask for help or support." And you follow it. . . . You stay quiet and don't tell other people what is going on with you. You make it seem like you are always fine and ask about the other person. . . . How is that for you?

CLIENT: Well, I know about all their lives, and they don't even know me.

THERAPIST: So you continue to be unknown, unseen?

CLIENT: (*Appears sad.*) Yes.

THERAPIST: And that's hard, to feel unknown? The good news is that once we see that we are following rules [a script or a playbook], then we can decide whether to follow it . . . or whether to try other actions that might be more effective. (*pauses for discussion*)
    I wonder, what it would be like if you started talking more about yourself [to your friends]?
    I know it might be scary to do that, but I also wonder what might be in there for you, too, like if you might experience more emotional closeness, for example?

CLINICAL GOAL 4: *Identify Choice and Reinforce the Person as a Choice-Maker*

The therapist helps the client to isolate thoughts in a stream of mental activity and to notice the space between thoughts and actions, or "the choice point" (the moment that they get to choose how to respond). The individual's agency in actively choosing the direction of her life is highlighted. Acceptance is engaged to facilitate willingness to choose valued directions, even when it is hard. Sample dialogues and scripts are provided below. Table 9.1 (on pages 232–233) provides some additional strategies.

IN PRACTICE

Dialogue A (with the Mind Personified)

CLIENT: Last year, I was studying for hours and hours (three times as much as I needed to). Then I just gave up. I couldn't do it anymore.

THERAPIST: When you let go of school, you picked up AN instead . . . counting calories, losing weight, and being good at that. . . . It gave you something else to focus on and achieve.

CLIENT: Yeah, school just became awful.

THERAPIST: And now your mind gives you that [AN] any time you are feeling insecure or overwhelmed, and encourages you to invest in AN instead . . . as something that makes you feel better. Thank you, mind! (*pause*)

I wonder if we can begin to notice your mind saying, "Hey! Look over here! [at AN]" (*waves arms to the side, as if to get the client's attention*). (*pause*)

And just notice that point where you get to choose: Choose whether you turn toward AN . . . and away from these other things that matter to you.

CLIENT: I care about school, but I just can't do it . . .

THERAPIST: School was painful, in part, because of how you were treating yourself. I think it will be important for us to think about how you can engage things that matter to you in a kinder, gentler way . . . so you can choose to turn toward them (if you want to). So you have the option . . .

Dialogue B (with the "Reporter Sound Bite" and "Title of the Book" Metaphors)

CLIENT: I have been working on eating more, but it is just so uncomfortable.

What if I let go of AN and nothing is there? I don't know who I am anymore, or what I like.

I used to do silly things, but I don't anymore. Like go skating and wear mismatched socks. I think I would just feel so lost. . . .

THERAPIST: Your mind has a lot to say about what might happen if you keep going forward. . . . Sometimes it can be useful to identify a single thought in a stream of mental activity. If you were going to package this into one thought, what would that be? Imagine a reporter is going to write a story and is going to include a sound bite, something like "And then Abigail's mind said: "[ ]" . . . Or imagine that you have been reading from a book and then you flip it over to read the title. What would it be?

CLIENT: "You are nothing without AN."

THERAPIST: You are nothing without AN. . . . Let's just pause there. I can feel the significance of that . . . how painful an idea that is [if experienced literally] . . . and how hard that would be when that thought shows up . . . (*pause*)

   And maybe start to notice *the you* who is having that thought, and who chooses what you do (the actions that you take). Like, whether you listen to that thought and stay stuck, or whether you choose something else—something that might feel risky but is life giving.

CLIENT: It seems like it might be true [that I am nothing]. And then other times not. I just don't know what else is there, I guess . . .

THERAPIST: It feels scary and so you try to figure it out. . . . Is there anything to me or not?

CLIENT: (*Responds.*)

THERAPIST: Instead of trying to figure out if the thought is true or not, I wonder if you can use another metric altogether. Like whether getting hooked by the thought "I am nothing without AN" is helpful. Whether it expands or enhances your life (or not). . . . It seems that thought would suggest that you should cling tighter to AN. Is that helpful to you?

Therapist Script A
(with the "Signs on the Highway" Exercise)

The client is describing thoughts that derailed her this past week.

"On your drive here, you take the highway, don't you? You probably have noticed all the signs along the way—some provide information (e.g., an upcoming rest stop) and some are advertisements (e.g., trying to manipulate your behavior). I always notice the signs that encourage me to shop at the outlets or stop to see the rock formation or underground lake. Sometimes the signs will get increasingly insistent the closer you get to the exit—like 'You don't want to miss it, Exit now!' Our thoughts are like signs on the highway. Sometimes sort of politely reminding us about something (sometimes when it's not helpful or not what we are looking for) and sometimes being wildly insistent, full of warnings and such.

   "I wonder if, right now, you can imagine you are driving down the highway. Maybe it is a familiar one, one that you know. Maybe it is one that you can imagine.

   "Imagine that you are driving precisely where you intend to—in the direction that you intend—maybe you have the GPS set to your deepest values. Maybe you are on the road of being a 'present parent,' for example. (*pause*)

   "And now I want you to see if you imagine that the road signs have your thoughts on them. The things that show up in your mind . . . that might throw you off course. The thoughts that come up at the moment that it is hardest to be present with your kids; maybe the moment when it is most important to be present . . . like when they might need you fully there the most. Maybe the thought 'I have not done a good job as a parent; otherwise she would not be suffering like this' (*pauses for several minutes*). This sign might suggest that you give up, shut down. See if you can notice, that you are the driver . . . that in a very real way, you get to choose whether you notice the sign and keep driving, or whether you turn off . . . get off the road of present parenting . . . (and instead try to manage your feelings) . . . (*pause*)

"Now, I don't mean to suggest that we never make wrong turns. We all get hooked by thoughts, and listening to our thoughts often works. Like the thought, 'I should leave earlier to avoid traffic.' You listen to that thought and maybe you arrive on time. But sometimes our minds take us off track and have us driving down dead ends or stuck endlessly making the loop around a clover leaf . . .

"Our job is simply to find our way back, back to the road that we want to be on . . . with kindness, gentleness, compassion."

Therapist Script B
(with the "Pop-Up Advertisements" Metaphor)

Client is describing thoughts that derailed her this past week.

"It is like pop-up advertisements on websites. They might have an evocative image (e.g., fad diet before/after pictures) or inciting announcement, like 'Don't Miss this Great Event!' or something similar. You are completely minding your own business and there they are. . . . We did not ask for them to be there . . . they just show up. They are strangely compelling because they are matched to our interests and [search] history.

"Here's the important part, though: We get to decide what happens next, what we do: whether we click on the pop-up box and bury deeper in . . . or whether we gently redirect our attention/energy to what matters most to us.

"That thought 'You are a worthless piece of crap!'—flashing on the screen in bright letters. Can you imagine it? [pauses]

"What would it be like to choose whether to click . . . whether to get pulled in and lost for hours in pages of information (trying to figure out if it is true, or what to do about it) . . . or whether to simply notice it and orient to what matters to you (most deeply)."

Therapist Script C
(with the "Train Station" Metaphor)

"It's like a train station. There are many tracks, and new trains pull in all the time. I wonder if you can notice that *you* get to decide if you board . . . and this decision depends on whether the train is taking you in the direction that you would like to go. Like the thought "you are worthless" . . . is that the train you want to board?

"In some cases, the train may be down the track before you realize that you have hopped on. Like, imagine the "you are worthless" train pulls in. . . . Next thing you know, you are down the track, trying to figure out what is wrong with you, what you can do to be better, whether other people know and will leave.

"If you can notice that the train has "left the station" and you are on it, this is your new choice point, your new moment to get off the train and come back to the station (centered, grounded, and stable where it has always been)."

TABLE 9.1. Additional Strategies to Separate the Person from the Mind and Highlight Choice (Response-Ability)

Strategy

Reading a book

This metaphor highlights that the mind is constantly narrating, and that sometimes we will be compelled by the stories that it tells. As with an actual book, we can get forget that we are reading and become so lost in the story that we lose touch with the world around us. Whether to stay locked in is a choice.

Sample dialogue

CLIENT: I don't know what I would do [without AN]. I have nothing to offer . . .

THERAPIST: The mind is always narrating about us and our lives . . . has a story about how things are . . . or how they have been in the past or will be in the future.
   Some of the stories are old and familiar to us . . . like this one. . . . This story that you have nothing to offer, that you are nothing without AN . . . that is something that has come up for you a lot . . .
   (*pause*)
   Imagine that this shelf is full of books . . . and some have compelling titles . . .
   Like the book *I Am Nothing without AN.*
   That is one that you pick up. I get it, its title is compelling. Absolutely.
   It seems like you might be prone to pick up this book when you are scared.

CLIENT: (*Affirms.*)

THERAPIST: What other books might be there?

CLIENT: (*Describes.*)

THERAPIST: I wonder what it would be like to notice when you pick up that (or another) book . . . to notice when you are caught up in the story, completely lost in the words on the page, imagining the scenes and living the narrative, and look up. (*Gestures, looking up from book into client's face.*) To see the world around you. The world has people and things that you care about, and that are here, now. Can you imagine it?

Strategy

Conversation with "mind"

The therapist role-plays the client's mind, sitting in a chair alongside the client and chattering (saying things aloud that the client thinks; e.g., worries, judgments). The client is encouraged to respond to the therapist as her mind (e.g., listening, agreeing, debating).
   In engaging with her mind, the client may also be turned away from other things that matter to her.

Sample dialogue

The therapist moves to a chair next to the client.

THERAPIST: I am going to be your mind, OK? And across the way there (in the seat I was in), are your friends at lunch yesterday.

CLIENT: OK.

THERAPIST: (*Speech is rapid and indecisive.*) "Should I get the pasta or the salad? If I get the pasta, I'll be following the nutritionist's guidelines to eat more carbs. My friends will also be relieved if they see me eating something other than salad. But on the other hand, if I get the pasta, I'll feel disgusting and bloated and I'll gain weight and . . ."

CLIENT: (*Turns toward therapist and starts telling mind to just make a decision, etc.*)

THERAPIST: Notice how you turned toward me (turned toward your mind) . . .

CLIENT: (*Discusses this.*)

THERAPIST: And what happens to your friends across there?

CLIENT: I'm not really paying attention to them.

(continued)

TABLE 9.1. *(continued)*

THERAPIST: Yeah, you can't see them, connect with them, be part of things, because you are debating with your mind. What is that like for you?

CLIENT: *(Describes this.)*

THERAPIST: What if you could choose . . . to be entangled with your mind or not—choose to be present with your friends while your mind blah blah blahs . . . *(Makes a gesture as though his hand is talking in his ear.)*

CLIENT: How would I do that? I wouldn't be able to keep it up.

THERAPIST: Maybe it's a process of "turning back." Gently coming back to the conversation *outside* your head. Rejoining, as many times as it takes.

Strategy

Other active language

Using active language (e.g., listening, buying, hooked) delineates the individual from her mind and highlights that she can choose actions that are consistent or inconsistent with the literal content of her thoughts.

Sample dialogue

CLIENT: I am so stupid!

THERAPIST: Are you [listening to, buying, hooked by] that thought?

CLIENT: I guess, um . . . yes . . .

THERAPIST: I can feel how strong a hold that thought has right now. It's powerful. *(respectfully)*
Some thoughts are stickier than others because their content is threatening. They get our attention more than others. Like "Danger! Danger! Something is wrong with you! Pay attention!"

CLIENT: *(Discusses.)*

THERAPIST: If that thought "I am so stupid" were able to give advice, how would it advise you? What would it suggest that you do?

CLIENT: Shut my mouth for one thing!

THERAPIST: Yeah . . . And, I wonder . . . is that what you want to be doing in this situation?

CLIENT: Not at all . . . *(Discusses this.)*

THERAPIST: The good news is, you get to decide. You get to decide whether you listen to thoughts (or your mind) and the advice it gives . . .

CLIENT: But it is true. . . . I am stupid.

THERAPIST: I hear you—whether it's true [or not] feels important. I wonder what it would be like to use a different metric? Not whether a thought is true or not true, but rather whether it is workable . . . whether listening to its advice takes you where you want to go . . .

CLINICAL GOAL 5: *Practice Defusion with Thoughts Exerting Undue Influence over Behavior*

The therapist creates additional opportunities for clients to experience their most evocative or compelling thoughts as mental activity, reducing the "hooks." Clients are encouraged to engage with these thoughts nonliterally and in as many diverse ways as possible. For the individual with AN, target thoughts might include "I am fat," but more importantly, the painful content ("I am defective, disgusting, selfish, needy, etc.") that the individual avoids by focusing on body weight and shape, or by exerting rigid control over her behavior. We provide sample strategies in Table 9.2 on pages 237–238 and in the next illustrative dialogues.

IN PRACTICE

Dialogue A (with the "Role-Playing the Mind" and "Putting Thoughts to Music" Exercises)

The client is describing leaving a social situation abruptly.

THERAPIST: I am wondering if we can slow down into that moment that you are describing . . . the moment right before you left the room?

CLIENT: Well, I was thinking, I am such an idiot . . . so awkward . . . and . . . how will I ever make friends?

THERAPIST: Your mind was really giving you a hard time. Giving you a laundry list of what is wrong with you. Were you hooked by those thoughts?

CLIENT: Yeah, I guess. . . . All the other girls look relaxed . . . like they are having fun. . . . I wonder if I will ever feel that way . . .

THERAPIST: So there you are trying to connect . . . and your mind is blabbing in your ear about whether you are OK . . . (*Sits next to the client and plays the character of her mind; rambles about the other girls in the room, makes judgments and warnings.*) And so your attention is taken away from the situation . . . and you are just in this conversation with your mind. This is the opposite of the direction that you want to go. . . . You want to be with people.

CLIENT: It just feels so powerful in the moment.

THERAPIST: Yes, it can be so compelling! Even though you have heard it a thousand times, it still grabs you by the gut. I wonder if we can play around with this thought a bit . . . interact with it in a new way . . . so that you have a choice in that moment—to turn inward or not.

Are you game?

CLIENT: OK.

THERAPIST: If we were going to put this thought to a tune . . . something maybe unexpected for it . . . what might we use? . . . Maybe happy birthday or something . . .

CLIENT: (*Identifies a tune.*)

THERAPIST: Awesome! Let's sing it together . . .

CLIENT: Uh . . .

(*Therapist begins and client joins in or just listens.*)

THERAPIST: What if it was a rap, what might it sound like?

Dialogue B (with the "Tip of the Iceberg," "Guests in Your Home," and "Internal Traffic" Metaphors and a Mindful Observation Exercise)

CLIENT: I wanted to go, but I felt too fat. I tried on all these clothes . . . and nothing fit the way that I wanted . . . and so I just stayed home.

THERAPIST: The thought "I am fat" is something your mind gives you a lot, and sometimes it hooks you more than other times. It sounds like on this day, it was particularly compelling . . . and it changed the course of your day. Rather than going to X, you stayed home. I wonder if we can notice what else was going on (around and inside of you) when that thought showed up. Like maybe "I am fat" is the top layer that is really accessible, but there are other layers underneath? Like an iceberg, with some things that can be easily seen on the surface . . . but there is more below.

CLIENT: (*Sits quietly, thoughtfully.*) I called Julie to talk and I felt like she was in a hurry. . . . I feel like a burden to her. . . . I think I am just too much for people.

THERAPIST: So the top layer is the thought "I am fat," but just below that is the thought "I am too much" . . . like you are too much for people, and that you need to take up less space in their lives or the world or something. . . . And when this thought shows up, you pull back. . . . Am I getting that right?

CLIENT: Yeah, I did look really fat in my dress though, and it's embarrassing, you know? Everyone will notice . . . and maybe if I could just get my eating and weight under control. (*Goes on at length about eating and her body.*)

THERAPIST: Your mind makes it about "fat," but all of that sort of comes down to this fear of being "too much." . . . (*Therapist gives another example of this from the client's history.*)

Would it be OK if we go back to the thought "I am too much," and see what it is like to notice that thought . . . *as a thought* . . . that shows up when you care about a relationship and are afraid you might lose it . . . ?

CLIENT: Yes . . .

THERAPIST: (*Speaks slowly and deliberately, invites client to close her eyes.*) First, let's just get in touch with this as *the experience* of being too much: "I am too much." . . . Hear it just as you might in your head. Notice how it feels in your body. Notice any urges that you might have . . . (*pause*)

Now, let's see what it is like to notice it, like this, "I am having the thought that I am too much . . ." Maybe say that over in your mind several times . . . (*pause*)

And now, "I am noticing that I am having the thought that I am too much." Maybe say it over in your mind that way . . . just reminding yourself that this is a thought that you are having . . . (*long pause*)

Just taking a moment to notice that you are having a thought . . . and it is of this kind . . .

(*long pause*)

Maybe taking a moment to notice that there are other things in your experience, too. Other experiences that, like this thought, are like guests in your home . . . passing through, maybe staying a while. . . . (*long pause*)

Maybe you notice the sound of the air conditioner, for example . . . maybe other sounds, allowing yourself to be aware of this aspect of your experience too. . . . *I am noticing the sound of the air conditioner, and I am noticing the thought that "I am too much."* Notice the feeling of your breath moving through your body, the places where the breath feels strong and the places where it is barely detectable . . . *I am noticing the feeling of the breath moving through the body.* Notice the feeling of your feet touching the floor, or other places where your body contacts the world, noticing this aspect of your experience too. . . . *I am noticing my breath . . . and my feet touching the floor, and I am noticing the thought that "I am too much"* (as mental activity, words and images). (*pause*) Maybe now noticing what you can smell. *I am noticing the smell of* [blank]. . . . Noticing what you can taste . . . and *notice that you are having the thought "I am too much."* All of this is here, now . . . (*long pause*)

We tend to give our mental activity a special place. . . . Right now, we are sort of leveling things out. Noticing all there is to notice. Thoughts are part of our experience— not all of it. There is so much internal traffic. . . . All of it internal traffic. Thoughts, too.

Dialogue C (with the "Thoughts on Cards" Exercise and the "Old Friend" Metaphor)

Writing the thoughts on cards encourages "looking at" rather than "looking from" thoughts. It also isolates thoughts as discrete events, which can be particularly helpful if individuals have long and complex narratives. By summing up the experience into one characteristic thought (or theme), it might be more easily recognized and related to differently.

CLIENT: The lunch meeting was awful. I was sitting there like a fat waste of space with this huge sandwich in front of me.

THERAPIST: That sounds like a really uncomfortable experience . . . and that your mind has a lot to say about it . . .

CLIENT: Yeah, it does!

THERAPIST: I wonder if we could slow down and really unpack what your mind was saying. So you were sitting there at the lunch meeting . . .

CLIENT: I was thinking about how I'm so fat and ugly . . .

THERAPIST: Is it OK with you if we write these thoughts down?

CLIENT: OK.

THERAPIST: (*Hands the client notecards and suggests using quotation marks.*) So, you were having the thought "I'm fat and ugly" . . . and what else . . . ?

CLIENT: I mean, I don't even know what I'm doing and I'm sure my boss thinks I have nothing to offer. I can't ever think of anything to say . . . and I'm not an asset to the company . . . (*goes on and on*)

THERAPIST: These are familiar themes . . .

CLIENT: Yes, very much so . . .

THERAPIST: It's the hand your mind deals you in these situations. Every time. Doesn't even get creative about it (*smiles*).

CLIENT: (*Smiles.*)

THERAPIST: So "I don't know what I'm doing" . . . "I have nothing to offer" . . .

CLIENT: Yes, well and I guess, that I'm stupid.

THERAPIST: "I'm stupid." Can you put that one on a card, too? (*Client puts it on a card.*) OK,

TABLE 9.2. Defusion Strategies for Thoughts Exerting Undue Influence over Behavior

Strategy	Description
Adopt language conventions that decrease literality.	The client adopts language conventions that decrease literality. Rather than simply stating the content of thoughts, the client begins with "I am having the thought that . . ." or "I am noticing that I am having the thought that. . . ."
Change the auditory or visual cues.	The client is encouraged to change the auditory or visual cues to facilitate less literal engagement with thought content.
	Context cues that are unexpected or incongruent with the literal content will facilitate greater deliteralization (e.g., a self-deprecating thought put to an upbeat tune).
	Other examples include speaking thoughts aloud in funny voices (the voice of a radio commentator or infomercial) and difficult thoughts presented beautifully (e.g., in colorful, sparkly letters or as a piece of artwork).
Objectify the thought.	The client is asked to imagine the thought as an object and describe its properties, or otherwise interact with it (e.g., place it on her lap or on a nearby chair).
	Objectifying a thought separates the thought (there) from the individual (here). It also cues a repertoire of curiosity or observation.
Watch it form.	The client is asked to imagine that her thoughts are written with a sparkler (with a trace that fades and may be written again) or in smoke (that collects and dissipates again and again).
Personify.	The client's "mind" is personified to cue adaptive responses to evocative thoughts. This might include describing the mind as an advisor, a dictator, a critic, or a well-intentioned friend. Personification should be consistent with the client's experience and the behavioral repertoire that the therapist seeks to elicit (i.e., describing the client's mind as a friend will elicit more compassion than describing it as a dictator).
Level it.	Situating thoughts as one event in an internal landscape "levels it," such that it is equivalent to any other element of experience that might be observed (rather than special in some way).
	The client is invited to notice her "internal traffic." This includes not only thoughts but also other elements of her experience: what can be noticed via five senses (e.g., tingling sensations in the hand, temperature of the skin, the breath moving through the body).
	The client is invited to observe these experiences as they come into awareness—"I am noticing the thought that X, I am noticing the tingling sensations," "I am noticing the patches of warmth on my skin, the way my chest rises and falls," "I am noticing my feet on the floor, the sound of the clock . . . and I am noticing the thought X . . ."— and to hold these things simultaneously and lightly as aspects of experience.

(continued)

TABLE 9.2. *(continued)*

Strategy	Description
Call it what it is (labeling).	Thoughts may be labeled as a warning, prediction, judgment, worry, memory, and so forth (without engagement in the thought content). This may be practiced mindfully or playfully in session (see sample therapist scripts below).

Therapist Script A

"Your mind is always making judgments—mostly about you! I wonder what it would be like to notice it in the moment and call it what it is?

Imagine that each thought that arises is a memo passing over your desk (gestures taking a paper across a desk). Imagine that you have a stamp that says 'judgment' and that you can stamp the memo and move on to the next one (pretends to stamp a paper and pick up the next one).

Maybe it's another judgment, maybe its something else. Whatever arises."

Therapist Script B

"Imagine that you have a bell that you can ring when a judgment shows up [said in a light-hearted voice] 'Ding ding ding, judgment folks! We have a judgment!'

Just start to notice it . . . no need to engage it or its content. This is just noticing. . . . See how many you can catch."

Note. These strategies are also a practice of noticing the dynamic nature of thinking or that thoughts are products of an ongoing stream of mental activity, particularly, "Watch It Form," "Level It," and "Call It What It Is."

so now we have all these thoughts on cards in front of you. What's it like to have them out here . . . instead of back there (*gestures behind her head*)?

CLIENT: (*Describes what it is like.*)

THERAPIST: Now that they are out here in front of us . . . I wonder if we can check them out (*gestures as if looking at an object in her hand*) . . . be curious about them . . . maybe give them an age. How old is this one (*identifies a card*)?

CLIENT: Oh, that one is old. . . . I've thought that for a long time . . . maybe 15 years? (*Discussion continues.*)

THERAPIST: When these thoughts have hooked you . . . captured your attention . . . it seems it would be hard to see anything else. (*Invites the client to put one of the most compelling cards close to her face and see what else is available to her, what else can be seen.*) It would be hard to contribute that way . . . (*Therapist briefly role-plays being in a meeting and trying to show the client something while the client has the card close to her face.*)

I wonder what it is also like to have some distance; create some space. (*Invites the client to put the card out a little further, so that there is physical distance between her face and the card. The client can see the card, but she can also see the therapist and the room.*) Like, how is this different? Could you imagine choosing to speak under these conditions? Maybe you could give a nod to these thoughts (like, "hello old friend"), and then choose to speak?

CLINICAL GOAL 6: *Diversify the Psychological Functions of Food, Eating, and the Body or Meeting Needs*

For individuals with AN, food, eating, the body, and responding to the body's needs are aversives. In most cases, aversion has been conditioned through indirect (relational or verbal) learning. Sometimes this is intentional. For example, when individuals are trying to control their eating, they may condition aversion by equating foods to other stimuli that have disgust functions (e.g., describing rice as maggots). Other times, it is the result of a complex set of verbal interactions, which may not be clearly identified. For example, among individuals with AN, responding to one's emotional and physical needs (e.g., eating when hungry, resting when tired, seeking social support when lonely or upset) may correspond with being weak, lazy, needy, greedy, or selfish. As a result, clients are often motivated to avoid engaging in these behaviors. Defusion strategies can decrease the power of these verbally ascribed properties to allow other elements of experience to exert stimulus control. This includes, for example, the directly experienced benefits of responding to various forms of deprivation (e.g., the positive effects of fueling the body when it needs nourishment). The therapist may also facilitate new experiences with food, eating, or the body to broaden their psychological functions. Examples of strategies are listed in Handout 9.1 (at the end of this chapter); a copy can be downloaded and printed for use in your work with clients (see the box at the end of the table of contents).

CLINICAL GOAL 7: *Practice Being in the Present Moment*

The therapist helps the client practice being in the present moment, as illustrated in the dialogue and script below. This work builds on Clinical Goal 1, which teaches clients to discriminate mental activity from direct experience (or experiencing the world through the five senses). In the dialogue below, we return to Therapist Script E (with the "Driving on Autopilot" metaphor) from Clinical Goal 1; however, here the therapist explicitly aims to shape the client's capacity to "be here now." Often this practice has to be titrated slowly, given the discomfort of individuals with AN in contacting sensed experience (including their own breathing, etc.). More advanced practice in being present might include longer periods of sitting in stillness (in session or outside of session), being in nature, manipulating clay or another art without a product, or doing gentle movement (e.g., restorative yoga). An increased capacity for "being" without "doing" allows individuals with AN to engage in activities they enjoy even if they do not lead to a specific achievement, have more restful moments, and be more spontaneous (e.g., accepting an invitation from a friend).

IN PRACTICE

Dialogue (with the "Five Senses" Exercise)

THERAPIST: Our minds are rarely focused on what we are doing in the moment. Instead, they are running backward or forward in time (ruminating about the past, worrying about the future) . . . analyzing or problem-solving a situation. . . . Have you ever been driving somewhere and you arrive and have no idea how you got there (you didn't see anything along the way)? Your mind was somewhere else.

CLIENT: (*Discusses this.*)

THERAPIST: Even right now . . . your mind keeps running over what happened yesterday and whether you did something wrong . . . then thinking about the future, and planning how to prevent it from happening again. Do you notice that?

CLIENT: Yes.

THERAPIST: I wonder what it would be like for you to *be here now* . . . to not miss what is happening in the moment you are in . . . ?

CLIENT: How do I do that?

THERAPIST: One way to do it is with your five senses. What you can see, hear, smell, taste, feel . . . these experiences in the present moment.

Another way to come to the present moment is with your breath. You are breathing all the time, but are probably not aware of it (unless it becomes labored or something). When you start to become aware of your breath and notice each inhale and exhale, you are in the present moment . . .

Can we practice together now?

CLIENT: (*Agrees.*)

THERAPIST: (*Proceeds at a slow pace.*) First, let's just settle in . . . allow your body to grow still . . . soften the gaze . . . now I invite you to notice four or five things that you see . . . objects or colors, patterns or shapes in the room . . . no need to say them out loud, just notice them. . . . (*silently*) (*long pause*) Now, notice what you feel (for example, your feet against the floor, the temperature of your skin . . . or a feeling inside your body, like your chest rising and falling with breath). Notice what you taste. . . . Notice what you smell. . . . Notice what you hear. . . . (What is the smallest noise? The biggest . . . what noise is closest to you? What noise is furthest away? . . .) And also notice if your mind tries to take you somewhere else . . . and see if you can find your way back to this moment. You can use your breath as an anchor to be here now. Simply find your next inhale or exhale . . . [For some individuals with AN, or in some stages of treatment, feet on the floor or another anchor might be more appropriate than the breath.]

Therapist Script (with the "Mindful Receiving" Exercise)

"There is something really useful about being able to fully be in the present moment. We so rarely do that. Often we are some other time or place in our heads. This is particularly true in transitions, when we are walking or driving somewhere. Our bodies are walking or driving, but our mind is still where we were *before* or where we are going *next* (or what we have to do later).

"Another thing that we do is we judge or evaluate our experience, and so we are not experiencing the moment directly, but through labels, categories, and interpretations. I wonder if we can do a practice together that is about being in the present moment . . .

"If you are willing, I would invite you to take a moment and let your eyes fall closed or avert your gaze to your lap. . . . Put both feet on the floor . . . feeling the grounded, rooted energy where you contact the earth. The crown of your head lifts as your chin gently tucks . . . (*long pause*)

"Maybe notice the sounds around you . . . in this room and outside of this room. . . . Maybe the smallest noise that you can notice. . . . (*long pause*) Notice if your mind wants to tell stories about the noises, and see if, instead, you can come back to the direct sensory qualities. . . . (*long pause*) Let yourself become aware of your breathing. The rise and fall of your chest . . . the gentle inhale and exhale. Allowing your attention to rest on these sensations . . . and how the breath feels moving through the body. See if you can allow your shoulders to drop . . . let go of the need to be doing anything, including *holding things in* or *holding things out* . . . bracing against things. . . . (*long pause*) Just allowing things to be. Just being. Not doing. If thoughts show up (including judgments or interpretations), let them, but don't follow or chase them . . . or elaborate on them in any way . . . simply acknowledge them and gently redirect your attention back to your breath . . . as gentle as you might lead a lamb to water (or how you might take the hand of a toddler). . . . (*long pause*) If you are willing, I invite you to turn your palms up . . . opening your hands as if to receive a gift . . . the gift of the present moment. . . . Allowing whatever is here to be here as experiences of a conscious human being. Just being here now, for a few moments longer. You are here and you are alive. That simple. You are here and you are alive. . . . Take three or four more cycles of breath . . . (*long pause*) then allow your eyes to flutter open . . . coming back into the room. . . ."

CLINICAL GOAL 8: *Practice Broad and Flexible Attention*

Individuals with AN are vigilant to signs that they have failed to meet expectations. This may manifest as distracted ("scanning") or fixated attention on their bodies (e.g., sensations in their gut, the stomach pressing against a waistband, the spread of their thigh), the bodies of other people, or signs of interpersonal conflict or disapproval (e.g., a frown). Defusion interventions might have already helped clients "unhook" from these experiences and their interpretations. Additional present-moment interventions can build clients' capacity to flexibly attend to these events as they occur. Clients can practice choosing a focus for their attention and broadening attention to take in other aspects of the situation that might be useful in guiding behavior, or helping them situate events in their broader context to understand their meaning.

For individuals with AN, focused attention might first be practiced with events outside the body (e.g., attending to the sound of a clock) rather than internal experiences, which may be more challenging. The therapist might also use props such as clay to provide an external focus to practice purposeful attention (a clay exercise was described earlier, pages 222–223). The dialogue below illustrates how the therapist might guide the client to practice shifting attention flexibly between internal and external stimuli.

IN PRACTICE

Dialogue

THERAPIST: We've been talking a lot about how your attention gets captured by your gut, and as long as it is narrowly fixated there, you are missing all sorts of other things, including, for example, opportunities to connect with colleagues or your son. I would like us to practice flexible attention here together. Would that be OK? Attention is like a muscle. . . . It has to be worked . . . developed.

CLIENT: Yes, that seems like a good idea . . .

THERAPIST: Great! First, I am going to invite you to assume that dignified sitting posture that we have been practicing. (*Gives some instruction to settle the client into the exercise.*) For this exercise, let's leave the eyes open, but avert your gaze to the floor to minimize visual input. Now, simply allow your attention to move over your body, and when it "gets stuck," give me a wave.

CLIENT: (*Waves.*)

THERAPIST: Is it at your gut?

CLIENT: My waistline, yes.

THERAPIST: OK. Go ahead and allow your attention to be poured into that. That place where you can feel your waistline. (*long pause*) Now, I invite you to gently direct your attention to the sound of the clock. Like you are leading a lamb or a child. Not yanking or forcing. A really gentle offering. (*Proceeds at a slow and deliberate pace.*)

And now see if you can also direct your attention to your feet on the floor and that grounded sensation, and maybe you can hold your waistline and your feet simultaneously.

(*slow and deliberate pace*)

And now see if you can look up to find the painting on the wall. Noticing your waistline and then (gently) noticing the wall.

(*slow and deliberate pace*)

And maybe you can find me in front of you, too . . .

(*slow and deliberate pace*)

There are people in your life that you might be able to see, that you hadn't seen for a long time, with this sort of practice . . .

Looking Ahead

Self-as-context is engaged in all therapeutic work to some degree, and particularly in defusion, which separates the observer from what is being observed. However, psychological flexibility may be further enhanced by focused work strengthening the observer self or targeting other self-processes. In Chapter 10, we briefly discuss interventions that more directly engage self-as-context, as well as interventions that address issues in the knowing self (self-as-verbal process) and the conceptualized self (self-as-content) among individuals with AN.

Strategies to Recontextualize Food, Eating, or the Body

Instructions: Challenge yourself to broaden your relationship with food, eating, or your body with the strategies below. The goal is not to eliminate *old* associations but rather to create *new* ones, such that you have an array of options for how you might relate to food, eating, or your body in any given moment.

Strategy	Example
Shift the environmental cues.	Change the physical space in which eating takes place. Make it more appealing, less distracted, and so forth.
Pair food, eating, or the body with appetitives (e.g., personal values).	Make meals quality time with a loved one. Do something that is meaningful or engaging after eating.
Mindful eating or mindful movement	Eat (or move) in a slow, deliberate manner that engages all five senses. Observe the experience of eating/moving.
Exposure exercises	Eat a feared food or allow the body to be "exposed" or in its more natural state (rather than contracting the stomach, covering the thighs with a pillow, etc.). The goal is to be present with these experiences or interact with food or the body in a new way (habituation may be a side effect, but is not the goal per se).
Tell its story.	Narrate the life of a food (e.g., from seed to supermarket to plate) or one's body (e.g., scars, and so forth, that tell the body's unique history).
Observe the whole body instead of parts.	Practice observing the body as a whole unit rather than dismantling it into its component parts (thighs, stomach, etc.). This may be done while looking in the mirror, or in the mind's eye. This practice might also include sensing the full self, from the inside out, i.e., noticing the sensations of the body separately and then noticing all sensations at once, as an integrated whole.
Food play or adventures	Interact with food in a more playful manner: learning new recipes, taking a cooking class, making food faces in plates, plating food in an appealing manner, trying new or exotic foods.
Metaphor	Consider what it would be like to treat the body like a garden, a sunset, or a friend.

CHAPTER 10

Sensing the Self

If you listen to the body when it whispers,
you won't have to hear it scream.
—UNKNOWN

I am bigger than anything that can happen to me.
—CHARLES F. LUMMIS

The self is a complex construct with different meanings across therapeutic traditions. Thus, it is useful to first describe "the self" from a relational frame theory (RFT) or contextual behavioral science perspective, before elaborating on the application to AN. The observer self (self-as-context) is identified as a core functional dimension of psychological flexibility. However, there are other elements of our self-experience. First, there is self-as-verbal process, or the *knowing self*, in which we verbally describe (or label) our ongoing internal experiences. This includes identifying a fuzzy collection of internal events as an emotion (e.g., "I notice that I am feeling anxiety") or other interoceptive cue (e.g., "I notice that I am feeling hunger"). The ability to verbally describe our internal experiences is helpful. Verbal labels relate to other training about what to do when one feels a particular way. If an individual is able to label her feelings, then she might also know what actions may be helpful to meet her needs.

Second, there is the *conceptualized self*, or the content dimensions of ourselves, in which we describe ourselves in relation to a variety of characteristics, categories, or roles. This is perhaps the most familiar "self" and in other traditions may be referred to as *self-concept*. A flexible conceptualized self is adaptive. Coherent narratives of ourselves and our lives can give us a sense of identity and allow us to predict and control our own behavior. However, we can also be overly attached to our self-narratives, which can make it difficult to deviate even when it would be effective. Attachment to the conceptualized self is encouraged by our language conventions that provide contextual cues for equating ourselves to our content (e.g., "I am").

Finally, the *observer self* is the constant vantage point from which all internal and external events are observed. It is the "I, Here, Now" perspective, or that perspective that emerges as we discriminate "I" from "You," "Here" from "There," and "Now" from "Then." Interventions that strengthen the observer self increase an individual's capacity to experience the self as stable and immutable across time, and as "more than" any experience that one might have. Observer-self interventions may also increase an individual's capacity to flexibly take perspective: their own perspective at another time or place, or the perspective of another individual. Flexible perspective taking allows the individual to appreciate the impact of situational factors on behavior and experience empathy and/or compassion (for oneself or other people).

Among individuals with AN, self-processes may be engaged to further:

- Enhance awareness of what one is feeling (and the need that is conveyed by that feeling) (knowing self skills).
- Decrease attachment to particular self-content (e.g., achievements or the body) and broaden identity (aspects of the conceptualized self).
- Increase capacity for empathy and self-compassion (observer self).

Clinical Goals

We outline five clinical goals and strategies.

CLINICAL GOAL 1: *Enhance Self-Awareness (or Strengthen the Knowing Self)*

The therapist helps the client enhance self-awareness and build self-knowledge. This includes improving the client's ability to know what she is feeling moment to moment (e.g., emotions, hunger, satiety, pain, fatigue) and recognize the needs conveyed by her feelings. It also includes the ability to identify personal preferences.

As mentioned previously, interventions that focus on emotional or interoceptive clarity should be appropriately timed and sensitive to the impact of low BMI on signals arising from the body (e.g., muting of hunger or somatic correlates of emotion with underweight), and reversing starvation should be prioritized above appetite awareness.

Identifying Emotions

Understanding how we feel is essential for meeting our physical and emotional needs. It is also important for communicating with others and building connection through shared emotional experiences and empathy. Individuals with AN often have difficulty labeling their emotions and use vague terms such as "bad" or "upset." They might also describe emotions in only somatic terms (e.g., feeling heavy or "fat"), or have difficulty discriminating emotions from other body signals (e.g., hunger/satiety). The therapist helps the client verbally describe her internal states, building an emotional vocabulary.

When training emotional awareness, the therapist provides descriptions of each of the basic emotions (e.g., anger, fear, sadness, guilt, shame), including the typical thoughts, feelings (physiological changes), urges, and behaviors associated with these emotion labels. It can be particularly useful to highlight how emotions impact the experience of the body, body weight, or the gut. For example, some emotions may make the individual feel heavy, weighted, or sluggish (e.g., sadness); others may be associated with a pit or knot in the stomach (e.g., guilt, shame). For some individuals, pictures can be useful. This might include "emoticons" or images that depict somatic constitutes or correlates of emotion (e.g., butterflies in the stomach). Other resources that might be used include emotion regulation handouts from DBT (Linehan, 2014) and emotion wheels.

The ability to label an emotion can be shaped by first identifying an internal experience that is known to the client (e.g., sensation in the gut), and then expanding the client's awareness to other corresponding internal events (e.g., co-occurring thoughts, feelings, body sensations, urges), and potentially, situational factors that might provide information about what she is feeling. This might be described as *data gathering* or, for younger clients, *detective work* (i.e., gathering clues to form a hypothesis about a likely emotion), which shifts the context from avoidance/control to curiosity. Emotional labeling might also be shaped using a diary card with multiple-choice responses that are phased out over time. Handout 10.1 (at the end of this chapter) is a blank version of a multiple-choice diary card. A version you can download and use in your work with clients is provided on the publisher's website (see the box at the end of the table of contents).

In addition to labeling emotions, clients may be taught to notice varying degrees of emotional intensity and the natural rhythm (or rise and fall) of emotions. In doing so, the therapist does not suggest that any level of intensity is "too much" or that return to baseline affect is the desired outcome, simply that emotional experiences are dynamic, and observing these dynamics can be helpful. It can build self-knowledge (e.g., this is how my body feels at a low level of anxiety, this is how it feels at a high level) that informs the client's actions.

Finally, the therapist might also help the client appreciate the context in which her emotions arise. Identifying factors influencing mood increases the predictability of emotional experience and can help the individual come to know herself and what she might need or prefer.

Initially, the therapist may be more active in providing emotion labels; however, over time, the client will increasingly produce these labels herself. Sample dialogues below illustrate emotional awareness skills training (Dialogue A) and shaping emotional awareness in the moment using client content (Dialogues B and C).

IN PRACTICE

Dialogue A

THERAPIST: How are you feeling right now?

CLIENT: I don't know . . .

THERAPIST: This is something that comes up for you a lot . . .

CLIENT: Yes! How do people know how they are feeling? Ugh.

THERAPIST: You wish there was a manual or something.

CLIENT: Yes!

THERAPIST: I don't have a manual. (*Smiles.*) But we can talk about what emotions tend to feel like. Then we can practice the "cueing in" part: observing what is going on inside of you and using that information to identify what you are feeling and what you might need.

Emotions are labels used to describe a fuzzy collection of experiences that tend to cluster together. . . . This includes thoughts, feelings (body sensations), physiological changes, urges, and so forth. Some emotions feel activating (like excitement or anxiety), while others feel deactivating (like sadness). Some you might feel more in your chest and others in your gut. Emotions also vary in intensity, and sometimes we use different words to express differences in intensity. We might say that we are annoyed if we feel a low level of anger and that we feel rage if we feel a very high level of anger. Common emotions include sadness, happiness, anger, frustration, fear, guilt, shame, and jealousy.

I think it might be helpful if we unpack this a bit. Is it OK if I write on the board?

CLIENT: (*Agrees.*)

THERAPIST: OK, let's start with sadness. What is sadness like? (*Elicits some from client and then elaborates.*) Yeah, sadness often feels heavy. That's why people say things like "I have the weight of the world on my shoulders." When we feel sad, we might feel as though we are dragging our legs through mud. We might feel really tired or sluggish. Our body language will often convey this too: We might slump or look down when we are feeling this way. We often have the urge to withdraw when we are sad, even though this often creates more feelings of sadness because we are away from people and things that we care about.

Can you think of a time when you felt sad? What else did you notice?

CLIENT: (*Describes feeling sad.*)

THERAPIST: Sometimes people might feel as though they are fatter when sad . . . and this could be because sadness directs our attention to things that we don't like (about ourselves, etc.).

However, it might also be because sadness feels heavy in the body, and so we think that we are "fat" or "lazy."

CLIENT: (*Discusses this.*)

THERAPIST: Feelings exist for a reason. They serve a function in our lives and are adaptive and useful—even as they are also painful and hard, at times. Sometimes our emotions will be a signal to us—a communication. In this case, they may convey a need that we have. For example, if we are feeling sad, this might suggest that we need to grieve a loss, that we need comfort, or that we need to make a change in our lives.

Taking these actions is not to make the feeling go away (although it might, as the communication is no longer necessary), but rather to be responsive to our needs. Sometimes emotions are not communicating anything but are simply cued up by some contextual feature, or aspect of the situation. For example, I might feel sad when I smell the fall leaves because this reminds me of a difficult time in my life/history. How does this apply to your experience?

CLIENT: (*Describes.*)

THERAPIST: OK, next up, fear . . . (*Therapist works through all the primary emotions.*)

Dialogue B

The therapist notices a change in attention to body weight/shape and is shaping emotional awareness in the moment. The focus is on providing an emotion label.

THERAPIST: What happened there?

CLIENT: Huh?

THERAPIST: Well, we were talking about your work, and then you brought up weight. I am wondering if something showed up for you in that conversation . . .

CLIENT: I was just noticing how my thighs felt.

THERAPIST: Were you noticing your thighs before that moment?

CLIENT: Um . . . I guess not.

THERAPIST: I'm wondering what else was happening at that moment? Did you notice any other thought or feeling . . . ? At the same time, or even before you noticed your thighs . . . ?

CLIENT: (*Fidgets.*)

THERAPIST: I appreciate your willingness to slow down and reflect on your experience . . . I know that it is difficult. (*long pause*)

CLIENT: I just feel fat . . . heavy and gross . . .

THERAPIST: (*Notices light tearing.*) I am wondering if you might also be feeling sad. . . . Sadness can feel heavy . . . and it can bring tears . . .

CLIENT: Yes, I guess so . . . I didn't notice it before.

THERAPIST: Maybe this is what sadness feels like for you (in this moment, maybe other moments)? Knowing what we are feeling, we can choose how to respond rather than react . . .

Dialogue C

The therapist notices a change in body language and is shaping emotional awareness in the moment. In addition to labeling the emotion, the client is also practicing discriminating the intensity of an emotion and the events that give rise to it.

THERAPIST: You seem to be collapsing into yourself . . . drawing in. . . . I am wondering what you might be feeling?

CLIENT: I don't know. Nothing.

THERAPIST: Would it be OK if we took a minute to check it out?

CLIENT: Yes.

THERAPIST: Do you feel that . . . that experience of drawing in?

CLIENT: Yes. . . . I just want to disappear.

THERAPIST: Do you notice anything else? Any other thoughts or feelings, or anything in your body . . . ?

CLIENT: Nothing else really. Well, I guess, my stomach is upset. But it feels like that a lot.

THERAPIST: What is it like?

CLIENT: A pit. Right in the center.

THERAPIST: How strong is the sensation? If 1 is slight, and 10 is the most intense experience like this you have ever had . . .

CLIENT: An 8.

THERAPIST: It is really present. (*long pause*) You started pulling in when we started talking about your mom.

CLIENT: I've worried her so much. I am such a bad daughter.

THERAPIST: The thought "I am a bad daughter." . . . That is another aspect of your experience. . . . If you were going to give this emotion a label, what might you call it?

CLIENT: Umm . . . I don't know. (*long pause*)

THERAPIST: Do you think you might be experiencing guilt or shame . . . ?

CLIENT: Yes, I wouldn't have thought of it, but shame sounds right. . . . I feel ashamed of myself . . . for not doing better . . .

THERAPIST: Putting words to our experience . . . labeling our emotions can be helpful. We can come to know them and what gives rise to them. So this is what shame at an 8 feels like. . . . I wonder if you can tell me more about what is important to you in this situation . . . what kind of daughter you want to be . . . ?

CLIENT: (*Describes.*)

THERAPIST: And the urge to hide is coming from shame . . . it is the advice that shame gives . . . and I wonder if going with that urge is helpful to you . . . helpful in building the life you want . . .

Discriminating Hunger/Satiety

Clients sometimes need explicit training to learn (or relearn) their signals of hunger and satiety as weight is restored and, potentially, to discriminate hunger/satiety from emotions. Clients might need to be taught to use hunger/satiety signals to initiate eating before they are overly hungry and to stop eating when they are satisfied (rather than overly full). Appetite awareness can be shaped by having clients rate hunger and satiety before, during, and after a meal (e.g., using a 7-point Likert scale, 1 = *ravenous*, 7 = *overly full*), with the aim of spending more time in zones 3, 4, and 5 (Craighead, 2006). It is important not to do this work too early, as difficulties in discriminating hunger and satiety are exacerbated with starvation, and hunger/satiety signals sometimes need to be defied during nutritional rehabilitation (i.e., the individual may need to eat when she does not feel hungry or eat past comfortable satiety).

Identifying Needs Conveyed by Feelings

Feelings have adaptive value and serve as communication to others and to ourselves about what we need. Knowing the needs that our emotions (or other internal experiences) convey allows us to be responsive and attuned. Clients can practice this by asking the question: "What am I feeling, and what does this tell me about what I need right now?" Taking action to meet our needs is not to reduce the feeling (although it might), but rather to behave in a manner that respects our feelings. Knowing the needs conveyed by our feelings also allows for an accumulation of self-knowledge ("I am a person who needs time to recharge after social interactions"). Self-knowledge helps us build a life that is vital or meaningful and brings joy.

Handout 10.2 (at the end of this chapter) lists some examples of feelings and the needs that they may convey; a copy can be downloaded and printed for use in your work with clients (see the box at the end of the table of contents).

Importantly, the need conveyed by a feeling (as well as the workable responses) is context-specific. For example, when the body has been in motion, fatigue may convey the need to rest and restore. However, if the body has been very *inactive*, fatigue might convey the need to move or activate. When determining the need conveyed by a feeling, a client might be encouraged to consider the signal arising from the body *and* the context in which it is occurring.

Identifying Personal Preferences

Individuals with AN may have difficulty knowing their personal preferences. This might be due to a long history of basing decisions on the opinions or perceived expectations of others or the emergence of AN at a key period of identity development. The capacity to identify preferences can be shaped by gentle insistence that the client check in with her experience as a guide, and by blocking reassurance seeking, as illustrated in Dialogue A. Personal preferences (or *preferencing*) can also be shaped through questioning. Clients can be presented with repeated prompts to consider personal preferences (that vary in degree of challenge, complexity, and content). The key is for the client to develop a general capacity for preferencing rather than reveal some particular information about herself. Prompts may include personal preferences related to food (e.g., preferred textures or tastes), but this should occur later in treatment, when AN has less influence. We provide a therapist script with some examples of prompts for personal preferences, as well as an example of this exercise in session (Dialogue B).

IN PRACTICE

Dialogue A

The client is describing trying to make a decision.

CLIENT: I asked my mom, and she said that I should take the job that offered the most money. What do you think I should do?

THERAPIST: I guess I am wondering how *you* feel about this situation. . . . What do *you* want to do?

CLIENT: I don't know. I just want someone to tell me what will be best.

THERAPIST: This seems like other times when you have felt really unsure, and start looking to other people for the answer; trying to figure out the "right" thing to do. . . . (*long pause*) I wonder if there is not a *right* thing . . . and trying to figure that out (by asking other people) has kept you stuck a bit, feeling dissatisfied in life and in your decisions. I'd like to see if we can help you check in with how *you* feel; what you want or prefer (in this situation, but other ones too) . . .

Therapist Script (Practice Preferencing)

"I wonder if we might practice identifying personal preferences. This is something you haven't done much [because of AN, rule following, or compliance], and this is a skill that can be developed with practice . . .

"Let's start with some general sensory experiences (*therapist takes a playful tone and conveys that there are no wrong answers*):

- Do you like red or blue?
- Do you like the texture of this sofa or this chair?
- Do you like the smell of this lotion or that one?
- Do you like this tone or that one?

"Over the next week, I would like you to go on a bit of a scavenger hunt and see if you can identify a color, smell, or sound that you like. As you are on your hunt, I encourage you to check in to consider how you knew that you preferred one over the other. Try not to over-think this (don't think at all!); rather, check in on your experience. Be mindful of the urge to choose something because someone else would, or because you think it is the 'right' answer, and try to choose from your heart (or your nose!).

"OK, let's do a few more. . . . These are a bit more complex . . .

- Do you prefer a river or a lake?
- Do you prefer sunrise or sunset?
- Do you prefer mysteries or autobiographies?
- Do you prefer cats or dogs?
- Do you prefer the city or the country?

"And how about some open-ended questions:

- What did you like about *X* activity?
- How would you like *X* to be different?"

Dialogue B

THERAPIST: I wonder if we can play around with identifying your personal preferences. . . . It is easy for our heads to get overinvolved in this process. . . . Instead of cueing in to what we like or dislike, we might find ourselves trying to figure out what is right or trying to match other people's preferences or expectations of us.

CLIENT: I do that!

THERAPIST: Well, if you are willing, let's see what it is like to freely choose. Sound good?

CLIENT: I'll try.

THERAPIST: Here's one: Do you prefer sunrise or sunset? See if you can find the answer inside you. Not based on me or ideas of what you should like.

CLIENT: I don't know. (*Smiles.*) Maybe I don't want to do this! (*pause*)

THERAPIST: Try choosing from your heart or your gut, instead of your head. There are no wrong (or right!) answers. (*pause*)

CLIENT: Sunset . . .

THERAPIST: Did that come from your head or somewhere else?

CLIENT: You told me not to use my head! (So I didn't.)

THERAPIST: Fabulous! What was it like to choose, to have a preference?

CLINICAL GOAL 2: *Decrease Attachment to a Narrow Conceptualized Self and Build Self-Content*

Individuals with AN are overidentified with outward appearance. This includes their physical bodies, as well as other accomplishments that can be observed (or are visible) to themselves or other people (e.g., academic or professional achievements). They might also be overidentified with AN and have little competing content (i.e., ideas of who they are beyond the eating disorder). Overidentification with these elements of the conceptualized self, and the relative poverty of other content, increases the threat of relinquishing rigid control over eating and restoring weight, or experimenting with a kinder, gentler approach to managing themselves.

Overidentification can be addressed by (1) creating a context in which the individual can experience herself as separate, distinct, and "more than" her content (or things about her) (illustrated in the therapist scripts and Dialogue A below) and (2) expanding or diversifying self-content. Self-content is diversified as individuals with AN open up to experience and try new things, potentially facilitated via behavioral challenges (described in Chapter 7). Self-content is also expanded as clients articulate personal values and engage in value-guided behavioral activation (described in Chapter 8). The therapist may explicitly highlight this new and emerging content to encourage more varied identification ("It seems you care about X and that is part of you too"). The goal is for clients to have a *diverse array* of "things about them" but also to hold these things *lightly* (i.e., not be *overly* attached to any particular aspect of the self or identity). An additional exercise to expand or diversify self-content is provided in Dialogue B.

IN PRACTICE

Therapist Script A

"You are a person experiencing AN, but you are not only that. There is more to you . . . much more."

Therapist Script B

"There is a person who was there before AN . . . and will be here after. . . . It is the same person who is here now."

Therapist Script C

"That part of you that cares about *X* [value] . . . that is not AN. You have both of those things, and are neither . . ."

Therapist Script D

"When did *you* get reduced to your body (a gold ribbon, etc.)? What about all the elements of you that cannot be seen?"

Dialogue A (with the "Observer Self" Exercise, Focus on the Body)

THERAPIST: It seems you have been reduced to your body or outside appearance . . . how you look to others, your successes. . . . This happens to all of us in some way. We get attached to things *about us* and start to confuse our*selves* with those things.

In a very real (experienced) way there is a you who is "more than" anything *about* you . . . that transcends momentary thoughts or feelings, or even the body, which has changed and been different across time. . . . A *you* who "has" these things . . . this body . . . but is not those things.

CLIENT: I sort of understand what you mean, but it all sounds strange.

THERAPIST: I wonder if we can do something . . . to see if we can experience it to be so. Would that be OK?

CLIENT: Umm . . . OK.

THERAPIST: (*Leads a brief centering exercise.*) And now I want you to see if you can imagine a much younger "you." The "you" before you had to be anything in particular . . . the you before you had to prove your worth. Before you worried about whether you were attractive or smart. . . . "You" when you were freer to be you.

See if you can look through the eyes of that younger you.

Embody that "you" that it is in that moment. Embodying is different than looking *at you*. It is looking through your own eyes. See if you can look through your eyes rather than looking at you or seeing yourself from a more distant vantage point.

[The therapist pauses to allow for this.]

Do you have it?

CLIENT: Yes.

THERAPIST: See if you can look from those eyes and notice who and what is around you, what you are thinking, what you are feeling, how it feels in your body. . . . (*pause*) Now see, if just for a moment you can also notice that the "you" that is behind those eyes is the same "you" who is here now. (*pause*) And can notice who and what is around you *now*, what you are thinking and feeling, and how it feels in your body. The same "you" who can notice these things now, was noticing those other things then. . . . All of those things were different and yet in a really deep way, as a matter of experience, this is the same you. The same you is behind those eyes.

Now, I know that a lot *about* you has changed. You have been through a lot. . . . You have thought things and felt things, and your body has been different. It has been sick and well. It has been fed and starved. And yet, in a very real way, the "you" behind the eyes is the same. You have not changed. That hasn't changed, even as your body has changed. Your body is actually always changing, in every moment. . . . Cells are regenerated, repeatedly. . . . Things are changing all the time inside of you without your awareness. You have grown completely new hair. Your skin has replaced itself over and over. You have lost your teeth and gotten new ones.

And you are the same. You have always been you. You will always be you. Your body has actually been changing in every moment . . .

And yet you remain you. Not in a logic way, but as a matter of experience. . . . The you behind the eyes is/has been the same. . . .

Dialogue B (with the "I Am" Exercise)

In this exercise, the therapist encourages the client to generate varied content in response to the prompt "I am." If the client gets stuck, the therapist might give a suggestion that opens up another category. For example, if the client is providing roles ("daughter," "student," "friend," etc.), the therapist might offer characteristics ("spiritual," "reserved"). The therapist might also offer things that are seemingly in contradiction to highlight how content might vary in accordance with the situation. For example, the client might be "reserved" in one context and "outgoing" in another. This encourages clients not to be too attached to any particular aspect of the self. The therapist also observes with the client that she is not really any of these things (she is the "I" in "I am").

THERAPIST: I hear that it is scary and it feels vacuous in a sense: that without AN, you are not sure what is there. I guess the question is: What do you want to be there, like, maybe in some sense it is a choice. You have said you value X. What would it be like to start to build that out a bit . . . to make that more a part of who you are or who you choose to be?

(*Client engages for a few minutes, but quickly feels blocked.*)

THERAPIST: Can we do something together? It is about flexing the mind. We can do it out loud or on paper, whichever you prefer.

CLIENT: OK.

THERAPIST: I want you to complete this sentence stem as many times as possible. Ready? "I am _____."

CLINICAL GOAL 3: *Increase Capacity to Experience the Self as Transcending Any Particular Experience*

Clients may benefit from additional interventions that facilitate a separation between the individual and her momentary thoughts and feelings. The aim is to create a hierarchical, rather than equivalence, relation (such that the individual experiences herself as "bigger than" any thought/feeling that she may have). The result is that all experiences may be held (or allowed), including *unwanted* thoughts/feelings. Metaphors to facilitate this relation are provided in the next therapist scripts. A sense of self that transcends momentary experiences might also be strengthened by adopting language conventions that explicitly identify the observer, for example, reporting "I am noticing X [e.g., the feeling of anger]" rather than "I am X [e.g., angry]." Interventions might also include relevant meditations such as the Mountain Meditation by John Kabat-Zinn (1994, p. 135).

IN PRACTICE

Therapist Script A (with the "Guests in Your Home" Metaphor)

"These feelings are like guests in your home. . . . Guests come and go. . . . (*pause*) Maybe some of them stay a while . . . put their feet up. . . .

(Even if you don't want them to stay . . . you can't really force them to go. In fact, the more that you insist, perhaps the more comfortable they become. . . .)

"The guests are not the home. They are simply visitors. I wonder if you can sense that their presence does not impact the integrity of your home. . . . (*long pause*) It (you) stays intact . . . as guests come and go . . ."

Therapist Script B (with the "Clouds in the Sky" Metaphor)

"Can you bring to mind the sky—imagine it expanding in all directions—maybe a beautiful blue? Clouds may be there, or they may come in. Clouds of different shapes and sizes and colors. Some clouds are dark and stormy and may sit there longer than we would like. . . . At times, we may resist these clouds, resist the rain (noticing, too, that resisting doesn't change whether the rain falls).

"Whether clear, cloudy, or stormy . . . the sky behind the clouds (that holds the clouds) is the same. . . . (*long pause*) As the weather changes, as clouds move in and out . . . the sky behind the clouds remains intact . . . the sky, the backdrop for the changing weather . . ."

CLINICAL GOAL 4: *Practice Flexible Perspective Taking*

Individuals with AN have difficulties discriminating *their own* perspective from the perspective of *other people*. Thus, they may report that they do not know if they *genuinely* feel a particular way or have taken on the feelings of other people. They might also assume other people share their judgments and criticisms. As a result, the world may seem dangerous and rejecting. Difficulty discriminating self–other perspectives may also make it difficult for clients to appreciate how their actions (e.g., severe weight loss) affect other people (e.g., family).

Individuals with AN might also have difficulty taking *their own* perspective *at another time and place*. This might impact their ability to appreciate the impact of situational factors on their behavior or experience self-compassion.

The therapist helps the client build skills in flexible perspective taking. This is accomplished through repeatedly asking questions that require the client to consider her own perspective or the perspective of others, and how they might differ from one another or across time and place. Sample prompts are provided below, along with in-session dialogues. In some cases, flexible perspective taking might need to be shaped in the context of less emotional valence; for example, by the client imagining that the situation is not self-relevant or by making it less so (e.g., imagining the same scenario happening to another person, or to a much younger version of themselves).

IN PRACTICE

Therapist Script

Prompts to practice perspective taking in session include:

> "What are you feeling now? What were you feeling then?"
> "How might someone feel in this situation? What about that situation?"
> "What do you think she was feeling then? What about now?"
> "What do you think might be contributing to how you (or she) feels? How might *X* influence how one feels in this situation?
> "You are thinking and feeling *X*; however, what might she be thinking and feeling?"

Dialogue A

CLIENT: I'm sure she was thinking that I am a fat pig . . .

THERAPIST: Those are your thoughts and feelings. . . . Aren't they . . . ? Rather than looking from your eyes, can you look from hers? Can you imagine what her experience might have been in that moment?

Dialogue B

CLIENT: My mom and I got into a fight last night. . . . She was just being so mean! She said I couldn't stay over at my friend's house for the sleepover and we just got into it. . . . She ended up leaving my room in the middle of it.

THERAPIST: How did that make you feel?

CLIENT: I felt sad . . . like I'm being left out of what my friends are doing again. It's just so annoying that my mom won't let me go. I'm so mad at her.

THERAPIST: Yeah, I get why you feel sad and annoyed—I know how important your friends are to you. I wonder what you think was going on for your mom in that moment? What was she feeling?

CLIENT: I don't know. She just wants to make my life miserable. . . . Well, I guess she said that I wouldn't eat if I stayed over there . . . so that was why, too.

THERAPIST: What do you imagine she was feeling then? See if you can drop into your mom's eyes for a moment . . . and what it would be like to be her . . .

CLIENT: I guess she is scared. She doesn't want me to end up in the hospital again.

THERAPIST: She loves you a lot.

CLIENT: Yes, and I know that I have worried her. I am sure she feels pretty desperate to keep me from going down that road again. . . . Really, she doesn't get to decide though.

THERAPIST: Yeah.

CLIENT: And so maybe she feels helpless, too. I don't know.

THERAPIST: That would be hard. It's hard on both sides.

CLINICAL GOAL 5: *Help the Client Practice Self-Compassion*

Clients' ability to take their own perspective at another time or place, or to see themselves through another person's eyes (rather than their own) allows for greater self-compassion. As a result, clients suffer less and may choose a gentler way of regulating themselves and their behavior. Self-compassion work is extremely challenging with individuals with AN, but it is also deeply meaningful. Below, we provide a therapist script for an exercise that guides the client in imagining a younger version of herself and choosing a compassionate rather than punitive approach. This is followed by a brief dialogue that highlights shaping self-compassion in the moment as an opportunity arises in session.

Therapist Script (with the "Younger You" Exercise)

"I wonder if you can bring up this younger version of you in your mind's eye. See if you can really see her—imagine what she is wearing and the way her hair falls around her face . . . the way that she moves in the world. Imagine talking to this younger version of you the way that you talk to yourself now. Imagine saying 'You don't deserve it' to that young girl, and imagine what you might notice in her eyes when she receives that. (*pause*) See if you can sense in this moment that that girl is you.

"That the pain is your pain.

"I wonder if you can imagine choosing kindness toward her. As a choice. Not as a feeling, and not based on whether she's earned it or something. Just because she is a human being and has inherent worth. Just because that is the way you choose to treat people, and her."

(*Clients with children might be asked to imagine speaking to their own child in this manner or to imagine their child speaking to herself in this manner to build self-compassion.*)

Dialogue B

CLIENT: I'm just such a sh*tty person. Why do I keep making mistakes?

THERAPIST: I get that your mind tells you that—that you are a bad person. It says that quite a lot. This asking "why?" . . . "Why do I do things?" This is also familiar. (*pause*)

   I wonder if right now, in this moment, you can allow some kindness or compassion toward yourself . . . ? You might bring to mind something or someone that you have deep compassion and warmth toward . . . (*long pause*) and imagine giving that to yourself.

   Maybe you could allow your hand to come to you heart and your eyes to fall closed. Allow some warmth, some kindness . . .

   (*The therapist models hand to heart, eyes closed.*)

Looking Ahead

In the final chapter, we provide a brief discussion of issues related to treatment progress and termination. We also provide some final thoughts for the AN therapist, including guidance on recognizing therapist psychological inflexibility.

Multiple-Choice Diary Card (with Workability Assessment)

Instructions: Awareness of our internal experiences is a skill that can be built over time. This form guides you in identifying your thoughts, feelings, and bodily sensations. It also helps you reflect on how you are relating to these experiences and the workability of your behavioral responses (or actions). Complete this form when you feel the urge to engage in an eating disorder behavior or when you notice a change in your mood, and use that as an opportunity to reflect on what else you might be experiencing. Later, practice without the multiple-choice options (Part B).

A. SITUATION OR EVENT

Where are you?

☐ Classroom ☐ Kitchen ☐ Family room

☐ Cafeteria ☐ Bedroom ☐ Locker room

☐ Friend's house ☐ At practice ☐ Outside

☐ _____

What is happening?

I am ☐ alone ☐ with other people

_____

(e.g., practicing trumpet)

Thoughts: What thoughts do (or did) you notice?

☐ People are mean, ugly. ☐ I am so boring.

☐ This is confusing. ☐ No one understands me.

☐ No one will ever like me. ☐ This is not fair.

☐ I'll never be good enough. ☐ I don't want to be doing this.

☐ Why can't I be more like her? ☐ I am going to fail.

☐ The future is scary. . . . It won't work out. ☐ _____

☐ _____ ☐ _____

On a scale of 0–10, how hooked are you by your thoughts?
(0 = *Not at all*; 10 = *Completely*)

_____

(continued)

Urges: What do you feel like doing?

☐ Running away   ☐ Leaving

☐ Speaking up   ☐ Not eating

☐ Hiding   ☐ Hitting

☐ Asking for help   ☐ Giving up

☐ Working harder   ☐ Exercising

☐ Jumping up and down   ☐ Apologizing

☐ Hurting myself   ☐ Crying

☐ Asking a question   ☐ _____

☐ Yelling   ☐ _____

☐ Getting quiet   ☐ _____

What sensations do you notice in your body?

☐ Tightness in the chest   ☐ Tension

☐ Butterflies in the stomach   ☐ Pit in my stomach

☐ Heart racing   ☐ Edgy

☐ Lightheaded   ☐ _____

☐ Heaviness in the arms or legs   ☐ _____

☐ Nausea

What emotion are you experiencing?

☐ Angry   ☐ Jealous

☐ Ashamed   ☐ Afraid/anxious

☐ Sad   ☐ Excited

☐ Embarrassed   ☐ Happy

☐ Guilty   ☐ Lonely

☐ Bored   ☐ _____

On a scale of 0–10, how strong are your emotions?
(0 = *Barely noticeable*; 10 = *Extremely strong*)

_____

On a scale of 0–10, how much are you fighting or struggling with your emotions?
(0 = *Not at all*; 10 = *Completely*)

_____

On a scale of 0–10, how much are you allowing the emotion to take over and rigidly determine your actions? (0 = *Not at all*; 10 = *Completely*)

_____

(continued)

Workability Assessment

What did you do in this situation?

What were the results?

Were your actions consistent with your values?

B. SITUATION OR EVENT

Where are you?

What is happening?

What are you doing?

Thoughts

What thoughts do you notice?

On a scale of 0–10, how hooked are you by your thoughts?
(0 = *Not at all*; 10 = *Completely*)

_____

(continued)

Urges

What urges do you notice?

Sensations

What sensations do you notice in your body?

Emotions

What emotions are you experiencing?

On a scale of 0–10, how strong are your emotions?
(0 = *Barely noticeable*; 10 = *Extremely strong*)

_____

On a scale of 0–10, how much are you fighting or struggling with your emotions?
(0 = *Not at all*; 10 = *Completely*)

_____

On a scale of 0–10, how much are you allowing the emotion to take over and rigidly determine your actions? (0 = *Not at all*; 10 = *Completely*)

_____

Workability Assessment

What did you do in this situation?

What were the results?

Were your actions consistent with your values?

Internal Experiences and the Need That They May Convey

Instructions: Signals from our bodies (including our emotions) provide valuable information about what we might need. Learning our needs, and how best to meet our needs, requires practice. Below is a list of signals from the body and the needs that they *might* convey. Consider the signal that is arising from your body *and* the context in which it is occurring to determine your needs. For example, when the body has been in motion, fatigue may convey the need to rest and restore. However, if the body has been *in*active, fatigue might convey the need to move or "get the blood pumping."

Signals	Need
Hunger	To eat
Satiety	To stop eating
Fatigue	To rest or restore the body
	To move
Pain	To monitor
	To treat (with medical attention, movement, or rest)
Loneliness	To be in the presence of others
	To relate/affiliate
	To be connected
	To be known (to reveal oneself)
	To be part of something larger than oneself
Sadness	To grieve
	To be comforted or supported
	To contact meaning
	To activate
	To "play"
Fear (afraid or nervous)	To preserve or protect ourselves or our relations
	To approach something meaningful
	To build skills
	To ask for help
Guilt	To clarify values
	To align behavior with values (e.g., amend)
	To practice self-kindness or self-compassion

(continued)

Signals	Need
Shame	To treat self with respect or assumed worth
	To be effective (i.e., competent)
	To receive love
	To practice self-kindness or self-compassion
Anger	To preserve or protect someone or something
	To set boundaries or limits
	To get our legitimate rights
	To be vulnerable
Boredom, Dullness	To be stimulated
	To learn
Resentment	To set boundaries
Disappointment	To review or communicate expectations
Overwhelmed	To do less
	To ask for help

CHAPTER 11

Treatment Progress and Termination, and Final Thoughts for the Therapist

with **Ashley A. Moskovich**

Although, by necessity, treatment focuses heavily on restoring weight, the issue in AN is not eating per se but rather a broader lack of attunement to one's needs: to eat, to stop eating; to move, to rest; to relate, to be alone; and to work, to play. The overarching aim of treatment is to help individuals with AN shift from rigid rules that deprive the individual to a kind, flexible approach to managing themselves and their behavior.

Parenting styles provides a useful frame for this shift. There are two dimensions to parenting (demands/expectations and warmth), and each may be high or low. The intersection of these two dimensions results in four different parenting styles or approaches (adapted from Baumrind, 1991): authoritarian (high demands, low warmth), neglectful (low demands, low warmth), authoritative (high demands, high warmth), and permissive (low demands, high warmth).

Individuals with AN have adopted an *authoritarian* approach to self-parenting, imposing oppressive rules and structure and punishment for being out of bounds. Adopting a more *authoritative* style can improve client functioning and adaptability; that is, choosing to self-parent in a way that is accepting and supportive of herself and her needs and appropriately flexible. This style of parenting is associated with positive outcomes, including high self-esteem (Baumrind, 1991). Among individuals with AN, self-parenting in a responsive, attuned manner allows weight to be restored and maintained at an adaptive level (based on the individual's age, sex, and growth curves) and more adaptive flexibility in eating (e.g., variation in the amount, content, and timing of food consumed, based on energy needs and the demands of the situation). It also results in general improvements in self-care and more time invested in activities that are personally meaningful.

The shift from authoritarian to authoritative self-parenting might not be a straight line. Sometimes during the course of treatment, clients might become *permissive self-parents*:

nondirected, open-ended, and without limits. This may be because they have difficulty finding the "middle ground" between punitive overcontrol and overindulgence. Permissiveness might also be a reaction to the trauma of starvation, which can make it psychologically difficult for clients to impose even healthy limits due to fear of returning to a starved state. For some clients, permissive parenting is simply a phase that needs to be monitored to avoid the onset of binge eating or other impulsive behavior or transition to bulimia nervosa. For others, and somewhat paradoxically, permissive parenting may necessitate interventions to increase willingness to allow limits.

Treatment Duration and Decreasing Therapeutic Support

Treatment duration can be highly variable, but it is generally longer for AN than for other problems due to the unique challenges that low weight presents. This includes the ego-syntonic nature of dietary restraint and the need to devote therapeutic time and resources to reversing starvation, particularly early in treatment. Although there is a lot of variability in AN treatment duration (Watson & Bulik, 2013), among adolescents and individuals with AN with BMIs higher than 17.5, a common treatment dose is 20 sessions (Fairburn et al., 2009, 2015; Lock & Le Grange, 2015). For low-weight individuals, treatment duration might be twice as long (e.g., 40 sessions over 40 weeks; e.g., Fairburn et al., 2013).

The appropriate time to decrease the frequency of therapeutic contact (or end treatment) is not an exact formula. However, one marker of readiness is the ability to maintain weight at an acceptable level over a period of months with minimal use of external contingencies. Readiness for termination might also be reflected in significant reductions in clients' scores on standard eating disorder measures, such as the Eating Disorder Examination—Questionnaire (EDE-Q; Fairburn & Beglin, 1994). However, because thoughts/feelings are not directly targeted for change in ACT, it might be useful to assess changes in eating disorder behaviors separately from changes in attitudinal or cognitive items. Clients may report a decrease in the frequency or intensity of eating disorder thoughts/feelings, but not necessarily so. The presence of these internal experiences is not a problem in and of itself and, in fact, the ability to behave consistently with one's values in the presence of these thoughts/feelings would suggest greater psychological flexibility.

Measures of adaptability or functionality (particularly evidence that the client is able to effectively respond to her physical and emotional needs, adequate sleep, etc.) might be most informative of treatment progress, as well as process measures of psychological flexibility. This includes measures such as the Acceptance and Action Questionnaire–II (AAQ-II; Bond et al., 2011) and the Body-Image Acceptance and Action Questionnaire (Sandoz, Wilson, Merwin, & Kellum, 2013). Progress might also be quantified by change in clients' scores on the assessment of their capacities in the six ACT core process domains, as outlined in Chapter 3. Ultimately, whether to end treatment may come to these questions: Has the client been liberated in a sense? Is she able to live inside her own skin (as it is), free to pursue that which is meaningful to her and life-giving, even when it is difficult or uncomfortable at times? This does not suggest that she chooses to do this all the time, but that she has the capacity to and is not caged by uncertainty and fear.

Premature Decrease in Support or Termination

Relief or Fatigue

For individuals with AN, it may be tempting to decrease support prematurely, before eating and weight changes have been maintained for a sufficient period of time, or after the most life-threatening behaviors have remitted (but before the other areas of life have expanded in a way that effectively competes with AN). This may be driven by the client, the family, or the therapist, all of whom might be reacting out of relief or fatigue. Decreasing support too soon may result in a reemergence of AN behavior. It might also lead to clients feeling punished for improvements. Decisions to reduce therapeutic support may be approached as *experimental*, with the therapist monitoring the impact of less frequent sessions on eating and weight.

Topographical Change Misperceived as Functional Change

Clients may also seem to be functioning better, but they have actually exchanged one problem behavior for another. This might include, for example, increasing caloric intake but adopting vomiting or excessive exercise, cutting, substance use, or severe withdrawal to manage the resulting emotional upheaval. Ongoing, careful assessment can reveal this issue.

Delayed Termination

There are also instances in which termination with a client might be unduly delayed. This may be more common among clients with dependent personality features or those who are more socially isolated. In this case, finding other sources of social support (other people with whom the client can be vulnerable, express emotions, or allow perceived imperfections) and terminating treatment are key therapeutic goals. Delayed termination might also reflect fear (that the individual will return to dangerously low weight) on the part of the client, the therapist, or the family. Generally, when termination is delayed, the therapist should explore the function of not terminating, which will inform intervention.

Preventing and Responding to the Reemergence of Problem Behaviors

As treatment comes to a close, it is important that the client have a framework to understand the work and carry it forward into life without ongoing therapeutic support. This may include reviewing (1) thoughts/feelings that are evocative or compelling; (2) behaviors that tend to function as experiential avoidance (e.g., excessive planning or list making, excessive compliance); (3) client values and intentions; and (4) skills or practices that are helpful in maintaining change. It may also be helpful for the client to have a clear plan of what to do (e.g., initial changes to make, when to enlist the help of others) if she is engaging in behaviors that are not effective or value-guided. Clients might be reminded to monitor the Eating

Disorder Volume and use this as a signal to "check in" (with what they are thinking and feeling, and the situation, to determine their needs). Identifying upcoming challenges to maintaining behavior change (e.g., upcoming transitions) is often helpful, along with a plan for additional supports at those times.

It may be noted that the urge to restrict eating and lose weight (or engage in other punitive overcontrol) will return, particularly in times of stress. This should be expected. The presence of the urge may be discriminated from *acting on* urges (for which the client is *response*-able).

The therapist might also discuss the possibility that the client will engage in AN behavior (or other rigid control strategies) sometime in the future. In doing so, the therapist encourages the client to be compassionate and to appreciate that the reemergence of old patterns is part of being human. Rather than a goal to "never get off-track," the goal is to recognize when we have re-engaged old behavior patterns, and find our way back. The ability to recognize when this happens (and get back on-track more quickly than in the past) is celebrated as a victory. In this discussion, the therapist might also highlight that life offers continuous opportunities to realign behavior with personal values. These concepts are illustrated in the dialogues below.

IN PRACTICE

Dialogue A

THERAPIST: Most of our work has focused on the thought that you are a failure, and how that feels deep in your gut . . . and sends you scrambling to do and be better. This scrambling often looks like working more and more . . . until you are depleted.

I wonder how you might notice if you are being pulled by this thought/feeling (in the future, when we are not meeting)? . . . So that you can unhook and come back to the moment and the life you would choose.

CLIENT: I'm not sure . . .

THERAPIST: Maybe we could make a list of the things that would be a signal to you (that you are hooked) . . . like the thought "I need to lose weight" or more subtle things, like cutting back on your portions or missing lunch . . .

Dialogue B

THERAPIST: Eating disorder thoughts and feelings might always be there, playing in the background. . . . When things are going well and you are really engaged in your life, they might be so quiet that you can barely detect them. At other times, they might be louder. If the Eating Disorder Volume is turned up (louder than it had been), you might take that as a sign . . . a signal to check in with what might be bothering you.

You might notice, for example, that you have overextended yourself, and need to let go of some things, or that you are not speaking up about an important issue in a relationship, or that you are doing something that you don't want to be doing to make someone else happy and it's time for a change. . . . Ultimately, the aim is to see if you can sense what you are struggling with and what you need . . . and rather than channel energy into trying to change your body, find a way to honor those hard feelings and take action (if there is an action to take).

CLIENT: I just don't want to have the eating disorder anymore—I want to move on. Are you telling me that these thoughts and feelings are going to be there forever?

THERAPIST: We don't really get to decide whether you have particular thoughts or feelings. . . . We do get to decide what we do in response to them, whether we get caught up in them, and for how long. It may be a continual process of noticing (when you are hooked), and coming back to yourself and your values . . . as often as you need to, with kindness, compassion . . .

Dialogue C (with the "Mary Had a Little Lamb" and "Remember the Numbers" Exercises)

The client is describing the reemergence of eating disorder thoughts.

CLIENT: I thought I was past this, but I keep thinking about skipping dinner or throwing up or something. I'm not acting on it, but I keep thinking about it.

THERAPIST: It comes back up for you . . . even when you feel like you're "past it." Learning is cumulative, you know, it never really goes away. . . . Remember Mary had a little . . .

CLIENT: Lamb.

THERAPIST: Twinkle, twinkle, little . . .

CLIENT: Star.

THERAPIST: Absolutely! And you haven't heard these rhymes in how long . . . and there was zero latency. You knew the answer right away. Let's try something else, OK? I want to see if we can also create new content, and this is particularly relevant because of the importance of numbers in your life.

Remember these numbers: 1 2 1. Got it? I'm going to ask you in a month, 6 months, or 6 years. Do you think you will remember?

CLIENT: Oh yeah!

THERAPIST: These things are just not going anywhere. Something is different though . . . how you relate to them. You *have them* instead of them *having you!*

Dialogue D

The client is talking about a recent meal that included challenge foods.

CLIENT: I was so worried that I would have the urge to throw up.

THERAPIST: This is something that has been difficult. It has felt as though the presence of the urge *means something* (deeply). . . . You found yourself watching the door, to make sure one doesn't show up . . .

CLIENT: (*Affirms.*)

THERAPIST: Maybe it doesn't mean anything at all, other than the fact that old learning doesn't really go away. Nothing you can do short of a lobotomy. (*Smiles.*) The great thing is, you get to choose. You get to choose whether you respond to the urge by vomiting (whether you take its advice). You get to choose whether to move toward or away from the life that you want in each moment. And it might be that sometimes you feel like you are losing your footing, and that is the time to reach out for support.

CLIENT: I'm just afraid that I will do it, especially if I keep eating these challenging foods.

THERAPIST: The feared future shows up and it is hard to sit with the uncertainty (of whether you will do it or not). It seems this might also point to how important reclaiming your life has been to you . . . and I know how hard you have worked.

CLIENT: Yes!

THERAPIST: This is such a human thing, you know? . . . There is always the possibility of falling back into old patterns of behavior or making choices that are not value-guided. Choices that take us down a different path.

CLIENT: (*Discusses.*)

THERAPIST: One thing that we have noticed before is that when you are compassionate and gentle with yourself, you are better able to find your way back (to return more quickly to your intention).

We can also make a plan for what to do if urges do show up, and how you will know that you need to reach out for help (either in that moment, or more broadly, by reengaging therapy, etc.).

Treating Individuals with AN: Final Thoughts for the Therapist

What is most personal is most universal.
—CARL ROGERS

Treating individuals with AN can be incredibly rewarding and meaningful for the therapist; however, it can also be extremely challenging. Sitting with another human being who is waging war against her body (against herself) can feel painful. Knowing the potential life-threatening and devastating consequences of AN behaviors can create a context of pressure and urgency to compel change. And, at the same time, experiencing the grip of AN and our clients' resistance to change can lead to feelings of frustration, helplessness, and even inadequacy. In holding all of these experiences, we appreciate not only that we coexist with our clients in the broader context of the human condition, but also that we are both working from a parallel space of great uncertainty and lack of control.

We, just like our clients, may struggle with these thoughts and feelings, and at times find that our actions are not aligned with our personal values (as therapists). This provides many opportunities for us to practice and model a flexible, adaptive relationship to our internal experience, both in and outside of the therapy room. Self-care and self-compassion are essential interventions, as treatment is often long, with improvements in client behavior waxing and waning.

TABLE 11.1. Behaviors Common to Therapists Treating AN that May Function as Experiential Avoidance

- Attempting to convince the client (e.g., "You are not overweight!").
- Failing to implement appropriate and previously discussed therapeutic contingencies (e.g., minimum weight required for outpatient care).
- Excessively seeking consultation or guidance from other sources.
- Choosing not to seek consultation or guidance from other sources.
- Functional apathy (choosing to be less connected or present with the client or therapeutic work).
- Blaming the client for poor outcomes.
- Overreliance on psychoeducation in the therapy room.
- Choosing not to challenge the client when doing so would be workable (e.g., staying at the level of eating disorder content rather than exploring underlying emotional experience).
- Over- or underreaction to behaviors or therapeutic outcomes (e.g., weight loss).
- Overreliance or insensitive application of the therapeutic protocol or other planned therapeutic interventions in the therapy room.

Ongoing awareness of our own internal experience, and the function and workability of our behavior, can help us respond flexibly to the ever-changing environment of the therapeutic space. Table 11.1 lists common avoidant behaviors among therapists working with individuals with AN. Table 11.2 lists therapist barriers through the lens of the six core ACT processes. While these lists are not exhaustive or applicable to all therapists all the time, we offer them as a guide for continuous self-assessment and intervention, to maximize our ability to be useful to our clients.

TABLE 11.2. Common Targets in the Six Core Process Domains *for the Therapist*

Target	Description/examples
Common targets for acceptance	
Anxiety	• Fear that the client will experience severe health consequences or early death. • Fear of doing something wrong/harmful. • Fear of being ineffective.
Guilt/shame	• A feeling of being at fault for absent or slow therapeutic gains. • A feeling of disappointing others (the client, the client's caregivers, other providers working with the client, the therapist's supervisor or clinical team).
Uncertainty	• Feeling unsure about one's clinical skill/ability to help the client. • Feeling unsure whether interventions will be successful.
Lack of control/helplessness	• A feeling of limited influence over the client's progress, behaviors, and outcomes (e.g., weight, restrictive behaviors, health consequences).
Feeling overwhelmed	• Feeling challenged by the limited time available to coordinate care, make decisions (e.g., treatment planning).
Hopelessness	• Feelings arising from fusion with thoughts that nothing has worked/will work to help the client change behavior, or that the client is incapable of change.
Anger/frustration	• Feelings arising from fusion with thoughts that others are not doing enough (e.g., feeling like the client is able, but unwilling, to make behavior change or try things, that one is working harder than the client, or that caregivers are unwilling to provide adequate support to the client).
Common targets for defusion	
Thoughts about one's own body or the client's evaluation of one's own body	• "She thinks I'm fat."
Thoughts about the impact of one's behavior	• "It's my fault she's not getting better." • "I'm going to do something that makes her worse." • "If I am direct with her, she will never come back to therapy."
Thoughts about one's acceptability or worth as a therapist	• "I'm a bad therapist." • "A better therapist would . . ."
Fusion with stories about outcomes	• "She's been struggling with AN too long and will never improve." • "Since her weight isn't up this week, she has to be restricting again."
Fusion with stories about the client's intention	• "She doesn't want to get better." • "She's being manipulative."
Fusion with rules	• "She must eat six times a day." • "I should blind-weigh all of my clients."

(continued)

TABLE 11.2. *(continued)*

Target	Description/examples
Common areas of narrow or rigid attention	
Past mistakes	• Something one did or said that the client responded to negatively. • Making a faux pas.
The feared distant future	• The client's "failure" in treatment or health consequences.
Evaluation/feedback	• The client, caregiver, or other providers' comments about the client's progress, or lack thereof.
Interpersonal threat cues	• The client's scanning of the therapist's body. • Signals of disapproval or dislike from the client.
Common issues of overattachment or impoverished self	
Success as a therapist	• The client's progress/outcome defines the therapist.
Narratives of being a flawed therapist	• "I'm a bad therapist." • "I have no idea what to do."
Limited emotional self-knowledge	• Limited awareness of thoughts/feelings that one is experiencing in response to the client (e.g., blaming the client for lack of progress rather than contacting one's own sense of felt inadequacy as a therapist).
Common difficulties with values clarity	
Avoidance of valuing because of potential for discomfort	• Disconnecting from the client and therapeutic work.
Common difficulties in committed action	
Interventions remain at the level of content.	• Overreliance on psychoeducation. • Trying to convince a client out of her thoughts/feelings/experience.
Actions are persistent despite unworkability.	• Insisting that a client must change a particular behavior (and not honoring the client's choice or willingness to take smaller steps).
Actions are overstructured.	• Rigidly and insensitively adhering to a therapeutic protocol.
Inaction	• Providing only supportive psychotherapy.

References

Agras, W. S., Brandt, H. A., Bulik, C. M., Dolan-Sewell, R., Fairburn, C. G., Halmi, K. A., et al. (2004). Report of the National Institutes of Health workshop on overcoming barriers to treatment research in anorexia nervosa. *International Journal of Eating Disorders, 35*(4), 509–521.

American Psychiatric Association. (2006). *American Psychiatric Association practice guidelines for the treatment of psychiatric disorders: Compendium 2006.* Arlington, VA: Author.

American Psychiatric Association. (2013). *Diagnostic and statistical manual of mental disorders* (5th ed.). Arlington, VA: Author.

Anderson, L., Reilly, E., Berner, L., Wierenga, C., Jones, M., Brown, T., et al. (2017). Treating eating disorders at higher levels of care: Overview and challenges. *Current Psychiatry Reports, 19*(8), 1–9.

Arcelus, J., Mitchell, A. J., Wales, J., & Nielsen, S. (2011). Mortality rates in patients with anorexia nervosa and other eating disorders: A meta-analysis of 36 studies. *Archives of General Psychiatry, 68*(7), 724–731.

Bailey, A., Ciarrochi, J., & Hayes, L. (2012). *Get out of your mind and into your life for teens: A guide to living an extraordinary life.* Oakland, CA: New Harbinger.

Bardone-Cone, A. M., Wonderlich, S. A., Frost, R. O., Bulik, C. M., Mitchell, J. E., Uppala, S., et al. (2007). Perfectionism and eating disorders: Current status and future directions. *Clinical Psychology Review, 27*(3), 384–405.

Baumrind, D. (1991). Effective parenting during the early adolescent transition. In P. A. Cowan & E. M. Hetherington (Eds.), *Advances in family research* (Vol. 2, pp. 111–163). Hillsdale, NJ: Erlbaum.

Berkman, N. D., Lohr, K. N., & Bulik, C. M. (2007). Outcomes of eating disorders: A systematic review of the literature. *International Journal of Eating Disorders, 40*(4), 293–309.

Berman, M., Boutelle, K., & Crow, S. (2009). A case series investigating acceptance and commitment therapy as a treatment for previously treated, unremitted patients with anorexia nervosa. *European Eating Disorders Review, 17*(6), 426–434.

Bond, F. W., Hayes, S. C., Baer, R. A., Carpenter, K. M., Guenole, N., Orcutt, H. K., et al. (2011). Preliminary psychometric properties of the Acceptance and Action Questionnaire–II: A revised measure of psychological inflexibility and experiential avoidance. *Behavior Therapy, 42*(4), 676–688.

Boutelle, K. N. (1998). The use of exposure with response prevention in a male anorexic. *Journal of Behavior Therapy and Experimental Psychiatry, 29*(1), 79–84.

Brockmeyer, T., Friederich, H.-C., & Schmidt, U. (2018). Advances in the treatment of anorexia nervosa: A review of established and emerging interventions. *Psychological Medicine, 48*(8), 1228–1256.

Brown, L. A., Gaudiano, B. A., & Miller, I. W. (2011). Investigating the similarities and differences between practitioners of second- and third-wave cognitive-behavioral therapies. *Behavior Modification, 35*(2), 187–200.

Brown, T. A., & Keel, P. K. (2012). Current and emerging directions in the treatment of eating disorders. *Substance Abuse: Research and Treatment, 6*, 33–61.

Bruch, H. (1962). Perceptual and conceptual disturbances in anorexia nervosa. *Psychosomatic Medicine, 24*(2), 187–194.

Bruch, H. (1982). Anorexia nervosa: Therapy and theory. *American Journal of Psychiatry, 139*(12), 1531–1538.

Bulik, C. M., Sullivan, P. F., Fear, J., & Pickering, A. (1997). Predictors of the development of bulimia nervosa in women with anorexia nervosa. *Journal of Nervous and Mental Disease, 185*(11), 704–707.

Byrne, S., Wade, T., Hay, P., Touyz, S., Fairburn, C. G., Treasure, J., et al. (2017). A randomised controlled trial of three psychological treatments for anorexia nervosa. *Psychological Medicine, 47*(16), 2823–2833.

Carter, J. C., Bewell, C., Blackmore, E., & Woodside, D. B. (2006). The impact of childhood sexual abuse in anorexia nervosa. *Child Abuse & Neglect, 30*(3), 257–269.

Carter, J., Blackmore, E., Sutandar-Pinnock, K., & Woodside, D. (2004). Relapse in anorexia nervosa: A survival analysis. *Psychological Medicine, 34*(4), 671–679.

Cassin, S. E., & von Ranson, K. M. (2005). Personality and eating disorders: A decade in review. *Clinical Psychology Review, 25*(7), 895–916.

Chen, E. Y., Segal, K., Weissman, J., Zeffiro, T. A., Gallop, R., Linehan, M. M., et al. (2015). Adapting dialectical behavior therapy for outpatient adult anorexia nervosa—a pilot study. *International Journal of Eating Disorders, 48*(1), 123–132.

Chesney, E., Goodwin, G. M., & Fazel, S. (2014). Risks of all-cause and suicide mortality in mental disorders: A meta-review. *World Psychiatry, 13*(2), 153–160.

Ciao, A. C., Accurso, E. C., Fitzsimmons-Craft, E. E., Lock, J., & Le Grange, D. (2015). Family functioning in two treatments for adolescent anorexia nervosa. *International Journal of Eating Disorders, 48*(1), 81–90.

Craighead, L. W. (2006). *The appetite awareness workbook: How to listen to your body and overcome bingeing, overeating, and obsession with food.* Oakland, CA: New Harbinger.

Crisp, A. (2006). In defence of the concept of phobically driven avoidance of adult body weight/shape/function as the final common pathway to anorexia nervosa. *European Eating Disorders Review, 14*(3), 189–202.

Dalle Grave, R., Calugi, S., Doll, H. A., & Fairburn, C. G. (2013). Enhanced cognitive behaviour therapy for adolescents with anorexia nervosa: An alternative to family therapy? *Behaviour Research and Therapy, 51*(1), R9–R12.

Dalle Grave, R., El Ghoch, M., Sartirana, M., & Calugi, S. (2016). Cognitive behavioral therapy for anorexia nervosa: An update. *Current Psychiatry Reports, 18*(1), 2.

Danner, U. N., Sanders, N., Smeets, P. A., van Meer, F., Adan, R. A., Hoek, H. W., et al. (2012). Neuropsychological weaknesses in anorexia nervosa: Set-shifting, central coherence, and decision making in currently ill and recovered women. *International Journal of Eating Disorders, 45*(5), 685–694.

Davies, H., Schmidt, U., Stahl, D., & Tchanturia, K. (2011). Evoked facial emotional expression and emotional experience in people with anorexia nervosa. *International Journal of Eating Disorders, 44*(6), 531–539.

Davies, H., Schmidt, U., & Tchanturia, K. (2013). Emotional facial expression in women recovered from anorexia nervosa. *BMC Psychiatry, 13*(1), 291.

Deep, A. L., Nagy, L. M., Weltzin, T. E., Rao, R., & Kaye, W. H. (1995). Premorbid onset of psycho-pathology in long-term recovered anorexia nervosa. *International Journal of Eating Disorders, 17*(3), 291–297.

Eddy, K. T., Dorer, D. J., Franko, D. L., Tahilani, K., Thompson-Brenner, H., & Herzog, D. B. (2008). Diagnostic crossover in anorexia nervosa and bulimia nervosa: Implications for DSM-V. *American Journal of Psychiatry, 165*(2), 245–250.

Eddy, K. T., Keel, P. K., Dorer, D. J., Delinsky, S. S., Franko, D. L., & Herzog, D. B. (2002). Longi-tudinal comparison of anorexia nervosa subtypes. *International Journal of Eating Disorders, 31*(2), 191–201.

Eisler, I., Dare, C., Hodes, M., Russell, G., Dodge, E., & Le Grange, D. (2000). Family therapy for adolescent anorexia nervosa: The results of a controlled comparison of two family interventions. *Journal of Child Psychology and Psychiatry and Allied Disciplines, 41*(6), 727–736.

Erdur, L., Weber, C., Zimmermann-Viehoff, F., Rose, M., & Deter, H.-C. (2017). Affective responses in different stages of anorexia nervosa: Results from a startle-reflex paradigm. *European Eating Disorders Review, 25*(2), 114–122.

Fairburn, C. G., Bailey-Straebler, S., Basden, S., Doll, H. A., Jones, R., Murphy, R., et al. (2015). A transdiagnostic comparison of enhanced cognitive behaviour therapy (CBT-E) and interper-sonal psychotherapy in the treatment of eating disorders. *Behaviour Research and Therapy, 70*, 64–71.

Fairburn, C. G., & Beglin, S. J. (1994). Assessment of eating disorders: Interview or self-report ques-tionnaire? *International Journal of Eating Disorders, 16*(4), 363–370.

Fairburn, C. G., Cooper, Z., Doll, H. A., O'Connor, M. E., Bohn, K., Hawker, D. M., et al. (2009). Transdiagnostic cognitive-behavioral therapy for patients with eating disorders: A two-site trial with 60-week follow-up. *American Journal of Psychiatry, 166*(3), 311–319.

Fairburn, C. G., Cooper, Z., Doll, H. A., O'Connor, M. E., Palmer, R. L., & Dalle Grave, R. (2013). Enhanced cognitive behaviour therapy for adults with anorexia nervosa: A UK–Italy study. *Behaviour Research and Therapy, 51*(1), R2–R8.

Fairburn, C. G., Cooper, Z., & Shafran, R. (2008). Enhanced cognitive behavior therapy for eating disorders ("CBT-E"): An overview. In C. G. Fairburn, *Cognitive behavior therapy and eating disorders* (pp. 23–34). New York: Guilford Press.

Farstad, S. M., McGeown, L. M., & von Ranson, K. M. (2016). Eating disorders and personality, 2004–2016: A systematic review and meta-analysis. *Clinical Psychology Review, 46*, 91–105.

Feldman, M. B., & Meyer, I. H. (2007). Eating disorders in diverse lesbian, gay, and bisexual popula-tions. *International Journal of Eating Disorders, 40*(3), 218–226.

Fox, J. R. (2009). A qualitative exploration of the perception of emotions in anorexia nervosa: A basic emotion and developmental perspective. *Clinical Psychology and Psychotherapy, 16*(4), 276–302.

Galsworthy-Francis, L., & Allan, S. (2014). Cognitive behavioural therapy for anorexia nervosa: A systematic review. *Clinical Psychology Review, 34*(1), 54–72.

Godart, N. T., Flament, M. F., Lecrubier, Y., & Jeammet, P. (2000). Anxiety disorders in anorexia nervosa and bulimia nervosa: Co-morbidity and chronology of appearance. *European Psychia-try, 15*(1), 38–45.

Golden, N. H., Katzman, D. K., Kreipe, R. E., Stevens, S. L., Sawyer, S. M., Rees, J., et al. (2003). Eating disorders in adolescents: Position paper of the Society for Adolescent Medicine. *Journal of Adolescent Health, 33*(6), 496–503.

Hall, A. (1982). Deciding to stay an anorectic. *Postgraduate Medical Journal, 58*(684), 641–647.

Halmi, K. A., Casper, R. C., Eckert, E. D., Goldberg, S. C., & Davis, J. M. (1979). Unique features associated with age of onset of anorexia nervosa. *Psychiatry Research, 1*(2), 209–215.

Halmi, K. A., Eckert, E., Marchi, P., Sampugnaro, V., Apple, R., & Cohen, J. (1991). Comorbid-ity of psychiatric diagnoses in anorexia nervosa. *Archives of General Psychiatry, 48*(8), 712–718.

Harrison, A., Sullivan, S., Tchanturia, K., & Treasure, J. (2009). Emotion recognition and regulation in anorexia nervosa. *Clinical Psychology and Psychotherapy, 16*(4), 348–356.

Hayes, S. C., Barnes-Holmes, D., & Roche, B. (2001). *Relational frame theory: A post-Skinnerian account of human language and cognition.* New York: Kluwer Academic.

Hayes, S. C., Strosahl, K. D., & Wilson, K. G. (1999). *Acceptance and commitment therapy: An experiential approach to behavior change.* New York: Guilford Press.

Hayes, S. C., Strosahl, K. D., & Wilson, K. G. (2011). *Acceptance and commitment therapy: The process and practice of mindful change* (2nd ed.). New York: Guilford Press.

Haynos, A. F., & Fruzzetti, A. E. (2011). Anorexia nervosa as a disorder of emotion dysregulation: Evidence and treatment implications. *Clinical Psychology: Science and Practice, 18*(3), 183–202.

Heffner, M., Sperry, J., Eifert, G. H., & Detweiler, M. (2002). Acceptance and commitment therapy in the treatment of an adolescent female with anorexia nervosa: A case example. *Cognitive and Behavioral Practice, 9*(3), 232–236.

Hildebrandt, T., Bacow, T., Markella, M., & Loeb, K. L. (2012). Anxiety in anorexia nervosa and its management using family-based treatment. *European Eating Disorders Review, 20*(1), e1–e16.

Hill, M. L., Masuda, A., Melcher, H., Morgan, J. R., & Twohig, M. P. (2015). Acceptance and commitment therapy for women diagnosed with binge eating disorder: A case-series study. *Cognitive and Behavioral Practice, 22*(3), 367–378.

Hill, M. L., Masuda, A., Moore, M., & Twohig, M. P. (2015). Acceptance and commitment therapy for individuals with problematic emotional eating. *Clinical Case Studies, 14*(2), 141–154.

Hoffman, E. R., Gagne, D. A., Thornton, L. M., Klump, K. L., Brandt, H., Crawford, S., et al. (2012). Understanding the association of impulsivity, obsessions, and compulsions with binge eating and purging behaviours in anorexia nervosa. *European Eating Disorders Review, 20*(3), e129–e136.

Hudson, J. I., Hiripi, E., Pope, H. G., & Kessler, R. C. (2007). The prevalence and correlates of eating disorders in the National Comorbidity Survey Replication. *Biological Psychiatry, 61*(3), 348–358.

Ivarsson, T., Råstam, M., Wentz, E., Gillberg, I. C., & Gillberg, C. (2000). Depressive disorders in teenage-onset anorexia nervosa: A controlled longitudinal, partly community-based study. *Comprehensive Psychiatry, 41*(5), 398–403.

Juarascio, A. S., Manasse, S. M., Schumacher, L., Espel, H., & Forman, E. M. (2017). Developing an acceptance-based behavioral treatment for binge eating disorder: Rationale and challenges. *Cognitive and Behavioral Practice, 24*(1), 1–13.

Juarascio, A., Shaw, J., Forman, E., Timko, C. A., Herbert, J., Butryn, M., et al. (2013). Acceptance and commitment therapy as a novel treatment for eating disorders: An initial test of efficacy and mediation. *Behavior Modification, 37*(4), 459–489.

Kabat-Zinn, J. (1994). *Wherever you go, there you are.* New York: Hyperion.

Katzman, D. K. (2005). Medical complications in adolescents with anorexia nervosa: A review of the literature. *International Journal of Eating Disorders, 37*(Suppl.), S52–S59.

Kaye, W. H., Bulik, C. M., Thornton, L., Barbarich, N., & Masters, K. (2004). Comorbidity of anxiety disorders with anorexia and bulimia nervosa. *American Journal of Psychiatry, 161*(12), 2215–2221.

Kaye, W. H., Wierenga, C. E., Bailer, U. F., Simmons, A. N., & Bischoff-Grethe, A. (2013). Nothing tastes as good as skinny feels: The neurobiology of anorexia nervosa. *Trends in Neurosciences, 36*(2), 110–120.

Keys, A., Brožek, J., Henschel, A., Mickelsen, O., & Taylor, H. L. (1950). *The biology of human starvation.* Minneapolis: University of Minnesota Press.

Lang, K., Stahl, D., Espie, J., Treasure, J., & Tchanturia, K. (2014). Set shifting in children and adolescents with anorexia nervosa: An exploratory systematic review and meta-analysis. *International Journal of Eating Disorders, 47*(4), 394–399.

Lavender, J. M., Wonderlich, S. A., Engel, S. G., Gordon, K. H., Kaye, W. H., & Mitchell, J. E. (2015). Dimensions of emotion dysregulation in anorexia nervosa and bulimia nervosa: A conceptual review of the empirical literature. *Clinical Psychology Review, 40*, 111–122.

Le Grange, D. (2005). The Maudsley family-based treatment for adolescent anorexia nervosa. *World Psychiatry, 4*(3), 142–146.

Le Grange, D., Eisler, I., Dare, C., & Hodes, M. (1992). Family criticism and self-starvation: A study of expressed emotion. *Journal of Family Therapy, 14*(2), 177–192.

Le Grange, D., Hoste, R. R., Lock, J., & Bryson, S. W. (2011). Parental expressed emotion of adolescents with anorexia nervosa: Outcome in family-based treatment. *International Journal of Eating Disorders, 44*(8), 731–734.

Le Grange, D., & Lock, J. (2005). The dearth of psychological treatment studies for anorexia nervosa. *International Journal of Eating Disorders, 37*(2), 79–91.

Le Grange, D., Lock, J., Agras, W. S., Moye, A., Bryson, S. W., Jo, B., et al. (2012). Moderators and mediators of remission in family-based treatment and adolescent focused therapy for anorexia nervosa. *Behaviour Research and Therapy, 50*(2), 85–92.

Le Grange, D., Lock, J., Loeb, K., & Nicholls, D. (2010). Academy for eating disorders position paper: The role of the family in eating disorders. *International Journal of Eating Disorders, 43*(1), 1–5.

Lindvall Dahlgren, C. L., & Rø, Ø. (2014). A systematic review of cognitive remediation therapy for anorexia nervosa—development, current state and implications for future research and clinical practice. *Journal of Eating Disorders, 2*(1), 26.

Linehan, M. M. (2014). *DBT skills training manual* (2nd ed.). New York: Guilford Press.

Lock, J. (2011). Evaluation of family treatment models for eating disorders. *Current Opinion in Psychiatry, 24*(4), 274–279.

Lock, J. (2015). An update on evidence-based psychosocial treatments for eating disorders in children and adolescents. *Journal of Clinical Child and Adolescent Psychology, 44*(5), 707–721.

Lock, J., Agras, W. S., Bryson, S., & Kraemer, H. C. (2005). A comparison of short-and long-term family therapy for adolescent anorexia nervosa. *Journal of the American Academy of Child and Adolescent Psychiatry, 44*(7), 632–639.

Lock, J., Garrett, A., Beenhakker, J., & Reiss, A. L. (2011). Aberrant brain activation during a response inhibition task in adolescent eating disorder subtypes. *American Journal of Psychiatry, 168*(1), 55–64.

Lock, J., & Le Grange, D. (2015). *Treatment manual for anorexia nervosa: A family-based approach* (2nd ed.). New York: Guilford Press.

Lock, J., Le Grange, D., Agras, W., & Dare, C. (2001). *Treatment manual for anorexia nervosa: A family-based approach.* New York: Guilford Press.

Lock, J., Le Grange, D., Agras, W. S., Moye, A., Bryson, S. W., & Jo, B. (2010). Randomized clinical trial comparing family-based treatment with adolescent-focused individual therapy for adolescents with anorexia nervosa. *Archives of General Psychiatry, 67*(10), 1025–1032.

Lopez, C., Tchanturia, K., Stahl, D., Booth, R., Holliday, J., & Treasure, J. (2008). An examination of the concept of central coherence in women with anorexia nervosa. *International Journal of Eating Disorders, 41*(2), 143–152.

Löwe, B., Zipfel, S., Buchholz, C., Dupont, Y., Reas, D. L., & Herzog, W. (2001). Long-term outcome of anorexia nervosa in a prospective 21-year follow-up study. *Psychological Medicine, 31*(5), 881–890.

Lynch, T. R., Gray, K. L., Hempel, R. J., Titley, M., Chen, E. Y., & O'Mahen, H. A. (2013). Radically open-dialectical behavior therapy for adult anorexia nervosa: Feasibility and outcomes from an inpatient program. *BMC Psychiatry, 13*, 293.

Maslow, A. H. (1943). A theory of human motivation. *Psychological Review, 50*(4), 370–396.

Masuda, A., Ng, S. Y., Moore, M., Felix, I., & Drake, C. E. (2016). Acceptance and commitment therapy as a treatment for a Latina young adult woman with purging: A case report. *Practice Innovations, 1*(1), 20–35.

Merwin, R. M., Moskovich, A. A., Wagner, H. R., Ritschel, L. A., Craighead, L. W., & Zucker, N. L. (2013). Emotion regulation difficulties in anorexia nervosa: Relationship to self-perceived sensory sensitivity. *Cognition and Emotion, 27*(3), 441–452.

Merwin, R. M., Zucker, N. L., & Timko, C. A. (2013). A pilot study of an acceptance-based separated family treatment for adolescent anorexia nervosa. *Cognitive and Behavioral Practice, 20*(4), 485–500.

Mitchell, J. E., & Crow, S. (2006). Medical complications of anorexia nervosa and bulimia nervosa. *Current Opinion in Psychiatry, 19*(4), 438–443.

Murphy, R., Straebler, S., Cooper, Z., & Fairburn, C. G. (2010). Cognitive behavioral therapy for eating disorders. *Psychiatric Clinics, 33*(3), 611–627.

Mustelin, L., Silén, Y., Raevuori, A., Hoek, H. W., Kaprio, J., & Keski-Rahkonen, A. (2016). The DSM-5 diagnostic criteria for anorexia nervosa may change its population prevalence and prognostic value. *Journal of Psychiatric Research, 77*, 85–91.

Noordenbos, G., Oldenhave, A., Muschter, J., & Terpstra, N. (2002). Characteristics and treatment of patients with chronic eating disorders. *Eating Disorders, 10*(1), 15–29.

Nunn, K., Frampton, I., Gordon, I., & Lask, B. (2008). The fault is not in her parents but in her insula—a neurobiological hypothesis of anorexia nervosa. *European Eating Disorders Review, 16*(5), 355–360.

O'Brien, K. M., & Vincent, N. K. (2003). Psychiatric comorbidity in anorexia and bulimia nervosa: Nature, prevalence, and causal relationships. *Clinical Psychology Review, 23*(1), 57–74.

Parling, T., Cernvall, M., Ramklint, M., Holmgren, S., & Ghaderi, A. (2016). A randomised trial of acceptance and commitment therapy for anorexia nervosa after daycare treatment, including five-year follow-up. *BMC Psychiatry, 16*, 272.

Pawlowska, B., & Masiak, M. (2007). Comparison of socio-demographic data of female patients with purging and restricting types of anorexia nervosa hospitalised at the Psychiatry Department of the Medical University of Lublin in the years 1993–2003. *Psychiatria Polska, 41*(3), 351–364.

Pinto-Gouveia, J., Carvalho, S. A., Palmeira, L., Castilho, P., Duarte, C., Ferreira, C., et al. (2017). BEfree: A new psychological program for binge eating that integrates psychoeducation, mindfulness, and compassion. *Clinical Psychology and Psychotherapy, 24*(5), 1090–1098.

Pitt, S., Lewis, R., Morgan, S., & Woodward, D. (2010). Cognitive remediation therapy in an outpatient setting: A case series. *Eating and Weight Disorders, 15*(4), e281–e286.

Pollatos, O., Kurz, A.-L., Albrecht, J., Schreder, T., Kleemann, A. M., Schöpf, V., et al. (2008). Reduced perception of bodily signals in anorexia nervosa. *Eating Behaviors, 9*(4), 381–388.

Pollice, C., Kaye, W. H., Greeno, C. G., & Weltzin, T. E. (1997). Relationship of depression, anxiety, and obsessionality to state of illness in anorexia nervosa. *International Journal of Eating Disorders, 21*(4), 367–376.

Pomeroy, C., & Mitchell, J. E. (2002). Medical complications of anorexia nervosa and bulimia nervosa. In K. Brownell & C. G. Fairburn (Eds.), *Eating disorders and obesity: A comprehensive handbook* (pp. 278–285). New York: Guilford Press.

Powers, M. B., Zum Vörde Sive Vörding, M. B., & Emmelkamp, P. M. G. (2009). Acceptance and commitment therapy: A meta-analytic review. *Psychotherapy and Psychosomatics, 78*(2), 73–80.

Preti, A., Rocchi, M. B. L., Sisti, D., Camboni, M. V., & Miotto, P. (2011). A comprehensive meta-analysis of the risk of suicide in eating disorders. *Acta Psychiatrica Scandinavica, 124*(1), 6–17.

Rhodes, P., Baillee, A., Brown, J., & Madden, S. (2008). Can parent-to-parent consultation improve the effectiveness of the Maudsley model of family-based treatment for anorexia nervosa?: A randomized control trial. *Journal of Family Therapy, 30*(1), 96–108.

Rhodes, P., Brown, J., & Madden, S. (2009). The Maudsley model of family-based treatment for anorexia nervosa: A qualitative evaluation of parent-to-parent consultation. *Journal of Marital and Family Therapy, 35*(2), 181–192.

Roberts, M., Tchanturia, K., Stahl, D., Southgate, L., & Treasure, J. (2007). A systematic review and meta-analysis of set-shifting ability in eating disorders. *Psychological Medicine, 37*(8), 1075–1084.

Roberts, M. E., Tchanturia, K., & Treasure, J. L. (2010). Exploring the neurocognitive signature of poor set-shifting in anorexia and bulimia nervosa. *Journal of Psychiatric Research, 44*(14), 964–970.

Robertson, A., Alford, C., Wallis, A., & Miskovic-Wheatley, J. (2015). Using a brief family-based DBT adjunct with standard FBT in the treatment of anorexia nervosa. *Journal of Eating Disorders, 3*(Suppl. 1), O39.

Rommel, D., Nandrino, J.-L., De Jonckheere, J., Swierczek, M., Dodin, V., & Logier, R. (2015). Maintenance of parasympathetic inhibition following emotional induction in patients with restrictive type anorexia nervosa. *Psychiatry Research, 225*(3), 651–657.

Salbach, H., Klinkowski, N., Pfeiffer, E., Lehmkuhl, U., & Korte, A. (2007). Dialectical behavior therapy for adolescents with anorexia and bulimia nervosa (DBT-AN/BN): A pilot study. *Praxis der Kinderpsychologie und Kinderpsychiatrie, 56*(2), 91–108.

Sandoz, E. K., Wilson, K. G., Merwin, R. M., & Kellum, K. K. (2013). Assessment of body image flexibility: The Body-Image Acceptance and Action Questionnaire. *Journal of Contextual and Behavioral Science, 2*(1–2), 39–48.

Schmidt, U., & Treasure, J. (2006). Anorexia nervosa: Valued and visible: A cognitive-interpersonal maintenance model and its implications for research and practice. *British Journal of Clinical Psychology, 45*(3), 343–366.

Serpell, L., Treasure, J., Teasdale, J., & Sullivan, V. (1999). Anorexia nervosa: Friend or foe? *International Journal of Eating Disorders, 25*(2), 177–186.

Sharp, C., & Freeman, C. (1993). The medical complications of anorexia nervosa. *British Journal of Psychiatry, 162*(4), 452–462.

Steinglass, J., Albano, A. M., Simpson, H. B., Carpenter, K., Schebendach, J., & Attia, E. (2012). Fear of food as a treatment target: Exposure and response prevention for anorexia nervosa in an open series. *International Journal of Eating Disorders, 45*(4), 615–621.

Steinglass, J. E., Albano, A. M., Simpson, H. B., Wang, Y., Zou, J., Attia, E., et al. (2014). Confronting fear using exposure and response prevention for anorexia nervosa: A randomized controlled pilot study. *International Journal of Eating Disorders, 47*(2), 174–180.

Steinhausen, H.-C. (2002). The outcome of anorexia nervosa in the 20th century. *American Journal of Psychiatry, 159*(8), 1284–1293.

Storch, E. A., Geffken, G. R., Merlo, L. J., Jacob, M. L., Murphy, T. K., Goodman, W. K., et al. (2007). Family accommodation in pediatric obsessive–compulsive disorder. *Journal of Clinical Child and Adolescent Psychology, 36*(2), 207–216.

Strandskov, S. W., Ghaderi, A., Andersson, H., Parmskog, N., Hjort, E., Warn, A. S., . . . Andersson, G. (2017). Effects of tailored and ACT-influenced internet-based CBT for eating disorders and the relation between knowledge acquisition and outcome: A randomized controlled trial. *Choice Reviews Online, 48*, 624–637.

Strober, M. (1980). Personality and symptomatological features in young, nonchronic anorexia nervosa patients. *Journal of Psychosomatic Research, 24*(6), 353–359.

Sullivan, P. F. (1995). Mortality in anorexia nervosa. *American Journal of Psychiatry, 152*(7), 1073–1074.

Tchanturia, K., Davies, H., Roberts, M., Harrison, A., Nakazato, M., Schmidt, U., et al. (2012). Poor cognitive flexibility in eating disorders: Examining the evidence using the Wisconsin Card Sorting Task. *PLOS ONE, 7*(1), e28331.

Tchanturia, K., Giombini, L., Leppanen, J., & Kinnaird, E. (2017). Evidence for cognitive remediation therapy in young people with anorexia nervosa: Systematic review and meta-analysis of the literature. *European Eating Disorders Review, 25*(4), 227–236.

Tchanturia, K., Lloyd, S., & Lang, K. (2013). Cognitive remediation therapy for anorexia nervosa: Current evidence and future research directions. *International Journal of Eating Disorders, 46*(5), 492–495.

Tchanturia, K., Lounes, N., & Holttum, S. (2014). Cognitive remediation in anorexia nervosa and related conditions: A systematic review. *European Eating Disorders Review, 22*(6), 454–462.

Tchanturia, K., Morris, R., Anderluh, M. B., Collier, D., Nikolaou, V., & Treasure, J. (2004). Set shifting in anorexia nervosa: An examination before and after weight gain, in full recovery and relationship to childhood and adult OCPD traits. *Journal of Psychiatric Research, 38*(5), 545–552.

Thoma, N., Pilecki, B., & McKay, D. (2015). Contemporary cognitive behavior therapy: A review of theory, history, and evidence. *Psychodynamic Psychiatry, 43*(3), 423–461.

Timko, C. A., Zucker, N. L., Herbert, J. D., Rodriguez, D., & Merwin, R. M. (2015). An open trial of acceptance-based separated family treatment (ASFT) for adolescents with anorexia nervosa. *Behaviour Research and Therapy, 69*, 63–74.

Toner, B. B., Garfinkel, P. E., & Garner, D. M. (1989). Affective and anxiety disorders in the long-term follow-up of anorexia nervosa. *International Journal of Psychiatry in Medicine, 18*(4), 357–364.

Treasure, J., Murphy, T., Szmukler, T., Todd, G., Gavan, K., & Joyce, J. (2001). The experience of caregiving for severe mental illness: A comparison between anorexia nervosa and psychosis. *Social Psychiatry and Psychiatric Epidemiology, 36*(7), 343–347.

Watson, H., & Bulik, C. (2013). Update on the treatment of anorexia nervosa: Review of clinical trials, practice guidelines and emerging interventions. *Psychological Medicine, 43*(12), 2477–2500.

Whitney, J., Murray, J., Gavan, K., Todd, G., Whitaker, W., & Treasure, J. (2005). Experience of caring for someone with anorexia nervosa: Qualitative study. *British Journal of Psychiatry, 187*(5), 444–449.

Wildes, J. E., & Marcus, M. D. (2011). Development of emotion acceptance behavior therapy for anorexia nervosa: A case series. *International Journal of Eating Disorders, 44*(5), 421–427.

Wildes, J. E., Marcus, M. D., Cheng, Y., McCabe, E. B., & Gaskill, J. A. (2014). Emotion acceptance behavior therapy for anorexia nervosa: A pilot study. *International Journal of Eating Disorders, 47*(8), 870–873.

Wildes, J. E., Ringham, R. M., & Marcus, M. D. (2010). Emotion avoidance in patients with anorexia nervosa: Initial test of a functional model. *International Journal of Eating Disorders, 43*(5), 398–404.

Wilson, K. G. (2009). *Mindfulness for two: An acceptance and commitment therapy approach to mindfulness in psychotherapy.* Oakland, CA: New Harbinger.

Wilson, K. G., Sandoz, E. K., Kitchens, J., & Roberts, M. (2010). The Valued Living Questionnaire: Defining and measuring valued action within a behavioral framework. *The Psychological Record, 60*(2), 249–272.

Wiseman, C. V., Sunday, S. R., Klapper, F., Harris, W. A., & Halmi, K. A. (2001). Changing patterns of hospitalization in eating disorder patients. *International Journal of Eating Disorders, 30*(1), 69–74.

Index